Trauma-Informed Occupational Therapy in Women's Health

I0127937

Trauma-Informed Occupational Therapy in Women's Health equips occupational therapy practitioners and allied healthcare professionals with the tools and knowledge needed to deliver trauma-informed care in women's health.

Across a lifespan perspective, it explores the impacts of trauma—from adolescence to older adulthood—while addressing critical topics such as birth trauma, intimate partner violence, and care for marginalized populations. Featuring practical strategies, evidence-based frameworks, and innovative interventions, this book empowers practitioners to foster resilience, recovery, and meaningful engagement in women's lives. Vignettes provide clear examples of how women's pain has too often been dismissed, misunderstood, ignored, overlooked, or misdiagnosed.

This book is an essential resource for advancing trauma-informed care in occupational therapy to empower health professionals to move beyond checklists and deliver care that is relational, inclusive, and truly healing.

Sabina Khan, PhD, OTR/L, is an award-winning women's health specialist, educator, and researcher who has published extensively on trauma-informed care and women's health, advancing access and equity in healthcare.

Trauma-Informed Occupational Therapy in Women's Health

Sabina Khan

Routledge
Taylor & Francis Group

NEW YORK AND LONDON

Designed cover image: Getty Images

First published 2026
by Routledge
605 Third Avenue, New York, NY 10158

and by Routledge
4 Park Square, Milton Park, Abingdon, Oxon, OX14 4RN

Routledge is an imprint of the Taylor & Francis Group, an informa business

ISBN: 978-1-041-11159-7 (hbk)
ISBN: 978-1-041-11158-0 (pbk)
ISBN: 978-1-003-65855-9 (ebk)

DOI: 10.4324/9781003658559

Typeset in Times New Roman
by Apex CoVantage, LLC

For every woman whose story was overlooked, whose pain was misunderstood, and whose healing was made harder by systems that failed to see her.

May this work be a step toward justice, belonging, and the restoration of what was always yours to keep—your voice, your dignity, and your power.

And to the occupational therapists walking alongside them, thank you for choosing care that heals at the root.

Contents

About the Author   *ix*

1 Foundations of Trauma and Occupational Disruption in
   Women's Health   1

2 Relational Stress and Trauma in Adolescents   33

3 Stress and Trauma in Young Adult Women   71

4 Trauma Associated with Perinatal Events   103

5 Navigating Trauma and Occupational Transitions Across
   Midlife and Aging   136

6 The Spectrum of Violence Against Women   160

7 Health Implications of Violence Against Women   180

8 Trauma in the Lives of Women of Color   210

9 Stress and Trauma in Women with Disabilities   238

10 Gender and Sexual Minority Women   262

11 Tools for Trauma-Informed Practice Across the
    Continuum of Care   288

12 Innovative Strategies in Trauma Care   307

13 The Future of Trauma-Informed Occupational Therapy in
    Women's Health   328

    Index   *343*

About the Author

Dr. Sabina Khan is a nationally recognized women's health specialist, occupational therapist, and award-winning educator and researcher. With expertise in maternal health, trauma-informed care, and neurological rehabilitation, her work bridges clinical practice and systems innovation. She has been honored for her leadership in promoting equity and expanding the role of occupational therapy in women's health across the lifespan.

Dr. Khan has published extensively on topics related to women's health and occupational therapy and presents regularly at national and international conferences. Her research and advocacy focus on dismantling systemic barriers in healthcare and amplifying the voices of historically underserved communities. Through her work, she continues to champion inclusive, trauma-responsive models of care that center dignity, agency, and access.

She lives in South Florida with her husband and their three children, and enjoys traveling, reading, and visiting art museums with her family.

Chapter 1

Foundations of Trauma and Occupational Disruption in Women's Health

Chapter Objectives

Upon completion of this chapter, the reader will be able to:

1. Describe the neurobiological foundations of trauma in women, including changes in brain structures and stress response systems, and explain how these affect occupational participation.
2. Recognize trauma-related behaviors, such as dissociation, avoidance, and vigilance, as adaptive survival responses that influence function across everyday activities and roles.
3. Apply principles of trauma-informed care, including the six core principles from the Substance Abuse and Mental Health Services Administration, and the foundations of polyvagal theory, to support safety, regulation, and participation in therapy.
4. Analyze the structural and institutional factors that sustain trauma in women's health, including diagnostic bias, limited access to care, and violations of occupational justice.
5. Integrate an intersectional perspective to understand how trauma is shaped by identity factors such as race, gender, class, and ability, and guide culturally responsive occupational therapy across the lifespan.

Sherryl Thompson was twenty-six when she began to feel like a stranger in her own life. She had always been the one others turned to: the dependable coworker, the mother who never missed a school form, the daughter who managed her mother's medications with military precision. But nothing felt steady anymore. After the birth of her

DOI: 10.4324/9781003658559-1

third child, things shifted. The labor had been long, painful, and chaotic. Sherryl lost a significant amount of blood and remembered yelling for help, only to be told to calm down. In the days that followed, friends and family asked how the baby was doing, but no one asked about her. She smiled when she handed over the baby, but inside, she felt like something had splintered. She could not explain why she flinched when nurses touched her abdomen or why her nights were now filled with racing thoughts and cold sweats. Her partner eventually left, saying she had changed. She agreed. She had.

In the years that followed, Sherryl stopped asking for help. She began missing appointments and avoiding phone calls. She kept a notepad to remember what to do after work, and repeated the same three meals because anything else felt overwhelming. At night, she stared at the ceiling while her chest pulsed with tension she could not name. When she finally disclosed to her occupational therapist that she had not felt like herself in years, it was not framed as trauma. It was framed as failure. Her therapist, however, did not begin with productivity or mood tracking. She began by slowing down the pace of daily tasks, reducing sensory triggers in the home, and building a care plan centered on emotional safety. Sherryl was not broken. She was responding exactly as a nervous system would when survival had become the only option. Therapy helped her name that, and begin the work of returning to herself.

In 2017, neuroscientists at Stanford University asked a deceptively simple question: how does trauma shape the developing brain? Their findings would echo far beyond the MRI scanner. Among the children studied, many of whom had experienced chronic abuse, violence, or instability, profound sex-based differences emerged. While trauma changed the brains of all participants, the direction of those changes diverged by gender. For girls, the data revealed something more than variation: it suggested a kind of neurological acceleration, a biological toll that looked like early aging.

This isn't just about the brain. It's about what happens when trauma becomes a developmental environment, training the body to remain in a constant state of vigilance, disconnection, or shutdown. And for girls and women, the long-term consequences often go unnoticed, misunderstood, or pathologized. What presents in a clinic as fatigue, chronic pain, or emotional detachment may be the echo of experiences the body hasn't been allowed to forget.

But trauma in women's lives does not end with the nervous system. It reaches into how a woman navigates institutions that were not designed with her needs in mind. It influences how she shows up for others while suppressing her own needs, how she fulfills roles such as worker, daughter, partner, friend, mother, sibling, or patient, while carrying the unrecognized burden of survival. Trauma affects not only how women feel, but how they function. It disrupts participation in everyday life, and reshapes engagement in the activities that define identity, connection, and well-being.

Despite this, clinical care remains fragmented. Health systems continue to separate the mind from body, psychology from biology, and individual experience from structural context. Women's trauma is often rendered as a private issue, disconnected from the societal forces that create and sustain it. What's missed is that trauma is not only an internal wound, but a relational and systemic phenomenon—reflected in housing policies, healthcare practices, diagnostic criteria, and professional biases. In occupational therapy, this disconnect can lead to missed opportunities: misinterpreting survival strategies as dysfunction, or pathologizing disengagement without understanding its origin.

To address trauma in women's health, we must reframe how we see it. We must move beyond symptom lists, and begin to understand the biological and systemic architecture that drives those symptoms. We must recognize how trauma reshapes the foundational systems that govern participation, especially the nervous system. And we must root our interventions not only in compassion, but in an accurate understanding of how trauma alters a woman's capacity to engage in daily life.

The Neurobiology of Trauma in Women

Kalina Benoit was 35 when she was referred to occupational therapy for chronic pain and daily function concerns that had resisted explanation. She had cycled through multiple providers over the years: pain management, rheumatology, gastrointestinal. Every time, her test results came back normal. "It is probably stress," they told her. But Kalina was not convinced that stress alone could cause her to forget conversations mid-sentence, leave the stove on, or feel her chest tighten in quiet places like the grocery store. During her first occupational therapy session, the therapist asked a simple intake question: "Can you describe your usual roles and routines, and how they have changed over time?" Kalina paused. Then she admitted she no longer went grocery shopping alone. She avoided cooking when her daughter was home because she could not focus. She had trouble getting through the morning without feeling overwhelmed. The therapist gently followed up: "Has there ever been a time when you felt unsafe in your body or environment for an extended period?" Kalina looked away, then said quietly, "It started in high school. My boyfriend back then . . . he was controlling. Sometimes violent. I used to sleep with my door locked, even after we broke up."

The nervous system holds stories that words often cannot. For women who have lived through trauma, these stories are not just emotional; they are biological. Trauma reshapes the brain's architecture, alters immune and hormonal function, and rewires how the body responds to the world. What may appear as anxiety, fatigue, or disconnection is often the signature of a nervous system that has learned to survive at all costs. These changes are visible in brain scans, echoed in case studies, and lived out daily in classrooms, clinics, workplaces, and homes. In women, they often look different than in men. That difference matters.

Although trauma is frequently framed as a psychological or emotional issue, its impact is profoundly biological (Hillcoat et al., 2023). Its effects are measurable, observable, and often enduring. Trauma changes hormone levels, disrupts immune responses, and rewires brain architecture—particularly in areas responsible for memory, emotion, bodily awareness, and executive functioning. In women, these alterations often mirror the distinct contours of their trauma: sexual violence, reproductive coercion, relational betrayal, and the chronic strain of being unseen in systems not built to hold them. These gendered patterns of exposure help explain why women are more likely to develop post-traumatic stress, why their symptoms are often misread or minimized, and why trauma-informed care must begin not with pathology, but with biology.

Research has consistently shown that trauma alters the size, function, and connectivity of key neural regions, including the amygdala, hippocampus, insula, and prefrontal cortex (McLean et al., 2011; Rosada et al., 2021). These changes are not theoretical; they appear in imaging studies, are replicated across diverse populations, and are tightly linked to symptoms that show up in daily life. The result is a nervous system often locked in survival mode, constantly scanning for threat, misreading safety cues, and struggling to return to a resting state. In occupational therapy, this dysregulation is not a background detail; it plays out in the most essential domains of living: work, caregiving, learning, social participation, and self-care.

In women, these neurobiological changes often follow different patterns than in men, shaped by hormonal cycles and by trauma exposures that disproportionately affect girls and women (Klabunde et al., 2017). For example, studies have shown that trauma can lead to increased amygdala volume in boys, associated with externalizing behaviors like aggression, while in girls, the same trauma is more likely to result in amygdala hyperreactivity and insular shrinkage, which are linked to emotional numbing, dissociation, and internalized distress. These differences are key to understanding why women experience more complex, chronic trauma responses and why their symptoms are so often dismissed, misdiagnosed, or pathologized as mood disorders or personality traits. Effective intervention must be grounded in a nuanced understanding of female neurobiology.

Understanding these brain-body mechanisms is essential for reframing trauma-related symptoms. These are not signs of weakness; they are adaptive responses to overwhelming experiences. From altered sensory processing to emotional numbing, these are not failures of resilience—they are evidence of survival. Recognizing them as such is the first step toward restoring not only function, but dignity and agency. The structural and functional brain changes most commonly associated with trauma are listed in Table 1.1, with a focus on how they manifest in women and how they may disrupt occupational engagement across daily life.

The amygdala, hippocampus, insula, prefrontal cortex, and HPA axis are particularly vulnerable to the effects of trauma because of their central roles in emotion regulation, memory, body awareness, executive functioning, and hormonal balance. These structures are highly sensitive to neurochemical fluctuations and become flooded with stress hormones during and after traumatic events. When trauma is prolonged or repeated, as it often is in the lives of women facing intimate partner violence, early developmental adversity, or systemic oppression, these regions undergo functional and structural changes.

The amygdala becomes hyperactive, triggering exaggerated startle responses, emotional reactivity, and chronic hypervigilance. Clinically, this may present as avoidance of crowds, discomfort in noisy or unpredictable settings, or difficulty participating in group-based occupations due to a persistent sense of danger. This threat sensitivity can also manifest as quick emotional shifts or panic in response to seemingly minor stressors, making it harder to maintain interpersonal stability or occupational presence in environments that feel uncontrollable.

The hippocampus, critical for memory and spatial orientation, often shows reduced volume. This contributes to forgetfulness, disorientation, and difficulty distinguishing past threat from present safety. Women may report missing appointments, losing track of steps in a routine, or feeling triggered in environments that bear even a subtle resemblance to earlier trauma. The hippocampus also affects narrative memory, which can lead to fragmented or non-linear recollection of traumatic events, complicating both therapeutic work and personal understanding of one's story.

The insula, which governs interoception and emotional self-awareness, may become underactive. This can lead to numbing, confusion around internal signals like hunger or fatigue, and difficulty identifying or naming feelings. Therapists may see clients who appear disengaged, overlook bodily discomfort, or

Table 1.1 Trauma-Affected Brain Regions and Potential Occupational Disruptions in Women

Brain Region	Primary Function	Trauma-Related Impact	Occupational Disruption
Amygdala	Threat detection, emotional salience	Hyperactivity → hypervigilance, emotional reactivity	Difficulty focusing, feeling unsafe in public, overreacting in social or caregiving roles
Hippocampus	Memory consolidation, contextualizing experiences	Reduced volume → impaired memory, disorientation	Trouble learning new tasks, navigating environments, recalling information
Insula	Interoception, empathy, self-awareness	Shrinkage → emotional numbing, disconnect from body	Poor emotional regulation, difficulty engaging in self-care or social participation
Prefrontal Cortex	Executive functioning, impulse control, decision-making	Impaired function → reduced regulation	Difficulty with planning, multitasking, work/study efficiency, frustration tolerance
Hypothalamus-Pituitary-Adrenal (HPA Axis)	Hormonal stress regulation	Chronic activation → fatigue, hormonal imbalance	Low energy, poor stress tolerance, missed occupational roles (e.g., work, parenting) (Khan, 2025)

struggle to describe emotional states even during meaningful activity. Insular dysfunction can also contribute to alexithymia, the inability to put feelings into words, which can impair self-advocacy and frustrate clinical encounters that rely on verbal emotional processing.

The prefrontal cortex, which enables complex decision-making, regulation, and task initiation, often loses control over the more reactive limbic system. The result is difficulty planning, organizing, or persisting through tasks—not due to lack of interest, but due to a system that has prioritized survival over sequencing. Clients may present as overwhelmed, unable to follow through, or easily frustrated in settings that demand structure and forward thinking. Even previously mastered executive skills can become unreliable, particularly when a client is under stress or sleep-deprived, leading to a sense of failure or learned helplessness.

The HPA axis, responsible for regulating the body's hormonal stress response, may remain chronically activated. This dysregulation can interfere with sleep, menstruation, digestion, and immune response. Women may experience fatigue, pain, irregular cycles, or autoimmune symptoms that impair function and limit engagement across roles. In some cases, the body's stress regulation system becomes so worn down that clients swing between hyperarousal and exhaustion, creating an unpredictable baseline that challenges daily routines and emotional regulation.

These are not isolated symptoms. They are the signatures of a system working overtime to protect itself. For occupational therapists, recognizing these patterns is essential not just for accurate assessment, but for designing interventions that meet women where they are: in their bodies, in their stories, and in their everyday lives. A woman who avoids driving may not lack motivation but may associate car travel with past harm. A mother who appears disengaged during play may be in a state of dissociation, not disinterest. A student who cannot complete assignments may be facing executive dysfunction rooted in survival mode, not laziness. When we understand these patterns as biologically driven adaptations, we shift from blaming behavior to building capacity—and from treating symptoms to restoring participation.

The Stress Response System in Chronic Survival Mode

Jasmine Pesci sat in the corner of the outpatient waiting room, waiting to be seen for a shoulder injury. Her leg bounced continuously, crossed tightly over the other, and her fingers tugged at the edge of the intake form she had barely filled out. Every few minutes, she checked the clock, then the hallway, then the clock again. Though the room was quiet, she wore earbuds without sound, as if to create a buffer. Her shoulders stayed lifted, even as she leaned back in the chair. When a staff member called her name, she smiled quickly, but her eyes didn't soften. The emergency contact section on her form was blank. She said she just wanted to "get this over with," then apologized for being "weirdly on edge." Nothing about her presentation seemed urgent, but her body told a more complex story. What looked like restlessness was not impatience. It was a nervous system that had been taught to stay vigilant, even in rooms that were supposed to be safe.

The human stress response is a finely tuned biological system designed to detect danger, mobilize resources, and return the body to equilibrium once safety is restored. At the center of this system is the HPA axis, a hormonal feedback loop that governs the release of stress chemicals like cortisol and adrenaline. Working alongside the autonomic nervous system, which includes the sympathetic branch that prepares for fight or flight, and the parasympathetic branch that supports rest and repair, the HPA axis activates the body's defenses when something feels unsafe.

In short bursts, this response is adaptive. It enables survival. But when the system is activated too frequently or for too long, such as in the context of ongoing trauma, the stress response begins to misfire. Instead of returning to baseline after a threat has passed, the body remains stuck in a state of hypervigilance or shuts down completely. Over time, this dysregulation alters both physical health and functional capacity. What may appear as procrastination, memory loss, fatigue, or irritability is often a nervous system trying desperately and automatically to survive in a world that does not feel safe.

Dysregulation in the Female Nervous System

Women are not just emotionally, but biologically wired to experience and express stress differently than men. Estrogen, progesterone, and oxytocin all interact with the HPA axis, altering how stress is processed and how quickly the body recovers. These hormonal fluctuations can intensify stress sensitivity and modulate memory encoding of traumatic events, making some experiences more vivid, visceral, and difficult to suppress.

Moreover, the types of trauma that disproportionately affect women, including interpersonal violence, reproductive trauma, and relational abandonment, often trigger attachment-based and body-based survival responses. These responses may not appear as overt panic or rage, but instead as withdrawal, dissociation, or emotional numbing. These responses are still protective, but they are often misinterpreted as apathy, depression, or noncompliance.

For many women, the stress response system doesn't turn off. Instead, it becomes their baseline. This chronic survival mode can present as

- **Hyperarousal**: insomnia, irritability, exaggerated startle response, hypervigilance.
- **Hypoarousal**: fatigue, emotional detachment, dissociation, slowed cognition.
- **Oscillation:** between both states—hyperarousal and hypoarousal—often triggered by seemingly minor stressors.

The body adapts in order to survive. This adaptation can be both protective and persistent. However, the cost to long-term health and daily functioning is often profound. In clinical settings, these patterns are often noted in documentation but not fully understood.

A therapist may write that a client is easily startled, appears guarded, or requires repeated prompts to initiate tasks without recognizing these as signs of elevated arousal. A woman experiencing this state may speak rapidly, report difficulty sleeping, or struggle to tolerate noise or crowded spaces. She may describe feeling constantly on edge but blame herself for being irritable or overly sensitive.

In contrast, a woman in a lowered arousal state may present as detached or lacking energy. She might sit still for long periods, speak in a flat tone, or have difficulty following the flow of conversation. Therapists may note that she seems unmotivated or distant, when in reality her nervous system is withdrawing to conserve energy in response to perceived danger. She may struggle with remembering instructions, initiating routines, or maintaining basic self-care. These behaviors are not signs of disinterest or defiance but are expressions of physiological collapse.

Some clients move between these states even within a single session. A woman may begin feeling overwhelmed, restless, and overstimulated, and then shift without warning into quiet withdrawal or emotional absence. These transitions are not mood swings or defiance. They are biological strategies for survival, shaped by experience.

Although men can also experience stress-related dysregulation, they are more likely to display it through outward behavior such as irritability, impulsivity, or physical agitation. Women, on the other hand, tend to express stress internally through withdrawal, emotional blunting, or self-blame. This difference reflects not only biological processes but also the specific kinds of trauma that women more frequently encounter, including violations related to the body, trust, and safety in relationships. As a result, women are more likely to be misunderstood, mislabeled, or missed altogether in clinical care.

Understanding these patterns as nervous system adaptations rather than personality traits allows occupational therapists to respond more effectively. It supports a shift from managing symptoms to restoring physiological and emotional safety through regulation, connection, and therapeutic presence.

Occupational Impact of Chronic Survival Mode

The physiological changes described earlier do not remain confined to the brain or body. They shape how women move through daily life. Chronic survival responses alter the way women parent, work, rest, connect, and care for themselves. These disruptions often go unseen or are misinterpreted as personal deficits rather than responses to persistent stress. Table 1.2 outlines how patterns of nervous system dysregulation manifest across key occupational domains and how these patterns interfere with meaningful participation.

These occupational disruptions are not random or incidental. They reflect consistent patterns that emerge when the nervous system is forced into

Table 1.2 Neurobiological and Functional Consequences of Chronic Survival Mode on Women's Occupational Performance

Occupational Domain	Manifestation of Survival Mode	Underlying Neurobiological or Stress Pattern	Implications for Occupational Engagement
Parenting and Caregiving	Inconsistent responses to children's needs, overprotectiveness, emotional outbursts or shutdowns	Amygdala hyperactivity; reduced prefrontal modulation; chronic HPA axis activation	Difficulty attuning to child cues, establishing routines, or maintaining emotional presence during caregiving
Work and Productivity	Difficulty concentrating, procrastination, frequent fatigue, poor task initiation or follow-through	Prefrontal cortex dysfunction; cognitive fatigue; cortisol imbalance	Missed deadlines, underperformance, increased absenteeism, decreased confidence or self-efficacy
Self-Care	Irregular hygiene, disrupted eating/sleeping, neglect of medical needs or wellness routines	Insula hypoactivity; autonomic dysregulation; disrupted interoceptive awareness	Poor maintenance of personal health, avoidance of medical care, increased vulnerability to chronic illness
Social Participation	Isolation, avoidance of intimacy, mistrust, shame-based withdrawal	Social engagement system shutdown; vagal nerve hypoactivity; trauma-related cognitive schemas	Loss of supportive relationships, diminished community engagement, heightened loneliness and alienation
Leisure and Play	Loss of interest in hobbies, inability to experience joy or spontaneity	Dopamine system suppression; anhedonia; reduced parasympathetic activation	Reduced creative expression, emotional flatness, limited access to restorative or pleasurable activities
Education and Learning	Impaired memory, test anxiety, difficulty absorbing or applying new information	Hippocampal volume reduction; attention dysregulation	Barriers to academic progress, low academic self-esteem, increased dropout risk
Rest and Sleep	Insomnia, nightmares, fragmented sleep, excessive fatigue	HPA axis overactivation; elevated cortisol; disrupted circadian rhythms	Daytime drowsiness, difficulty participating in occupations requiring sustained alertness or focus (AOTA, 2020)

long-term survival. A missed deadline may be the result of cognitive fatigue, not disorganization. Avoidance of touch may signal a collapsed engagement system, not emotional detachment. What appears externally as inconsistency, defiance, or apathy is often an internal strategy to stay safe in a world that does not feel safe.

For women affected by trauma, participation is not simply about willpower or motivation. It is a constant negotiation between engaging and protecting. This lens invites a shift in how therapists view behavior—from asking "What is wrong with her?" to asking "What has her nervous system had to navigate, and how can we support her return to safety and presence through occupation?"

For example, a mother who suddenly bursts into tears during her child's bath time may not be emotionally fragile. She may be experiencing sensory flooding, shaped by unresolved birth trauma or years of unpredictability in caregiving. Her reaction is not a sign of weakness; it is overload.

A student who avoids group projects and fails to meet deadlines may not be unmotivated. Her nervous system might be caught in a cycle of vigilance and shutdown, making sustained attention and initiation nearly impossible, especially in environments that feel evaluative or unpredictable.

A woman who cancels appointments at the last minute, then apologizes profusely, may be navigating a dysregulated system that cannot predict how she will feel hour to hour. Rather than assuming she lacks commitment, a trauma-informed lens helps us see how inconsistency can be a symptom of survival and not avoidance.

Trauma Responses as Adaptive Survival Strategies

Clinical language often labels trauma-related behaviors as symptoms of dysfunction. Terms like avoidance, hypervigilance, dissociation, and emotional numbness appear frequently in charts and assessments. But these are not signs of weakness or disorder. They are the expressions of a nervous system that has learned how to survive overwhelming stress. When the brain detects threat, it does not prioritize long-term goals, emotional connection, or social roles. It prioritizes staying alive. In this context, trauma responses are best understood not as maladaptive traits, but as protective strategies that once kept the person safe in an unsafe world.

Recent research supports this perspective. A 2023 study published in *Violence Against Women* examined how women responded during experiences of sexual assault, and how those responses related to later symptoms of post-traumatic stress. The study found that behaviors such as freezing, shutting down, or going still—often interpreted as passive or submissive—were strongly linked to trauma severity, especially among women with difficulty identifying emotions. These findings suggest that what is often seen as failure to act may actually be a biologically driven response to unmanageable threat.

For women, many of these adaptations are relational and deeply embodied (Mirabile et al., 2024). Freezing in the face of conflict may have once prevented escalation. Over-functioning or perfectionism may have helped maintain control in a chaotic home. People-pleasing may have served to keep caregivers or partners stable (Muñoz-Rivas et al., 2021). These patterns can persist long after the original threat is gone, especially when the body has not had a chance to feel safe again. Over time, what began as protection can become habit, shaping how a woman relates to others, how she organizes her day, and how she experiences herself in the world.

From an occupational therapy perspective, these strategies often show up in how women engage with roles, routines, and responsibilities (Cicchetti & Rogosch, 2009). A woman who cannot say no to extra tasks at work may not lack boundaries. She may be reenacting a long-standing strategy to avoid rejection or disapproval. A client who leaves sessions early or struggles to initiate shared activities may not be unmotivated. Her nervous system may still be choosing safety over connection.

Recognizing trauma responses as adaptive does not mean accepting suffering as inevitable (Mason & Stagnitti, 2023). It means beginning with respect for what the body has endured. It means understanding that behaviors like emotional detachment, overcontrol, or withdrawal are not character flaws. They are responses to conditions that once felt impossible to survive. This shift in perspective lays the foundation for trauma-informed care. The goal is not to eliminate survival strategies, but to help women reclaim access to choice, regulation, and meaningful participation in life.

Structural and Systemic Dimensions of Women's Trauma and Occupational Justice

Ava Barone, a 27-year-old graduate student, schedules a follow-up with her primary care provider after months of worsening fatigue, joint pain, and trouble sleeping. She explains that the symptoms began after a difficult breakup and the sudden loss of housing. The provider briefly skims her chart, notes a history of anxiety, and suggests her symptoms are likely stress-related. No physical exam is conducted. "Try to relax more," he says. Ava leaves with no plan, no diagnosis, and a quiet but familiar sense that she wasn't taken seriously. Months later, she is diagnosed by a different provider with an autoimmune disorder that could have been treated earlier.

This story is not rare. It is part of a larger pattern. Women's trauma is often misunderstood or overlooked, not because it is invisible, but because the systems built to respond to trauma were not designed with women's experiences at the center. From healthcare to education to criminal justice, many institutions rely on frameworks developed through research focused on men and their symptoms. For example, post-traumatic stress disorder was originally defined through the study of male combat veterans, emphasizing flashbacks, aggression, and emotional reactivity. These criteria often fail to reflect the more internal, relational, and body-based expressions of trauma that are common among women, such as dissociation, emotional numbing, chronic pain, or persistent fatigue.

This mismatch is not limited to diagnosis. For decades, medical research excluded women from clinical trials, even in studies related to hormones, reproduction, or pain (Sinko et al., 2022). According to the National Institutes of Health, women were significantly underrepresented in research until the early twenty-first century. The effects of that exclusion continue today. Women's symptoms are more likely to be dismissed as emotional, their pain undertreated, and their diagnoses delayed. These are not isolated incidents. They reflect structural bias woven into how care is defined, funded, and delivered.

In both clinical and community settings, trauma responses that result from long-term stress are often mislabeled as dysfunction. Withdrawal, emotional numbing, or difficulty maintaining routines are commonly seen as signs of weakness rather than responses to threat. Brown et al. (2024) describe this mislabeling through an autoethnographic account of life after traumatic brain injury, where shifts in occupational identity were pathologized rather than understood as adaptations to trauma. Coping strategies are misread as personality flaws. When providers fail to explore the environmental or relational roots of these behaviors, women are more likely to be misdiagnosed, disbelieved, or pathologized. Instead of being viewed as adaptive responses to unsafe conditions, their behaviors are interpreted as instability or failure.

To fully understand women's trauma, we must also understand the systems that shape and sustain it. Many of the behaviors observed in survivors, including vigilance, overcontrol, avoidance, and shutdown, are not just the result of personal history. They are shaped by ongoing encounters with institutions that fail to offer safety, respect, or agency. In hospitals, schools, courtrooms, and workplaces, women are often retraumatized when their pain is dismissed, their voices ignored, or their needs met with punishment rather than support. These patterns are not random. They are structural. Table 1.3 outlines examples of how trauma is reinforced by major systems that impact women's lives. Each example shows how system-level dynamics contribute to occupational disruption, and how this disruption affects core life roles and functions.

These systemic conditions do more than prolong trauma. They create barriers to occupational justice. **Occupational justice** is the right of every person to access meaningful activity that supports identity, connection, and well-being (AOTA, 2020). When institutions disempower women or punish them for the effects of trauma, they do not simply interfere with mental health. They limit access to essential roles like caregiver, student, worker, advocate, and community member. These limits are not individual weaknesses. They are violations of rights.

Table 1.3 Structural Systems That Contribute to and Sustain Trauma in Women

System	Common Structural Dynamics	Trauma-Related Consequences for Women	Occupational Implications
Healthcare	Historical exclusion of women in research; non-sex-specific diagnostic tools; dismissal of gendered symptoms (e.g., pain, reproductive distress)	Medical gaslighting, mistrust of providers; chronic underdiagnosis	Avoidance of medical settings; disrupted routines for wellness/self-care; health-related occupational disengagement
Mental Health	Diagnostic models based on male symptoms; limited integration of relational, cultural, and trauma-informed perspectives	Mislabeling of trauma responses as personality disorders; stigma and ineffective care	Loss of occupational identity; barriers to emotional regulation skills needed for role performance (e.g., parenting, work)
Education	Behavior policies uninformed by trauma history; inadequate support for grief, violence, instability at home	School disengagement, dropout; developmental delays in identity formation	Interruptions in learning trajectory; reduced access to educational roles and social development opportunities
Justice System	Victim-blaming in sexual violence cases; low conviction rates; lack of trauma-informed practices	Re-traumatization; legal system avoidance; survivor silencing	Disempowerment in advocacy roles; erosion of safety in public spaces; social withdrawal
Workplace	Lack of trauma accommodations; emotional suppression; punitive leave/caregiving policies	Burnout, job insecurity; concealment of trauma history	Inconsistent job performance; strained work-life balance; disrupted vocational identity
Child Welfare	Risk-focused policies with little maternal support; minimal trauma assessment in parenting evaluations	Family separation; loss of parental rights; intergenerational trauma	Loss of parenting roles; diminished self-efficacy; avoidance of support services due to fear of surveillance (Khan, 2025)

A trauma-informed approach in occupational therapy must do more than address symptoms (U.S. Department of Labor Women's Bureau, 2011). It must restore choice, access, and connection. It must support each woman's capacity to participate in the routines, relationships, and roles that shape her life. And it must take seriously the task of not only healing the body but also transforming the systems that have caused the harm.

Key Theoretical Frameworks for Trauma-Informed Care

In occupational therapy that responds to trauma, both models and frameworks are essential tools. Although the terms are often used interchangeably, they serve different but complementary purposes in practice. Imagine an occupational therapist working with a woman who avoids public spaces after experiencing a violent assault. The therapist needs to understand why this behavior developed, how it connects to trauma, and what can support recovery. A model can explain the disruption. A framework can guide the care.

Models help explain what is happening. They offer theoretical perspectives that clarify how trauma impacts identity, daily function, and participation in meaningful activity. Models help therapists understand how occupational roles and routines are shaped by stress, loss, and adaptation. For example, the Person–Environment–Occupation model highlights how trauma can interfere with the interaction between a woman's internal experience, her surroundings, and her capacity to engage in daily occupations (Strong et al., 1999).

Frameworks, by contrast, guide how care is delivered. They offer structured principles and processes to ensure that services are responsive, collaborative, and emotionally safe (Nakao et al., 2021). One of the most widely used frameworks comes from the Substance Abuse and Mental Health Services Administration (SAMHSA), a federal agency focused on behavioral health. Although not specific to occupational therapy, this framework outlines six core principles for trauma-responsive care that align closely with occupational therapy's focus on autonomy, trust, participation, and meaningful context. While models help us understand the why behind disruption, frameworks help us organize the how of care in ways that avoid harm and support healing.

Occupational Therapy Models and Trauma-Informed Frameworks

In trauma recovery work, occupational therapists must address both the consequences of trauma and the conditions in which care is provided. Conceptual models help therapists analyze how trauma disrupts occupational roles, habits, routines, and identity. Frameworks offer guidance for structuring the therapeutic relationship, making decisions, and designing environments that support safety, trust, and participation. These tools are most effective when used in combination.

A helpful metaphor is to imagine trauma-informed care as a road trip:

- A **model** is the map. It helps the therapist understand the terrain of a client's life, including detours, current obstacles, and future goals.
- A **framework** is the way of driving. It shapes how the therapist paces the process, responds to conditions, and ensures that the journey is empowering, safe, and collaborative.

In occupational therapy practice, several models are used to conceptualize the impact of trauma. These include the Person–Environment–Occupation model, the Model of Human Occupation, the Canadian Model of Occupational Performance and Engagement, and the culturally grounded Kawa model (Iwama et al., 2009). These guide how therapists assess disruption in roles and routines.

Alongside these models, a variety of frameworks are used to shape how care is delivered. The Occupational Therapy Practice Framework, the Canadian Practice Process Framework, and the American Occupational Therapy Association's Guidelines for Trauma-Informed Care help structure clinical processes. Other frameworks commonly used in mental health and trauma work include Dunn's Sensory Processing Framework, the Recovery Model, the Biopsychosocial Framework, and the Cognitive Behavioral Frame of Reference (Kirsh & Cockburn, 2009). These tools are summarized in Table 1.4 and demonstrate how theory and application work together to support trauma-responsive care.

While these models and frameworks provide the foundation for effective trauma-informed occupational therapy, their value lies in how they are operationalized in everyday care. Among them, SAMHSA's six principles of trauma-informed care are particularly influential for structuring relationships, adapting environments, and delivering services in ways that reduce harm and promote healing. The following section explores each of these principles and their direct application to occupational therapy with women affected by trauma.

SAMHSA's Framework and the Six Principles of Trauma-Informed Care

The trauma-informed care framework developed by the Substance Abuse and Mental Health Services Administration (SAMHSA) has been widely adopted across health, education, and social service systems (Substance Abuse and Mental Health Services Administration, 2014). It is now increasingly applied in occupational therapy. This framework is based on four core assumptions: realize the impact of trauma, recognize the signs and symptoms, respond by integrating knowledge into all aspects of care, and resist re-traumatization. These assumptions are operationalized through six guiding principles.

Table 1.4 Models and Frameworks Used in Trauma-Informed Occupational Therapy

Tool Type	Name	Role in Practice	What It Helps With
Model	Person-Environment-Occupation	Analyzes how person, environment, and occupation interact to influence performance	Identifies environmental, task, or personal barriers to engagement following trauma
Model	Model of Human Occupation	Explores volition, roles, habits, and performance capacity	Helps understand how trauma disrupts motivation, occupational identity, and routines
Model	Canadian Model of Occupational Performance and Engagement	Emphasizes meaning-making through occupation, environment, and spirituality	Guides collaborative goal-setting and supports identity reconstruction after trauma
Model	Kawa Model	Uses metaphor of river flow to visualize life roles, barriers, and social supports	Enables culturally sensitive, narrative-based expression of trauma and recovery paths
Framework	Occupational Therapy Practice Framework	Outlines the domain and process of OT practice	Ensures trauma-informed care is grounded in standardized OT processes (assessment, goals, documentation)
Framework	Canadian Practice Process Framework	Provides a client-centered process for enabling occupation	Structures collaborative, respectful care across trauma-affected contexts
Framework	Dunn's Sensory Processing Framework	Explains sensory thresholds and modulation patterns	Helps tailor sensory-based strategies for regulation and participation after trauma

(Continued)

Table 1.4 (Continued)

Tool Type	Name	Role in Practice	What It Helps With
Framework	Cognitive Behavioral Frame of Reference	Focuses on changing maladaptive thoughts and behavior	Supports emotional regulation and reframing of trauma-related beliefs during occupational engagement
Framework	Biopsychosocial Framework	Considers biological, psychological, and social factors in health and function	Promotes holistic, non-pathologizing trauma care within occupational performance analysis
Framework	Recovery Model (Mental Health)	Emphasizes personal agency, hope, and individualized healing	Validates non-linear recovery, supports goal flexibility, and affirms survivor autonomy
Framework	Ecology of Human Performance	Focuses on context-task-person fit	Guides trauma-informed adaptations to reduce triggering environments and enhance occupational success

Although originally created outside of occupational therapy, the framework aligns closely with the profession's core values of context, autonomy, participation, and therapeutic relationship. For women affected by trauma, these principles resonate deeply. They speak directly to common experiences of systemic dismissal, disempowerment, and relational harm.

These six principles offer more than philosophy. They provide practical strategies for fostering safety, trust, mutual respect, and empowerment. In occupational therapy, they can be embedded into every phase of care, from assessment and planning to intervention and discharge. Whether supporting a woman navigating burnout, returning to work after intimate partner violence, or rebuilding routines following reproductive trauma, the principles provide a foundation for care that honors both identity and healing. Occupational therapists are uniquely positioned to apply these principles through activity analysis, use of self, and environmental design. Table 1.5 outlines how each principle translates to women's health and how occupational therapists can integrate them into practice.

Table 1.5 Operationalizing SAMHSA's Six Principles of Trauma-Informed Care in Occupational Therapy with Women

Principle	Description	Insight for Women's Health	Occupational Therapy Applications
Safety	Safety includes physical comfort, emotional security, and sensory regulation. It is established through predictability, consistency, and non-threatening environments.	Many women with trauma histories feel unsafe in clinical settings due to prior experiences of coercion, boundary violations, or emotional invalidation.	Design calming, low-stimulus environments; begin each session with grounding or regulation; clearly explain each step of an activity or evaluation. Avoid surprise touch, sudden changes, or ambiguous feedback.
Trustworthiness and Transparency	Clients must know what to expect and feel that the therapist is reliable, consistent, and clear in communication.	Distrust often develops from medical gaslighting, broken confidentiality, or trauma that occurred in institutional settings.	Use simple, transparent language about purpose, duration, and expectations. Follow through on stated plans. If something changes, explain why. Clarify the therapist's role and limitations early in care.
Peer Support	Healing is often strengthened through connection with others who have experienced similar trauma. Peer relationships reduce isolation and foster hope.	Women may feel alone or ashamed about their trauma, particularly in contexts like perinatal loss, IPV, or childhood abuse.	Recommend or co-facilitate support groups; incorporate client narratives into group OT when appropriate; collaborate with peer advocates or doulas in maternal health programs.
Collaboration and Mutuality	Therapeutic relationships should be built on shared decision-making, flattened hierarchies, and respect for each person's expertise.	Traditional healthcare often positions providers as experts and women as passive recipients, especially in reproductive care.	Ask clients what works for them before offering solutions. Co-develop treatment plans. Use collaborative phrases like "Let's figure this out together" rather than instructive commands. Name and check in on power dynamics when appropriate.

(Continued)

Table 1.5 (Continued)

Principle	Description	Insight for Women's Health	Occupational Therapy Applications
Empowerment, Voice, and Choice	Clients must be supported to identify their strengths, assert preferences, and regain a sense of agency. Empowerment is both a process and an outcome.	Trauma often involves a profound loss of control over one's body, choices, or environment. Rebuilding that control is central to recovery.	Offer options for activity pacing, location, or focus. Allow opt-outs without consequence. Frame feedback in terms of capability and growth. Normalize boundary-setting. Reflect back client strengths during goal setting.
Cultural, Historical, and Gender Responsiveness	Trauma must be understood within the broader context of identity, community, and history—including racism, sexism, colonialism, and heteronormativity.	Marginalized women often experience layered trauma that is invisible or misunderstood in clinical settings.	Validate identity-based trauma. Use culturally relevant occupations and examples. Educate oneself about historical harms in medical systems. Seek community partnerships and feedback to ensure interventions reflect cultural safety (SAMHSA, 2014).

While the SAMHSA framework offers a powerful structure for creating emotionally safe environments, it does not fully explain how safety is experienced within the body. For many women, trauma lives in the nervous system. It is expressed through chronic activation, emotional blunting, or physical shutdown that interrupts meaningful participation. To support healing at this level, therapists must understand how the body organizes experience in response to threat. Polyvagal theory provides a biological framework for understanding how trauma affects regulation, connection, and occupational performance. It helps explain how therapeutic presence, sensory experiences, and co-regulation can promote a return to safety, engagement, and self-agency.

Polyvagal Theory and Neuroception

Margot Petridis, 28, sat silently during her first occupational therapy session, her eyes fixed just past the therapist's shoulder, her body still but tense. Months earlier, she had resigned from a nonprofit she once believed in after learning that leadership had deliberately suppressed reports of harm within the communities they served. "Since then," she whispered, "I can't seem to do anything that matters." Though she appeared calm, her breath was shallow, her voice flat, and her posture folded inward. These were not signs of disinterest or apathy—they were markers of a nervous system caught in a state of shutdown. Margot's body was not resisting therapy; it was waiting for signs that this space was different. Rather than asking questions or introducing formal goals, the therapist invited her to sit on the floor with a weighted cushion, offered colored pencils and quiet music, and simply remained present while Margot slowly began to draw.

Polyvagal theory, developed by neuroscientist Stephen Porges, offers a powerful lens for understanding how trauma shapes the autonomic nervous system and, in turn, occupational engagement (Dana, 2018; Porges, 2011). Rather than viewing trauma responses as emotional reactions or behavioral choices, polyvagal theory describes them as physiological states involving automatic shifts in neural pathways that occur in response to perceived safety or threat. At the center of this theory is the vagus nerve, which helps regulate heart rate, digestion, facial expression, and social interaction.

The theory describes three primary patterns of autonomic response:

- The **ventral vagal state** supports social connection, communication, and occupational engagement when a person feels safe.

- The **sympathetic state** prepares the body for fight or flight when danger is perceived.
- The **dorsal vagal state** is associated with immobilization, shutdown, and dissociation when a threat feels inescapable or overwhelming.

A central concept in polyvagal theory is **neuroception**, or the body's unconscious process of scanning the environment for cues of safety or danger. Neuroception helps explain why a woman might dissociate during a medical exam, withdraw in a group setting, or struggle to engage in therapy even when she cognitively wants to participate. Her nervous system may detect cues that are not objectively dangerous, but that are deeply associated with past experiences of harm. These responses are not choices but adaptations shaped by the body's memory of what it had to do to survive.

These patterns are supported by research. A 2018 study by Dale and colleagues examined autonomic responses in 60 women with childhood trauma histories who did not meet the criteria for post-traumatic stress disorder. Compared to their peers, they showed lower baseline parasympathetic activity, higher resting heart rates, and stronger reactivity to physical and emotional stress. The findings suggested heightened physiological defensiveness, even in women without a formal diagnosis (Dale et al., 2018). In practice, this means that clients may appear calm on the surface while experiencing significant dysregulation internally.

For occupational therapists, polyvagal theory reframes trauma-related behavior not as resistance, avoidance, or emotional fragility, but as expressions of the nervous system's current state. The clinical question shifts from "Why is she not participating?" to "What does her nervous system need in order to feel safe enough to engage?" This perspective helps guide regulation-focused care that honors the body's wisdom rather than overriding it.

Strategies informed by this approach may include beginning with rhythmic movement, incorporating deep pressure or proprioceptive input, or offering familiar objects and consistent routines. Sometimes, the most therapeutic tool is a calm voice, an attuned posture, and the therapist's ability to stay regulated themselves. Co-regulation, the use of relational presence to help a client access safety, becomes just as important as any intervention technique.

Women may shift between different autonomic states more frequently or subtly due to the nature of their trauma. Relational betrayal, chronic invalidation, systemic oppression, and reproductive trauma can all lead to heightened sensitivity to context. A client may arrive alert and talkative, but fade into emotional numbness or fatigue mid-session. These changes are not signs of disinterest or failure; they are invitations to slow down, to listen more deeply, and to meet the nervous system where it is. Polyvagal theory does not replace frameworks like those from the Substance Abuse and Mental Health Services Administration. It complements them. While trauma-responsive frameworks guide how we build safe services, polyvagal theory helps us understand how safety is experienced in the body. Together, they support a more integrated and respectful approach to occupational therapy for women affected by trauma.

The Role of Occupational Therapy in Healing From Trauma

Occupational therapy is uniquely suited to support trauma healing because it addresses not just symptoms, but the restoration of daily rhythm, identity, and connection (Edgelow et al., 2019). Rooted in occupational science, the profession views trauma not simply as a diagnosis, but as a disruption in the capacity to engage in meaningful activity, sustain roles, and maintain a coherent sense of self. The therapeutic goal is not only to reduce distress, but to rebuild agency, routine, and purpose through occupation.

Grounded in occupational science, occupational therapy approaches trauma not solely as a clinical diagnosis, but as a disruption in the ability to participate in meaningful occupations, maintain coherent routines, and sustain one's sense of self in the world (Brown et al., 2024). The therapeutic goal is not merely symptom reduction; but the restoration of agency, rhythm, and purpose through occupation.

Trauma often fractures the continuity of daily life. Patterns that once felt automatic such as getting out of bed, preparing meals, caring for others, may become disjointed, effortful, or altogether inaccessible. For many, there is a collapse in occupational identity: roles such as mother, partner, worker, or artist become blurred or abandoned in the aftermath of overwhelming stress. This loss is not only functional, but existential. From an occupational science perspective, trauma disrupts not just what people do, but how they know who they are.

Emerging evidence also highlights gendered differences in how trauma impacts occupational engagement. In a study of emergency healthcare workers, women exhibited significantly higher levels of post-traumatic stress symptoms, particularly re-experiencing and hyperarousal, compared to men. These symptoms were closely tied to reductions in leisure participation and social functioning, pointing to the ways trauma constrains occupational choices and erodes restorative occupations. For women whose identities are often shaped around caregiving and emotional labor, the loss of leisure and self-directed time reflects a deeper disconnection from agency, embodiment, and recovery.

Occupational therapists are distinctively equipped to support this re-engagement. Through therapeutic use of self, environmental adaptation, sensory regulation, and goal-directed activity, occupational therapy provides a safe structure through which women can slowly re-enter the roles, spaces, and rhythms that define their lives. Rather than focusing solely on symptom management, occupational therapy fosters conditions under which healing becomes embedded in daily life—in the small decisions of a morning routine, the rhythm of shared mealtimes, or the quiet return to a previously abandoned creative pursuit. In this way, occupational therapy becomes a bridge between trauma and recovery, not by erasing what happened, but by helping women reshape how they engage with life moving forward.

Intersectionality and Trauma Across the Lifespan

Haylie Aguirre, a twenty-eight-year-old first-generation immigrant from Mexico, worked as a library clerk in a small public branch outside her neighborhood. Spanish was her first language, but she navigated most of her workday in English. Lately, she had started calling out sick more often. She told her supervisor it was migraines, but the truth was harder to name. Since giving birth six months earlier, Haylie had been waking in panic, crying between shelving tasks, and forgetting where she placed returned books. The quiet of the library, once comforting, now made her feel exposed. When she sought care, the intake paperwork was only available in English. No one asked about the traumatic birth, the nurse who ignored her distress, or the loneliness she felt navigating motherhood without extended family nearby. In her first occupational therapy session, someone finally asked about her lifestyle, her everyday routine, what caregiving looked like in her culture, and how her body responded to stress. That simple act of listening reframed everything. Her pain was not pathology; it was adaptation. For the first time, Haylie felt like her experience was valid. She felt seen.

Trauma is never experienced in isolation. Its effects are shaped by the social positions we hold, the systems we navigate, and the histories we carry. Intersectionality, a concept introduced by legal scholar Kimberlé Crenshaw, helps us understand how race, gender, class, age, ability, and sexuality combine to influence both exposure to trauma and access to support (Bauer et al., 2021). Intersectionality, a term introduced by legal scholar, Kimberlé Crenshaw, describes how systems of oppression intersect to shape the unique experiences of individuals based on race, gender, class, sexuality, age, and other social categories (King-Mullins et al., 2023; Philibert et al., 2022). Within trauma recovery, intersectionality is essential to understanding both exposure to trauma and the capacity to access support.

For women, trauma is frequently entangled with gender-based oppression, caregiving expectations, economic inequity, and structural invisibility.

Compared to men, women are more likely to experience interpersonal violence, cumulative microaggressions, reproductive trauma, and violations of bodily autonomy. These experiences are often compounded by racial discrimination, ableism, or heteronormative bias, resulting in trauma that is not only psychological but also systemic. Moreover, the occupational consequences of trauma, including withdrawal from roles, loss of routine, and diminished volition, often intersect with expectations placed on women to perform emotional labor, sustain caregiving, and remain resilient in the face of instability.

Occupational therapists must not only address trauma as a disruption in participation, but also consider how identity shapes both the expression of trauma and the possibilities for re-engagement. A trauma-informed occupational therapy approach requires practitioners to examine when the trauma occurred across the lifespan, who it happened to, and how intersecting systems may have intensified the occupational consequences. This includes examining how racism, classism, ageism, and other forms of structural inequity alter recovery trajectories. Table 1.6 outlines examples of how trauma may present differently across life stages and social positions, and how occupational therapists can respond using an intersectional, trauma-informed lens.

Understanding trauma through an intersectional lens highlights the complexity of each client's lived experience and reinforces the need for a principled, adaptable approach to care. While the contexts and consequences of trauma vary widely, occupational therapists must remain grounded in values that foster safety, participation, and dignity across diverse identities and settings. Research shows that women from marginalized communities, such as

Table 1.6 Applying an Intersectional Trauma Lens in Occupational Therapy Across the Lifespan

Life Stage	Common Trauma Experiences	Relevant Intersectional Factors	Implications for Occupational Therapy
Adolescence	Bullying, sexual coercion, identity-based violence, family instability	Gender nonconformity, racialized surveillance, foster care involvement, neurodivergence	Support identity development and self-efficacy through structured routines, creative engagement, and environments that affirm safety and belonging

(Continued)

Table 1.6 (Continued)

Life Stage	Common Trauma Experiences	Relevant Intersectional Factors	Implications for Occupational Therapy
Young Adulthood	Intimate partner violence, campus assault, immigration-related trauma, incarceration	Legal disenfranchisement, housing precarity, language barriers, underrepresentation in care systems	Promote autonomy through collaborative planning, address role loss and emerging adulthood transitions, create access to culturally relevant occupations
Pregnancy and Postpartum	Birth trauma, obstetric violence, loss, reproductive coercion	Medical racism, lack of support for single or queer parents, stigma related to perinatal mental health	Facilitate regulation and re-engagement with caregiving roles, validate shifting identities, adapt routines and environments to reduce overwhelm
Midlife	Workplace discrimination, caregiving exhaustion, chronic health trauma	Intersection of gender and economic marginalization, invisible labor, cultural expectations of caregiving	Reconstruct occupational balance, address burnout and identity fatigue, support access to rest and leisure without moral framing
Older Adulthood	Historical trauma, grief, intimate partner violence, institutional betrayal	Ageism, cumulative discrimination, isolation, fear of dependency	Use occupation to promote agency, process loss and meaning, and adapt environments to maintain connection, dignity, and routine

Hispanic, Black, or immigrant populations, often encounter greater barriers to accessing care, which can negatively influence mental health and functional outcomes.

For instance, a Hispanic woman recovering from birth trauma may experience reduced occupational engagement, increased anxiety, and difficulty accessing postpartum care—not only due to trauma symptoms, but also because of language barriers, cultural stigma, or systemic discrimination. An occupational therapist applying an intersectional lens would not only provide emotional regulation strategies, but also collaborate with culturally responsive birth workers, ensure educational materials are accessible in her preferred language, and validate family caregiving norms within her recovery plan. In doing so, occupational therapy becomes more than trauma responsive. It becomes a practice rooted in equity, a way of offering care that not only meets the individual in their lived reality, but actively works to transform the conditions that shape it. This is the future of occupational therapy: not simply treating disruption, but co-creating spaces where healing, identity, and belonging can be reclaimed through occupation.

Core Principles Guiding Trauma Responsive Occupational Therapy

Trauma-informed occupational therapy reflects more than a therapeutic preference—it embodies an ethical and relational stance. It aligns with occupational therapy's historical commitment to person-centered care, social inclusion, and meaningful engagement. While trauma may present as emotional dysregulation, avoidance, or disconnection, its deeper consequence is often occupational: a disruption in how one enacts identity, participates in routines, and sustains belonging.

To meet these disruptions with integrity, trauma-informed OT draws upon a core set of principles that shape not only what interventions are offered, but how therapeutic relationships are formed and sustained. These principles are particularly relevant when working with women, whose experiences of trauma are frequently compounded by systemic inequities, caregiving demands, and gendered expectations that shape both the experience of harm and the trajectory of recovery. The following six principles, adapted from SAMHSA and grounded in occupational therapy values, shape trauma-informed care across settings.

Safety

Safety is the foundation of trauma-informed occupational therapy. It extends beyond physical protection to include emotional, sensory, relational, and cultural dimensions. For many women, especially those with a history of interpersonal or medical trauma, environments that seem neutral to others may evoke vigilance, withdrawal, or discomfort. Therapists must cultivate safety through consistency, clear communication, and an awareness of both verbal and nonverbal indicators of distress. For example, a woman with a history of sexual assault may feel anxious when placed in vulnerable physical positions or when someone enters her personal space unexpectedly, even in a clinical setting. Rather than following a standardized sequence of interventions, the therapist begins by inviting the client to share what feels safe or uncomfortable, identifying preferred spatial boundaries and environmental factors such as lighting or background noise. The therapist explains procedures in advance, allows time to pause or opt out without justification, and checks in regularly. In doing so, safety becomes a shared and evolving process rather than a static condition.

Trustworthiness and Transparency

Trust is often compromised by trauma, particularly when harm occurred in institutional or relational settings. Occupational therapists promote trust by establishing clear expectations, being consistent in communication, and avoiding surprises during sessions. Transparency involves not only explaining what will happen, but also creating space for the client to ask questions, voice concerns, and know their input will be respected. Consider a therapist working with a woman who disengages mid-session without explanation. Instead of labeling this as noncompliance, the therapist reviews the structure of care together with the client, clarifies goals, and checks in about what aspects of the session feel manageable or overwhelming. Through this process, trust is rebuilt not by demanding participation, but by demonstrating respect for boundaries and offering predictable support.

Collaboration and Mutuality

Trauma-informed practice reframes therapy as a shared process between therapist and client. Mutuality emphasizes that healing happens through relationship, not instruction. The therapist brings clinical knowledge and tools, while the client contributes insight into her lived experience, preferences, and capacity. For instance, when supporting a woman with complex trauma who is working to return to community-based volunteer roles, the therapist avoids prescribing a rigid schedule. Instead, they explore options together, prioritizing sustainability and control. By checking in regularly and responding to feedback without judgment, the therapist reinforces that progress is not measured by compliance, but by the client's sense of ownership in her own recovery.

Empowerment, Voice, and Choice

Empowerment in trauma-informed occupational therapy involves restoring a sense of control over decisions, routines, and personal narratives. Many women who have experienced trauma describe losing the ability to speak up, set limits, or prioritize their needs. Therapy becomes an opportunity to practice agency in both small and significant ways. For example, a woman recovering from medical trauma might choose to begin each session with a grounding activity rather than a structured task. The therapist honors this decision as a legitimate therapeutic entry point, not a delay. Over time, offering choices such as how to begin, what to focus on, or whether to pause supports the client in reclaiming voice within a system that may have silenced her before.

Cultural, Historical, and Gender Responsiveness

Trauma does not occur outside of culture. Clients arrive with identities shaped by their history, community, and the systems they have navigated. For women, trauma is often entangled with expectations about caregiving, silence, endurance, and service to others. Cultural responsiveness in occupational therapy demands more than surface-level competence—it requires deep reflection on one's own position, an understanding of social determinants of health, and a willingness to adapt care to reflect the client's values and lived context. A therapist working with an Indigenous woman healing from intergenerational trauma might integrate storytelling, land-based routines, or community rituals into intervention plans. Rather than assuming these elements are tangential to recovery, the therapist affirms that cultural practices are often central to occupational meaning and regulation. A culturally responsive approach invites the client to bring their full identity into the therapeutic space.

Peer and Community Support

While occupational therapy has historically focused on individualized treatment, trauma-informed care recognizes that healing often unfolds in the community. For many women, trauma is compounded by isolation, secrecy, or social disconnection. Peer support provides opportunities for validation, co-regulation, and the sharing of strategies that feel authentic and relevant. In a program supporting women survivors of intimate partner violence, an occupational therapist may coordinate with peer mentors or community health workers to co-facilitate a life skills group. Within this setting, participants exchange coping tools, reflect on common challenges, and engage in occupations that affirm shared resilience. The therapist's role is not to lead from above, but to support an environment where occupational growth is supported through belonging and mutual care.

Looking Ahead

Trauma alters more than individual well-being. It reshapes participation in daily life, disrupts the organization of identity, and constrains access to roles and environments that foster health and belonging. For women, these disruptions are compounded by social, structural, and institutional forces that frequently render trauma invisible or misinterpreted. Understanding trauma requires more than recognizing psychological symptoms; it requires attention to the broader ecological, cultural, and neurobiological systems in which those symptoms emerge.

Trauma-informed occupational therapy offers a framework through which healing can be pursued as both a personal and collective process. By addressing the physiological imprint of trauma alongside its occupational and relational consequences, practitioners are positioned to support recovery that is both meaningful and sustainable. This approach demands careful attention to context, power, and the conditions that shape participation. It also calls for critical reflection on how care is delivered, whose voices are centered, and what systems are either upheld or transformed through clinical practice.

Moving forward, the principles and insights discussed here offer a foundation for clinical reasoning, intervention planning, and systems-level advocacy. They invite occupational therapy practitioners to reimagine care not only as a path to function, but as a practice rooted in dignity, agency, and justice.

References

American Occupational Therapy Association (AOTA). (2020). Occupational therapy practice framework: Domain and process (4th ed.). *American Journal of Occupational Therapy*, *74*(Suppl. 2), 7412410010. https://doi.org/10.5014/ajot.2020.74S2001

Bauer, G. R., Churchill, S. M., Mahendran, M., Walwyn, C., Lizotte, D., & Villa-Rueda, A. A. (2021). Intersectionality in quantitative research: A systematic review of its emergence and applications of theory and methods. *SSM—Population Health*, *14*, 100798. https://doi.org/10.1016/j.ssmph.2021.100798

Brown, A., Barth, D. C., & Leslie, A. R. (2024). "You're someone different now": An autoethnography on identity and occupational identity disruption after traumatic brain injury. *The American Journal of Occupational Therapy: Official Publication of the American Occupational Therapy Association*, *78*(2), 7802180110. https://doi.org/10.5014/ajot.2024.050411

Cicchetti, D., & Rogosch, F. A. (2009). Adaptive coping under conditions of extreme stress: Multilevel influences on the determinants of resilience in maltreated children. *New Directions for Child and Adolescent Development*, *2009*(124), 47–59. https://doi.org/10.1002/cd.242

Dale, L. P., Shaikh, S. K., Fasciano, L. C., Watorek, V. D., Heilman, K. J., & Porges, S. W. (2018). College females with maltreatment histories have atypical autonomic regulation and poor psychological wellbeing. *Psychological Trauma: Theory, Research, Practice and Policy*, *10*(4), 427–434. https://doi.org/10.1037/tra0000342

Dana, D. (2018). *The polyvagal theory in therapy: Engaging the rhythm of regulation*. W. W. Norton & Co.

Edgelow, M. M., MacPherson, M. M., Arnaly, F., Tam-Seto, L., & Cramm, H. A. (2019). Occupational therapy and posttraumatic stress disorder: A scoping review. *Canadian Journal of Occupational Therapy. Revue canadienne d'ergotherapie*, *86*(2), 148–157. https://doi.org/10.1177/0008417419831438

Hillcoat, A., Prakash, J., Martin, L., Zhang, Y., Rosa, G., Tiemeier, H., Torres, N., Mustieles, V., Adams, C. D., & Messerlian, C. (2023). Trauma and female reproductive health across the life course: Motivating a research agenda for the future of women's health. *Human Reproduction (Oxford, England)*, *38*(8), 1429–1444. https://doi.org/10.1093/humrep/dead087

Iwama, M. K., Thomson, N. A., & Macdonald, R. M. (2009). The Kawa model: The power of culturally responsive occupational therapy. *Disability and Rehabilitation*, *31*(14), 1125–1135. https://doi.org/10.1080/09638280902773711

Khan, S. (2025). *Occupational therapy and women's health: A practitioner guide* (1st ed.). Routledge.

King-Mullins, E., Maccou, E., & Miller, P. (2023). Intersectionality: Understanding the interdependent systems of discrimination and disadvantage. *Clinics in Colon and Rectal Surgery*, *36*(5), 356–364. https://doi.org/10.1055/s-0043-1764343

Kirsh, B., & Cockburn, L. (2009). The Canadian Occupational Performance Measure: A tool for recovery-based practice. *Psychiatric Rehabilitation Journal*, *32*(3), 171–176. https://doi.org/10.2975/32.3.2009.171.176

Klabunde, M., Weems, C. F., Raman, M., & Carrion, V. G. (2017). The moderating effects of sex on insula subdivision structure in youth with posttraumatic stress symptoms. *Depression and Anxiety*, *34*(1), 51–58. https://doi.org/10.1002/da.22577

Mason, J., & Stagnitti, K. (2023). Occupational therapists' practice with complex trauma: A profile. *Australian Occupational Therapy Journal*, *70*(2), 190–201. https://doi.org/10.1111/1440-1630.12846

McLean, C. P., Asnaani, A., Litz, B. T., & Hofmann, S. G. (2011). Gender differences in anxiety disorders: Prevalence, course of illness, comorbidity and burden of illness. *Journal of Psychiatric Research*, *45*(8), 1027–1035. https://doi.org/10.1016/j.jpsychires.2011.03.006

Mirabile, M., Gnatt, I., Sharp, J. L., & Mackelprang, J. L. (2024). Shame and emotion dysregulation as pathways to posttraumatic stress symptoms among women with a history of interpersonal trauma. *Journal of Interpersonal Violence*, *39*(7–8), 1853–1876. https://doi.org/10.1177/08862605231211924

Muñoz-Rivas, M., Bellot, A., Montorio, I., Ronzón-Tirado, R., & Redondo, N. (2021). Profiles of emotion regulation and post-traumatic stress severity among female victims of intimate partner violence. *International Journal of Environmental Research and Public Health*, *18*(13), 6865. https://doi.org/10.3390/ijerph18136865

Nakao, M., Shirotsuki, K., & Sugaya, N. (2021). Cognitive-behavioral therapy for management of mental health and stress-related disorders: Recent advances in techniques and technologies. *BioPsychoSocial Medicine*, *15*(1), 16. https://doi.org/10.1186/s13030-021-00219-w

Philibert, L., Simon, D. J., & Lapierre, J. (2022). L'intersectionnalité pour mieux comprendre la problématique de la santé des femmes [Intersectionality to better understand women's health issues]. *Soins; la revue de reference infirmiere*, *67*(865), 18–21. https://doi.org/10.1016/j.soin.2022.05.006

Porges, S. W. (2011). *The polyvagal theory: Neurophysiological foundations of emotions, attachment, communication, and self-regulation*. W. W. Norton & Co.

Rosada, C., Bauer, M., Golde, S., Metz, S., Roepke, S., Otte, C., Wolf, O. T., Buss, C., & Wingenfeld, K. (2021). Association between childhood trauma and brain anatomy in women with post-traumatic stress disorder, women with borderline personality disorder, and healthy women. *European Journal of Psychotraumatology*, *12*(1), 1959706. https://doi.org/10.1080/20008198.2021.1959706

Sinko, L., Hughesdon, K., Grotts, J. H., Giordano, N., & Choi, K. R. (2022). A systematic review of research on trauma and women's health in the nurses' health study II. *Nursing for Women's Health*, *26*(2), 116–127. https://doi.org/10.1016/j.nwh.2022.01.005

Strong, S., Rigby, P., Stewart, D., Law, M., Letts, L., & Cooper, B. (1999). Application of the Person-Environment-Occupation model: A practical tool. *Canadian Journal of Occupational Therapy. Revue canadienne d'ergotherapie, 66*(3), 122–133. https://doi.org/10.1177/000841749906600304

Substance Abuse and Mental Health Services Administration (SAMHSA). (2014). *SAMHSA's concept of trauma and guidance for a trauma-informed approach* [HHS Publication No. SMA 14-4884]. Rockville, MD: Author. http://store.samhsa.gov/product/SAMHSA-s-Concept-of-Trauma-and-Guidance-for-a-Trauma-Informed-Approach/SMA14-4884

U.S. Department of Labor Women's Bureau. (2011). *Trauma-informed care for women veterans experiencing homelessness: A guide for service providers.* Washington, DC: Author. www.dol.gov/wb/trauma/

Chapter 2

Relational Stress and Trauma in Adolescents

Chapter Objectives

Upon completion of this chapter, the reader will be able to:

1. Explain how chronic relational stress during adolescence impacts brain development, identity formation, and emotional regulation in girls.
2. Identify common occupational disruptions linked to trauma in adolescent girls, including disruptions in roles, routines, and volition across school, home, and peer contexts.
3. Distinguish trauma-related behaviors such as dissociation, emotional numbing, and self-harm from intentional misbehavior using a neurodevelopmental and trauma-informed lens.
4. Apply trauma-informed strategies that support co-regulation, identity exploration, and safe participation in meaningful occupations for adolescent girls.
5. Analyze the role of gender, environment, and systemic inequities in shaping trauma exposure and occupational vulnerability during adolescence.

At sixteen, Monisha Sullivan had already become an expert at disappearing. She knew when to stay quiet, when to leave without asking, and how to keep her thoughts to herself. Since her mother left, she had been passed between relatives and foster homes, never staying long enough to unpack. When she walked into the clinic in Bayview Hunters Point, she did not ask for therapy. She came because her stomach cramped most mornings, her head throbbed after school, and she could not sleep through the night. Teachers said she was lazy.

DOI: 10.4324/9781003658559-2

One nurse called her dramatic. But nothing about her felt loud. She just wanted her body to stop feeling like it was trying to warn her. The doctor did not find an infection or a clear diagnosis. What she found was something harder to name. Monisha was not making it up. She was worn down. Her pain was real, but it was not coming from one place. It was everywhere. And it had been building for years.

Across the United States and in many global contexts, adolescent girls are navigating stressors that exceed what their developing nervous systems are designed to manage (CDC, 2023). While this stage of life is often described in terms of identity formation, exploration, and growing autonomy, many girls experience adolescence as a period of constraint, confusion, or emotional shutdown. When trauma is present, especially chronic relational trauma, it shapes not only how a girl feels, but how she develops, how she learns, and how she participates in daily life.

Emerging research in developmental neuroscience shows that adolescence is a sensitive window of brain plasticity (Eder-Moreau et al., 2022). During this time, the limbic system, which is responsible for processing emotion and threat, becomes more reactive, while the prefrontal cortex, which supports regulation and long-term decision-making, is still under construction. This imbalance makes adolescents more susceptible to intense emotional responses and less able to modulate them. When trauma is layered onto this neurodevelopmental stage, the risk for long-term changes in brain structure and function increases significantly.

For girls, trauma exposure often occurs within relationships that should feel safe, such as with caregivers, peers, teachers, or romantic partners. When these relationships become unpredictable or harmful, the result is not just psychological distress but also a recalibration of the nervous system toward vigilance, withdrawal, or collapse. These shifts may look like disengagement in school, heightened emotional sensitivity, perfectionism, or social avoidance. In clinical and educational settings, these behaviors are frequently misinterpreted as defiance, laziness, or lack of motivation. This misunderstanding can lead to punitive interventions rather than supportive ones, deepening the sense of disconnection.

Occupational disruption at this stage often begins subtly. A girl may stop participating in activities she once enjoyed, struggle to maintain routines, or report somatic symptoms like headaches and stomach pain without an identifiable cause. These are not minor concerns. They are often the first indicators of deeper dysregulation. Without timely, trauma-informed support, these patterns can solidify, shaping identity, limiting engagement, and carrying forward into adulthood.

Understanding the relationship between trauma, identity development, and occupational participation during adolescence is critical for practitioners. It requires more than empathy. It demands an informed clinical lens that recognizes how survival strategies develop, how they affect participation, and how they can be addressed without reinforcing shame or blame. Trauma-informed occupational therapy offers the opportunity to rebuild routines, restore safety, and support the development of agency in girls whose experiences have taught them to expect the opposite.

Developmental Considerations in Adolescence

At twelve, Sienna Johnson was known as the calm one. She made her younger siblings' lunches, kept track of the appointments her mother forgot, and answered texts from her father without showing how much they rattled her. Teachers praised her for being organized and mature. In therapy, she smiled and nodded often, but rarely talked about herself. When asked what she liked to do for fun, she hesitated, then said, "I don't really know." Her therapist noticed how often she deferred to others. Before starting a new task, she would ask, "Is this okay?" Her body was always just slightly tense, her eyes scanning for approval. What looked like responsibility was really protection. Sienna was not thriving. She was bracing.

Her math teacher reported that Sienna had become overly sensitive to correction. One afternoon, when he pointed out a small mistake on her homework, she went completely silent. Her face turned red, her eyes dropped to the desk, and she stayed withdrawn for the rest of class. Later, she tore the page from her notebook and threw it away. When her therapist gently asked what had happened, Sienna replied, "I mess everything up." Her reaction was not about the math. It was about what correction felt like, an echo of the times she had been blamed, dismissed, or left to figure things out alone. For Sienna, feedback was not just information. It was a threat to her safety and belonging.

What appeared to others as a dramatic overreaction was, in fact, a well-rehearsed survival strategy. Years of relational stress had taught her that mistakes might lead to rejection or emotional distance. In response, her nervous system did what it was wired to do: it shut down. In occupational therapy, her therapist began building small routines that helped her feel predictable success, paired with co-regulation strategies that made it safe to try again. Over time, Sienna began to understand that being corrected did not mean being unsafe. With support, her body could unlearn what it once had no choice but to expect.

What Sienna experienced reflects a broader pattern of relational stress in development, a form of adversity that is often misunderstood because it unfolds quietly beneath the surface of daily life. Adolescence is a period marked by rapid neurobiological growth, identity formation, and increasing social complexity. It is also a time when the brain is especially sensitive to environmental input, both supportive and harmful. For girls navigating this stage while also experiencing trauma, the effects can be especially profound.

Relational stress refers to the chronic strain that arises from instability, neglect, or harm within key interpersonal relationships. This may include emotional unavailability from caregivers, rejection or betrayal by peers, exposure to intimate partner violence within the family, or repeated disruptions in attachment figures. Unlike single-incident traumas, such as a car accident, a natural disaster, or a sudden act of violence, relational stress often unfolds slowly over time. It is embedded in the girl's daily life and often delivered by the very people who are supposed to provide safety. As a result, it not only wounds but also reshapes how she interprets connection, trust, and her own sense of worth.

While not all adolescents exposed to relational stress go on to develop depression, research has shown that difficulties navigating autonomy and connection within parent–teen relationships can predict depressive symptoms later on (Chango et al., 2012). In a longitudinal study published in the *Journal of Research on Adolescence*, teens who struggled to balance independence with emotional closeness, especially within strained family dynamics, were more likely to report depressed mood over time. This finding supports what developmental theorists like Bowlby described decades ago: that adolescence requires a shift from dependence to what he called "goal corrected partnerships," or relationships where both parties adjust to maintain emotional connection. When this balance breaks down, when a girl must choose between being herself and being accepted, the emotional cost can accumulate quietly, shaping her sense of safety, identity, and emotional regulation in ways that are often misunderstood.

These experiences occur precisely when the brain is forming critical neural pathways related to attachment, self-regulation, and executive functioning. Unlike the more observable forms of physical or acute trauma, relational trauma often remains hidden. Its manifestations are subtle but pervasive: difficulty trusting others, disrupted self-concept, and emotional dysregulation that emerges in classrooms, at home, or in peer relationships. These experiences can interrupt the developmental tasks of adolescence, leaving girls vulnerable to long-term mental health challenges and difficulties in identity formation. See Table 2.1 for an overview of how typical developmental tasks in adolescence may be disrupted by relational trauma and how these disruptions can impact occupational functioning across roles, routines, and contexts.

These developmental disruptions reflect more than temporary challenges. Relational trauma during adolescence can alter how girls interpret themselves, navigate relationships, and participate in meaningful activities. When tasks such as identity development, autonomy, or emotional regulation are interrupted, the

Table 2.1 Disruption of Developmental Tasks in Adolescent Girls Due to Relational Trauma

Developmental Task	Typical Function	Impact of Relational Trauma	Occupational Consequences
Establishing Identity	Exploration of values, interests, and roles; formation of self-concept	Fragmented or unstable sense of self; internalized shame; difficulty asserting preferences	Occupational disengagement, role confusion, limited goal setting, over-identification with trauma-based roles
Building Autonomy	Developing independence from caregivers; decision-making and self-direction	Distrust in self or others; fear of failure or abandonment; overdependence or premature independence	Difficulty initiating tasks, reliance on external validation, challenges with self-care and time management
Forming Peer Relationships	Developing intimacy, empathy, and belonging with peers	Peer mistrust, social withdrawal, or overattachment; increased vulnerability to bullying or toxic dynamics	Avoidance of social occupations, risky or people-pleasing behaviors, disrupted group participation
Emotional Regulation	Learning to manage stress, emotions, and conflict	Heightened reactivity, dissociation, or shutdown; poor frustration tolerance	Behavioral outbursts or passivity in school/home, difficulty adapting to changes in routines, impulsivity

(Continued)

Table 2.1 (Continued)

Developmental Task	Typical Function	Impact of Relational Trauma	Occupational Consequences
Academic Engagement	Building skills for learning, problem-solving, and academic success	Impaired concentration, executive dysfunction, or school avoidance	Incomplete assignments, reduced classroom participation, low academic self-esteem, dropout risk
Exploring Interests	Engaging in leisure, creativity, and future planning	Loss of joy or curiosity; avoidance of activities once enjoyed	Limited leisure engagement, lack of future planning, restricted occupational exploration
Developing Moral Reasoning	Understanding fairness, ethics, and accountability	Cynicism, Black-and-White thinking, or internalized guilt/blame	Difficulty navigating social conflicts, low self-advocacy, rigid or withdrawn participation in group activities (Khan, 2025)

effects often persist in other areas of life. These patterns are shaped by both internal neurobiological changes and external relational environments. For many girls, trauma becomes embedded in their emerging sense of self, shaping how they engage with others, how they make choices, and how they envision their place in the world.

Identity Formation and Vulnerability

During adolescence, identity is formed through a dynamic process of self-exploration, social comparison, and internal reflection. Girls begin to construct a sense of who they are by experimenting with roles, interests, values, and relationships. This developmental task requires a foundation of psychological safety and consistent interpersonal feedback. When relational trauma is present, such as abandonment, emotional neglect, or chronic invalidation, this foundation becomes weakened or entirely absent. Instead of developing a coherent and integrated self-concept, girls may internalize confusion, shame, or self-blame.

These disruptions are not always visible. A girl may excel in school or appear socially connected while privately struggling with a fractured sense of self. Others may adopt rigid roles, such as caretaker or high achiever, to create structure and predictability in emotionally unpredictable environments. These roles often reflect strategies for emotional survival rather than authentic identity development. Over time, trauma can obscure personal preferences, limit the ability to explore new activities, and foster dependence on external approval for validation.

From an occupational therapy perspective, disrupted identity development influences motivation, role performance, and participation in purposeful activities. When trauma distorts how a girl sees herself, it becomes difficult to engage in occupations that require initiative, self-direction, or decision-making. She may find it challenging to name her interests, express her needs, or take pride in accomplishments. Supporting identity formation in this context involves more than encouraging exploration. It requires the creation of emotionally safe environments where girls can reconnect with a sense of agency, experience consistent affirmation, and begin to build a narrative that reflects their strengths rather than their pain.

Gendered Exposure to Relational Trauma

Girls are more likely than boys to experience forms of trauma that are relational, prolonged, and rooted in power imbalances. These include emotional manipulation, body shaming, sexual harassment, and invalidation within close relationships. Such experiences often begin early and are reinforced through cultural messages that teach girls to prioritize others' needs, suppress their emotions, and tolerate discomfort to maintain connection. Over time, these patterns can erode self-trust and make it difficult to recognize or respond to harm.

Unlike acute trauma, which is often associated with a single event, gendered relational trauma tends to occur over extended periods of time and within trusted relationships. A girl who consistently receives the message that her voice does not matter, or that her boundaries can be ignored, begins to adapt in ways that help her survive emotionally. She may learn to appease others, avoid conflict, or disconnect from her own needs. While these adaptations are protective in the short term, they can limit long-term emotional development and restrict participation in meaningful activities.

These patterns are not isolated. National survey data reveal the widespread nature of this harm. According to the CDC's 2023 *Youth Risk Behavior Surveillance data*, one in five high school girls in the United States reported experiencing sexual violence in the past year, and one in ten had been forced to have sex. These experiences were strongly associated with depressive symptoms, suicidal ideation, and school disengagement. The study emphasized that girls who lacked access to safe environments and relational support were particularly vulnerable to long-lasting emotional and functional consequences.

In occupational therapy settings, the effects of gendered trauma often present subtly. A girl may appear compliant but disengaged, agreeable but emotionally distant, or focused on achievement while struggling with self-worth. These presentations are frequently misunderstood as personality traits rather than protective responses to persistent invalidation or relational harm. When these experiences are overlooked, interventions may focus on surface-level behaviors without addressing the deeper relational injuries that shape them (Miller, 2019).

Therapists working with adolescent girls must be attentive to the ways gendered trauma shapes identity, participation, and emotional safety. This includes recognizing how social expectations around caregiving, appearance, and emotional labor can reinforce harmful patterns. Effective support involves not only validating the impact of these experiences, but also helping girls reclaim agency in how they relate to others, make choices, and engage with the world around them.

Intersection of Puberty and Environmental Stressors

At thirteen, Janiya Alvarez started slipping out of view. Once known for her energy and bright smile in after-school dance, she now kept her hood up, avoided eye contact, and stopped turning in homework. When she was referred to occupational therapy through the school wellness team, she arrived at her first session silent and withdrawn. She folded her arms tightly and stared at the floor. When asked about her routines, she said flatly, "I don't do anything. I just feel gross all the time." Over time, pieces of her story came through. Janiya had recently started her period and was struggling with body-based routines. She had stopped showering regularly and refused to dress out for gym. Living with her grandmother after being removed from her mother's care, she described feeling judged in her neighborhood and out of place at school. Mirrors made her uncomfortable. Touch felt overstimulating. Her body no longer felt like hers.

Janiya's story reflects what many adolescent girls experience when multiple transitions collide. The onset of puberty does not occur in a vacuum. It often overlaps with environmental instability, shifting caregiving arrangements, and unresolved trauma. These overlapping stressors disrupt the formation of roles, routines, and body-based habits that are essential for identity development. What may appear as disengagement, moodiness, or poor hygiene is often the result of internal changes that feel confusing and overwhelming, especially in contexts that lack safety, affirmation, or consistency. For girls with trauma histories, this stage often marks the beginning of occupational withdrawal, not because of disinterest, but because of physiological and emotional overload.

Puberty represents a complex neuroendocrine transformation that influences emotional regulation and sensory processing, often intensifying the impact of prior trauma. For girls who have experienced relational stress or environmental adversity, these changes do not occur in isolation. Hormonal surges heighten emotional reactivity, intensify body awareness, and alter rhythms of sleep, appetite, and energy. When layered on top of environments marked by neglect, violence, or instability, the result is often a nervous system overwhelmed by both internal and external changes.

A longitudinal study by Boynton-Jarrett and Harville (2012) examined the relationship between childhood social hardships and age at menarche in a cohort of over 4,500 girls. They found that cumulative adversities, such as caregiver neglect, family dysfunction, paternal absence, and lack of supportive caregiving, were significantly associated with variations in the timing of menarche. Interestingly, while the presence of two or more early-life hardships increased the risk for later menarche, exposure to childhood sexual abuse was most strongly linked to early onset. These findings suggest that the type, timing, and chronicity of adversity shape biological development in different ways. The stress response system plays a critical role; chronic activation may disrupt hormonal balance, body composition, and developmental timing, influencing how girls enter and experience puberty.

These biological shifts are not without consequence. Early or delayed menarche has been linked to increased risk for depression, low bone mineral density, cardiovascular issues, and behavioral health problems. From an occupational perspective, girls whose puberty is shaped by hardship may withdraw from age-appropriate roles or feel emotionally unprepared for the changes in their bodies. They may avoid physical activity, disengage from hygiene routines, or feel discomfort in social spaces where gendered expectations are heightened.

Occupational Therapy Approach

Occupational therapy can play a vital role in supporting adolescent girls through the occupational disruptions that often accompany trauma and puberty. Rather than focusing solely on hygiene compliance or participation in school-based routines, therapists can reframe body-based occupations as entry points for co-regulation, sensory processing, and identity integration (AOTA, 2020).

For hygiene routines, the use of sensory-friendly products, such as unscented soap, low-foaming shampoo, and microfiber towels, can reduce overstimulation for girls who experience touch or smell as intrusive. Pairing these with environmental modifications, such as dimmable bathroom lighting, warm water presets, soft-close cabinet doors, or non-slip shower mats, can help create a more calming and predictable context that reduces sensory defensiveness and improves follow-through. A regulation break before or after bathing might include three minutes of deep pressure input using a weighted lap pad, a guided breathing app while seated on a closed toilet lid, or proprioceptive input like squeezing a therapy ball to reduce internal activation and support body awareness.

When girls refuse to change for physical education or other school-based activities, layered clothing strategies can serve as transitional tools. For example, a girl might wear compression shorts under looser gym clothes to maintain proprioceptive input and preserve modesty. A lightweight, breathable long-sleeve shirt may be worn under a school uniform to minimize direct tactile input from fabrics that feel scratchy or revealing. These strategies allow the girl to gradually build tolerance while maintaining a sense of safety and control.

Narrative-based tools, such as visual mapping of body experiences or reflective journaling prompts focused on "what my body helps me do," can support emotional processing while reinforcing positive body identity. For menstruation-related avoidance, occupational therapists can incorporate self-care kits into routine planning—complete with preferred pads or menstrual products, a private storage pouch, scent-neutral wipes, and access scripts girls can use to request help from school staff discreetly. These supports do more than facilitate hygiene. They help girls rebuild a sense of ownership over their bodies and reduce the shame and confusion that often accompany pubertal transitions in the context of trauma.

Neurological and Psychological Changes

During adolescence, the brain undergoes extensive remodeling. Emotional and reward-processing centers, such as the amygdala and ventral striatum, develop earlier than the prefrontal cortex, the region responsible for impulse control, long-term planning, and emotional regulation. This uneven maturation leaves adolescents especially sensitive to emotional inputs and vulnerable to impulsivity, particularly in contexts of stress or trauma.

What makes this stage especially complex for girls with trauma histories is not only what is developing, but also what is still under construction. Regulatory strategies like cognitive reappraisal rely heavily on prefrontal structures, which are still maturing throughout the teen years. According to a recent review by Sahi et al. (2023), adolescents are often less able to regulate emotions using traditional top-down strategies because the relevant neural systems are still in development. For girls who have experienced early adversity, this gap between emotional intensity and regulatory capacity may be even more pronounced.

However, the same review points to a promising opportunity: adolescence is also marked by increased sensitivity to peer input. The brain becomes finely attuned to social cues, particularly those from friends and trusted peers. Sahi et al. (2023) propose that regulation supported by peers, also referred to as social reappraisal, may be especially effective during this window. When adolescents receive validation or reframing from a friend, their emotional responses often soften. In essence, peers can act as co-regulators, offering real-time buffering against stress and dysregulation.

This insight is especially relevant to occupational therapy. Peer influence is often framed negatively in trauma-informed work, particularly in settings like group homes or schools where maladaptive behaviors can spread. However, this research invites a reframing: trusted peer relationships can be leveraged therapeutically to build self-regulation, reduce isolation, and enhance emotional processing.

In practice, this might look like:

- Pairing students for structured co-occupations that require reciprocal support, such as preparing a shared snack, planning a simple event, or co-leading a class warm-up. These tasks should include role-sharing, built-in feedback, and opportunities for positive peer affirmation. The focus is not just task completion but co-regulation through shared responsibility.
- Designing dyadic narrative activities where girls co-create a timeline or "day in the life" storyboard of each other's routines, then reflect on what emotions or challenges came up. This builds perspective-taking and strengthens social mirroring, which supports emotional self-awareness and validation.
- Embedding peer check-ins into existing group routines using tools like color-coded emotion cards or brief prompts (e.g., "What helped you feel calm today?"). These check-ins can be guided by an occupational therapist or peer mentor and offer low-pressure ways to name internal states while witnessing emotional patterns in others.
- Facilitating collaborative sensory regulation stations where girls rotate in pairs through calming activities—such as weighted lap pads, resistance bands, music selection, or lavender-scented lotion—while discussing which ones help and why. This allows peers to share strategies, compare preferences, and normalize nervous system support as part of daily life.
- Co-leading psychoeducational modules where older or more experienced participants introduce body-based coping strategies to younger peers. This builds self-efficacy for the mentor while reinforcing trust and belonging for the mentee. The occupational therapist provides the scaffold and structure, but the relational modeling happens peer-to-peer.

Rather than focusing solely on individual coping strategies, occupational therapists can create opportunities for relational scaffolding. These are interactions that help adolescents co-regulate and feel seen within safe and supportive contexts. These experiences do more than shape behavior. They influence how the developing brain interprets safety, connection, and threat. At the same time, adolescents are managing internal stress systems that are significantly affected by chronic adversity. The body's neuroendocrine pathways, especially the hypothalamic-pituitary-adrenal axis, play a key role in how stress is processed and retained. For girls with trauma histories, increased hormonal sensitivity can contribute to emotional dysregulation, persistent fatigue, and inconsistent participation in daily roles. Understanding these physiological mechanisms is essential for supporting regulation, engagement, and long-term recovery. For adolescent girls who have experienced adversity, recognizing how hormonal shifts affect emotional function and occupational participation is foundational to providing trauma-responsive care.

HPA Axis and Hormonal Sensitivity in Adolescent Girls

The HPA axis is a central component of the body's stress-response system, regulating cortisol and other hormones that influence energy levels, immune functioning, attention, sleep, and mood. During adolescence, this system becomes more active and more reactive, influenced by both hormonal changes and environmental context. For girls with a history of trauma, especially chronic relational stress or neglect, the HPA axis may not develop typical patterns of activation and recovery. Instead, it may remain in a heightened or blunted state, leading to physiological and behavioral patterns that are often misunderstood.

Girls with trauma exposure may experience **hyperactivation** of the HPA axis, where even minor stressors trigger exaggerated physiological responses such as racing heart, nausea, and emotional flooding. Others may show **hypoactivation**, where their cortisol output becomes blunted due to prolonged stress exposure. These individuals may appear disengaged, flat, or chronically fatigued. In both cases, the internal stress systems are working outside of typical regulatory bounds, making it difficult to respond adaptively to challenges in everyday life.

Recent research has shown that adolescents with trauma histories often display **dysregulated diurnal cortisol rhythms**, meaning their cortisol levels fail to follow the typical high-in-the-morning, low-in-the-evening pattern. This irregularity can result in poor sleep quality, low morning alertness, emotional lability, and diminished capacity to recover from stress throughout the day. These biological disruptions influence how girls participate in routines, interact with peers, and perform in academic or therapeutic settings.

From an occupational therapy perspective, understanding HPA axis dysregulation provides a critical framework for interpreting behaviors that might otherwise be labeled as defiance, laziness, or disinterest. Instead of focusing solely on behavior correction, OT practitioners can support regulation through routines, environmental modifications, and sensory-based strategies tailored to the girl's physiological profile. Table 2.2 presents an overview of common HPA axis response patterns, their functional impact, and considerations for occupational therapy.

These stress response patterns are not theoretical concepts. They unfold in real time as girls attempt to participate in daily routines, engage socially, or manage academic and personal demands. Hormonal changes during adolescence,

Table 2.2 Patterns of HPA Axis Dysregulation and Occupational Implications

HPA Axis Pattern	Physiological Characteristics	Occupational Presentation	Occupational Therapy Considerations
Hyperactivation	Heightened cortisol response to minor stressors	Emotional outbursts, restlessness, avoidance of performance-based tasks	Calming sensory input, predictable routines, co-regulation strategies
Hypoactivation	Blunted cortisol, low physiological arousal	Fatigue, passivity, reduced initiation, flat affect	Rhythmic movement, gradual activation strategies, environmental stimulation
Delayed Recovery	Prolonged stress response after stressor is removed	Sustained irritability, difficulty shifting from distress to calm	Scaffold transitions, extended processing time, post-activity recovery periods
Irregular Rhythms	Inconsistent cortisol levels throughout the day	Variable mood, sleep disturbances, low endurance for sustained engagement	Emphasize morning activation, embed rest periods, establish day-long regulation anchors

including shifts in estrogen, progesterone, and cortisol, amplify the sensitivity of the HPA axis and influence how emotions are processed and expressed. Estrogen, for example, can increase cortisol reactivity and heighten emotional responses, while fluctuations in progesterone are linked to mood variability and sleep disturbances. These hormonal rhythms interact with trauma-related stress responses, making emotional and behavioral regulation even more unpredictable. When the nervous system is functioning outside of its typical range, what appears to be moodiness or disinterest may reflect an internal environment struggling to maintain balance.

Understanding these interactions allows occupational therapists to recognize dysregulation as a biologically driven pattern, not a character flaw. These physiological shifts often emerge as patterns of emotional volatility, withdrawal, or inconsistent engagement, shaping how adolescent girls respond to daily demands and participate across roles, routines, and environments. Trauma during adolescence leaves a neurobiological imprint, but it is also lived through routines, roles, and relationships. By understanding these patterns through a trauma-responsive lens, occupational therapists can offer not just coping tools but also healing environments that restore dignity, identity, and choice.

Dysregulation Patterns in Adolescent Girls

For many adolescent girls with trauma histories, dysregulation is not constant, but episodic and unpredictable. A girl may appear calm and focused in one moment and completely shut down in the next, not because of mood instability alone, but because her nervous system is constantly recalibrating in response to both internal cues and environmental demands. These fluctuations are often invisible to others, making the girl's responses appear inconsistent, inappropriate, or disproportionate.

What is often overlooked is that trauma-related dysregulation is context-dependent. A girl might "hold it together" at school, only to release pent-up tension at home. Others may comply with adult requests while dissociating internally, disengaging from the emotional or sensory demands of the moment. Many teens describe feeling "numb but tense," or "angry for no reason," without understanding that these are survival-based adaptations rooted in physiological overload and emotional exhaustion.

This mismatch between external expectations and internal capacity can lead to a cascade of consequences: punitive discipline at school, ruptures in peer relationships, or feelings of self-blame. From an occupational perspective, dysregulation disrupts rhythm, flow, and identity. A girl may be unable to sustain daily routines, lose interest in meaningful activities, or cycle through roles that feel inauthentic or misaligned.

Importantly, dysregulation is not always loud. Some girls move through the day with minimal affect, flat tone, and a smile that conceals disconnection. Others appear driven, overachieving, or perfectionistic—until they collapse. These contrasting presentations can make it difficult for educators, therapists, or caregivers to recognize that support is needed.

Occupational therapists are uniquely positioned to decode these patterns, not through observation alone, but by asking: "What is the nervous system trying to protect?" and "What roles or routines feel unsafe, overwhelming, or unavailable?" Rather than trying to regulate the behavior, the role of occupational therapy is to help girls reconnect with regulation through co-regulation, occupational rhythm, and relational safety.

Marisol Fernandez, a fifteen-year-old quiet girl, was widely regarded by her teachers as a model student. She arrived on time, turned in her assignments, and never caused disruptions. In group settings, she smiled often but rarely contributed. Her school file noted "shy-ness" and "low participation," with no history of behavior concerns. It wasn't until an occupational therapy screening for academic fatigue flagged consistent late-afternoon shutdowns, such as long bathroom breaks, head down on the desk, and complaints of nausea, that any-one noticed something was off. When gently approached during a follow-up session, Marisol admitted she felt exhausted by lunchtime nearly every day. She described intense pressure to appear "normal" and "together" so no one would ask questions. At home, she often spent hours alone in her room with music or sleeping as her only form of relief. She had stopped dancing, something she once loved, and often forgot to eat. "It's like I'm always pretending to be in my body," she said, "but I don't feel like I'm really here."

Marisol's case highlights a dysregulation pattern that does not present with outbursts or defiance but rather with withdrawal, perfectionism, and emotional exhaustion masked as high-functioning compliance. Her nervous system was not dysregulated because she lacked coping skills, but because it had learned to survive by blending in. Without a trauma-informed lens, her distress might have continued unnoticed.

Marisol's behaviors, such as compliance, emotional flatness, and fatigue, may appear functional on the surface, but from an occupational therapy perspective, they reveal significant nervous system distress. Her ability to mask discomfort and meet external expectations suggests a pattern of functional dissociation, a state in which the body continues performing tasks while the emotional self detaches for safety. This strategy often develops in individuals who have learned that emotional expression or vulnerability leads to invalidation or harm. The loss of meaningful engagement in preferred activities like dance, the inconsist-ent participation later in the day, and her disconnection from basic routines such as eating reflect a broader pattern of occupational withdrawal. While Marisol is fulfilling performance roles (e.g., student), her volition, identity, and emotional presence within those roles are fragmented.

Unless dysregulation is explicitly identified and addressed, it will remain a persistent barrier to therapeutic progress across all occupational domains. Mari-sol's case illustrates that performance without regulation is not sustainable. From a clinical perspective, no intervention focused on executive function, academic achievement, health routines, or social participation will yield meaningful results if the nervous system remains in a protective state. A dysregulated system com-promises goal-directed behavior, limits access to memory and decision-making, and interferes with motivation and task initiation. This has direct implications for school-based goals, participation in ADLs and IADLs, and broader health management.

Occupational therapists are not only well-positioned to recognize these patterns but to respond with precision (Dowdy et al., 2022). Intervention should begin with co-regulation and sensory safety, establishing baseline routines that promote interoceptive awareness and emotional presence. For example, before initiating executive functioning strategies, the therapist might first introduce body-based regulation tools such as guided breathing paired with proprioceptive input during transitions. Before focusing on hygiene routines or academic productivity, it may be necessary to build emotional literacy and predictability into the daily schedule. Addressing dysregulation is not an adjunct; it is central to care planning. Once the nervous system begins to experience safety, other goals become more accessible. Only then can girls like Marisol begin to engage not just with tasks, but with themselves.

Trauma Responses in Adolescent Girls

Trauma rarely announces itself in straightforward ways. In adolescent girls, it often shows up as behaviors that seem confusing, disruptive, or inconsistent, especially to those unfamiliar with the inner workings of trauma (Danzi & La Greca, 2021). What appears to be defiance, attention seeking, or emotional instability may, in fact, be a survival strategy shaped by years of unpredictability, invalidation, or harm. These responses are not personality flaws or conduct issues. They are nervous system adaptations that emerge when safety is uncertain and regulation is inaccessible (Danzi & La Greca, 2021).

Occupational therapists play a critical role in recognizing the difference between protective responses and intentional misbehavior. The ability to differentiate between survival-based behavior and more typical acting out can guide intervention strategies that center safety, co-regulation, and occupational engagement, rather than punishment or compliance.

Survival-Based Behaviors vs. Acting Out

It is easy to misread trauma responses in adolescent girls as disrespect, apathy, or lack of motivation. A teen who refuses to engage in group activities may be labeled defiant, while one who becomes emotionally overwhelmed during a seemingly minor transition may be viewed as immature. Yet, these same behaviors often reflect attempts to protect the self, not acts of disobedience, but adaptive responses to environments that feel unsafe or unpredictable.

The distinction between survival-based behavior and intentional acting out lies in the function rather than the form. Survival responses are driven by the nervous system's effort to avoid perceived threat, manage emotional overload, or maintain a sense of control. These patterns are typically reactive, repetitive, and emotionally intense. In contrast, acting out, while still deserving of compassion, tends to be more deliberate and responsive to boundaries, consequences, or incentives. Understanding the underlying function of behavior can help therapists respond with compassion and clarity. Table 2.3 outlines key clinical indicators that can help distinguish survival-based responses from more intentional behavior patterns.

Table 2.3 Differentiating Survival-Based Responses from Intentional Acting Out

Area of Observation	Survival-Based Response	More Typical Acting Out
Consistency Across Contexts	Behavior varies depending on perceived safety; may appear regulated in structured classrooms but dysregulated at home or in unstructured settings	Behavior is more stable across settings; oppositional or attention-seeking behaviors are present in most environments
Response to Structure	Escalates or shuts down with rigid rules, time pressure, or unpredictable transitions (e.g., becomes tearful, freezes, or refuses altogether)	Responds to clear expectations, especially when paired with logical consequences; may argue, but eventually complies
Emotional Triggers	Strong reactions to subtle cues such as neutral tone, peer proximity, or facial expressions; may misinterpret guidance as threat	Emotional responses are tied to clear, observable triggers such as loss of privilege, being told no, or peer confrontation
Body-Based Symptoms	Frequent complaints of stomach pain, headaches, nausea, or fatigue, particularly before stress-inducing tasks; avoids sensory input like noise or bright lights	Physical symptoms are infrequent or clearly used to avoid a specific task (e.g., test, chore) without broader sensory sensitivities
Response to Feedback	May withdraw, shut down, or begin self-criticism when corrected or praised; often appears overwhelmed or dissociative	Typically adjusts behavior based on praise or consequence; may talk back, deflect, or express frustration openly
Level of Awareness	Often unable to name triggers or reasons for behavior; gives vague responses like "I don't know" or "nothing happened"	Can explain motive behind actions, even if impulsive (e.g., "I didn't want to," "I was upset") and may engage in negotiation

Survival-based behaviors are not deliberate choices, but patterned responses shaped by histories of unmet needs, perceived threat, and disrupted safety. These responses often emerge in environments that unknowingly mirror earlier relational harm, such as rigid authority, unpredictable transitions, or emotional invalidation. For many adolescent girls, especially those navigating structural inequities, these settings are part of their daily lives. When they are labeled as difficult, dramatic, or resistant, the underlying function of their behavior is missed. This misinterpretation not only fractures therapeutic relationships but also deepens the sense of invisibility and powerlessness that the behavior was meant to guard against.

Occupational therapy creates space for a different response—one that begins with observation, not correction. When therapists ask what the behavior is trying to communicate, what internal state is being protected, or what feels threatening about the current demand, they open the door to trauma-responsive care. This approach emphasizes safety over compliance and presence over performance. It centers the nervous system as a guide for intervention and recognizes that dysregulation often precedes words. As the next section explores, many girls do not act out at all. Instead, they disappear into themselves—numbing, avoiding, or disconnecting when presence feels unsafe. These quieter trauma responses are no less urgent, and they require a therapeutic lens attuned to what remains unseen.

Dissociation, Self-Harm, and Emotional Numbing

Trauma does not always result in visible distress. While some girls externalize emotional pain, others turn inward, distancing themselves from sensations, relationships, and even their own sense of identity. These responses are often mischaracterized as withdrawal, inattention, or manipulation. In reality, they reflect the body and mind working to survive conditions that have become intolerable.

Dissociation is a state in which a person becomes disconnected from the present moment. This can include a loss of bodily awareness, gaps in memory, or a sensation of floating outside of oneself. For adolescent girls who have experienced chronic emotional invalidation or violation, dissociation becomes a protective strategy. It allows them to remain physically present while emotionally escaping a situation that feels overwhelming. This response may look like zoning out in class, becoming nonresponsive during conflict, or appearing distant and unaffected in moments of high emotional intensity. It is often mistaken for apathy or noncompliance, rather than understood as the nervous system withdrawing to preserve psychological safety.

Self-harm is another misunderstood trauma response. Behaviors such as cutting or scratching are not usually about seeking attention. They are often attempts to cope with internal chaos, emotional numbness, or intense distress that cannot be expressed verbally. For many girls, self-harm is the only way they know to feel something, or to reestablish a sense of control over their bodies. When systems respond with punishment, surveillance, or isolation, the underlying distress remains unaddressed and may even deepen. What is needed instead is a response that prioritizes safety, relational attunement, and access to regulating occupations.

Emotional numbing refers to a reduced capacity to feel or express emotion. It is not an absence of care, but a sign that feeling has become too dangerous or overwhelming. Girls experiencing emotional blunting may withdraw from activities they once loved, stop responding to praise or conflict, or express disconnection from both positive and negative experiences. This emotional flatness is often interpreted as depression or lack of motivation, when in fact it is a trauma response rooted in survival. The nervous system narrows its emotional range to avoid further pain.

Occupational therapists can support regulation and reconnection by creating consistent, emotionally safe spaces where girls can gradually rebuild trust in themselves, their bodies, and others. These interventions are not about fixing behavior, but about restoring agency, presence, and capacity for meaningful participation (Fialkowski et al., 2022). Trauma-informed care begins with understanding that numbness, dissociation, and self-harm are not resistance to therapy—they are evidence of what the nervous system has endured. See Table 2.4 for occupational therapy approaches to support girls experiencing dissociation, numbing, or self-harm.

Table 2.4 Occupational Therapy Approaches to Support Girls Experiencing Dissociation, Numbing, or Self-Harm

Occupational Therapy Focus Area	Purpose and Therapeutic Function	Example in Practice
Sensory-based occupations	Reconnect with the body and build internal awareness without overwhelming the nervous system	Weighted lap pads during virtual learning; scented putty sculpting in a quiet room; self-directed walks with nature-based sensory kits
Creative or movement-based expression	Provide outlets for emotional release that do not rely on verbal processing or direct confrontation	Cultural dance forms; expressive journaling with music; creating zines or storyboards using recycled or personal materials

(Continued)

Table 2.4 (Continued)

Occupational Therapy Focus Area	Purpose and Therapeutic Function	Example in Practice
Structured, predictable routines	Reduce unpredictability and create opportunities for felt safety and regulation through rhythm	Consistent start and end-of-session rituals, routine-based scheduling, visual daily planners using icons; a morning sensory activation menu; OT-led group sessions with rhythmic breathing starts
Pleasure and joy re-engagement	Gradually reintroduce occupations that bring meaning and satisfaction to rebuild emotional range	Low-stakes community-based outings (e.g., art museum visits); digital photography scavenger hunts; art/drawing clubs
Co-occupation and relational safety building	Foster connection through shared activity that supports regulation through relationship	Cooking with a trusted adult, partnered crafts, co-created vision boards with a caregiver, peer mentoring through crafting or music or parallel play in early sessions

When a girl begins to reconnect with her body and emotions through safe, supported occupation, the path toward reengagement slowly opens. Yet, even as internal regulation improves, external environments, particularly classrooms, peer groups, and public spaces, can continue to feel unsafe, invalidating, or disorienting. Behaviors such as school refusal, social withdrawal, or shutting down during group activities are often not signs of apathy but deeply protective adaptations. To support reentry into these spaces, occupational therapists must understand both the perceived threats and the functional roles these adaptations play. Safe pathways back into participation may include transitional occupations such as volunteering in a low-stimulation school role before returning to class, using virtual attendance as a bridge to in-person learning, or establishing a quiet retreat space within school settings. Occupational therapists might also collaborate with teachers to modify participation demands, support peer pairing with trusted friends, or co-develop safety scripts girls can use when they feel overwhelmed. Reengagement is not a return to normal. It is a carefully scaffolded restoration of agency, voice, and belonging.

School Refusal, Avoidance, and Peer Withdrawal

Avoidance is one of the most misunderstood trauma responses in adolescent girls. When a teen repeatedly misses school, avoids social spaces, or withdraws from group activities, these behaviors are often seen as defiance, attention seeking, or a lack of motivation. Yet, for many girls with trauma histories, avoidance is a form of emotional self-protection, a way to reduce exposure to environments that feel overwhelming, unsafe, or invalidating. From a neurobiological perspective, avoidance is often the output of a nervous system that has shifted into a threat response. In the presence of chronic stress or relational trauma, key brain regions involved in emotional regulation such as the amygdala, insula, and prefrontal cortex become dysregulated. The amygdala becomes hypervigilant, detecting threat where there may be none. Meanwhile, reduced prefrontal control limits a girl's ability to reflect, reappraise, or remain engaged when overwhelmed. In this state, avoidance is not a passive behavior. It is a neurologically driven survival strategy aimed at reducing internal overload.

School refusal is not simply about disinterest in academics. It may reflect anxiety about being misunderstood, fear of social judgment, or a learned pattern of withdrawing when power feels imbalanced. A girl who appears oppositional may be navigating unspoken social dynamics, teacher bias, or overstimulation in crowded or noisy spaces. For others, peer withdrawal may serve as a boundary to prevent rejection, bullying, or exposure to situations that mimic earlier relational harm. The refusal is not about avoiding growth; it is about avoiding further harm.

These responses are often compounded by punitive or performance-based systems. When absences lead to truancy interventions or when avoidance is met with pressure to "push through," the nervous system becomes more activated. Girls may begin to associate occupational participation—especially in school and social contexts—with shame, failure, or exposure. Without intervention, a cycle of disengagement begins to form: the more they avoid, the less supported they feel, and the harder it becomes to reenter.

Occupational therapists can help disrupt this cycle by reframing avoidance as communication rather than resistance. Rather than forcing participation, the goal becomes uncovering what feels unsafe and working collaboratively to create a bridge back to meaningful engagement. This includes identifying the sensory, relational, emotional, or cognitive demands that may overwhelm the girl's capacity, and using occupation to reintroduce participation in a way that honors both readiness and agency. Table 2.5 outlines occupational therapy strategies for navigating avoidance and withdrawal in teen girls.

Reengagement is not achieved through force or compliance. It begins with a deeper understanding of the reasons behind a young person's withdrawal and the environmental or relational factors that have made school feel unsafe. However, a trauma-informed approach does not mean removing all challenges or exempting students from necessary social development. Rather, it means shaping the *how* of participation with care, flexibility, and transparency.

For example, when classroom assignments require group work, the goal is not to bypass participation entirely but to scaffold the experience in a way that honors readiness. A girl who feels overwhelmed by peer dynamics may benefit

Table 2.5 School-Based Occupational Therapy Strategies for Supporting Avoidance and Withdrawal in Adolescent Girls

Barrier to Participation	Therapeutic Focus	Occupational Therapy Strategy Example
Sensory overload in classroom or group	Create sensory regulation options in shared environments	Use of classroom calm kits, permission to use fidget items, dimmed lighting or sunglasses, flexible seating options, outdoor breakout zones
Social anxiety or peer mistrust	Rebuild safety in shared spaces through low demand social occupations	Collaborative art boards, audio-only shared playlists, gardening with a peer, group cooking with defined solo roles
Academic overwhelm or fear of failure	Support executive function and reduce performance pressure	Choice boards for assignment formats (video, drawing, audio), executive function coaching, visual scaffolds, flexible due dates
Emotional exhaustion or avoidance cycle	Use rhythm and routine to gently scaffold reentry	Hybrid school plans, "soft start" school days, OT-led morning prep sessions, wellness journaling with check-in rituals
Loss of agency or voice in system	Rebuild control and participation through shared decision-making	Co-writing classroom support plans, selecting their own seating or partners, designing their own self-regulation strategies

from a slow entry point such as being allowed to observe first, working alongside a trusted peer, or contributing asynchronously.

Occupational therapists can advocate for flexible grouping structures, co-develop scripts for navigating social tension, or coach students on how to assert boundaries during collaboration. If avoidance is rooted in past relational trauma, exposure to group work should not be forced but also not indefinitely postponed. With the right supports, students can gradually rebuild trust and confidence in their ability to contribute meaningfully, even in imperfect environments.

True trauma-informed care is not about removing every discomfort. It is about reducing harm, restoring agency, and helping students reenter roles with a renewed sense of safety and choice. In this way, participation becomes not just a classroom requirement but an act of healing.

Environmental and Systemic Influences on Occupational Disruption in Adolescents

When fifteen-year-old Nyla Auguste was suspended for skipping class and "talking back" to a teacher, the school labeled her as defiant. What they didn't see was that Nyla had started the day with no clean clothes, no phone charger, and no adult at home. She had moved in with a relative two weeks earlier after her mother's incarceration, sleeping on a pull-out couch in a living room that never really went quiet. Her mornings began at five, navigating two bus transfers across the city, often arriving at school without breakfast or a working pencil. She tried to stay invisible in class, but when her math teacher singled her out for not bringing her textbook, the frustration spilled out. Her tone was clipped. She rolled her eyes. It was not the math. It was the accumulation of being tired, unseen, and asked to meet expectations she had no resources to fulfill.

Stories like Nyla's are not rare. For many adolescent girls, especially those navigating trauma, daily life unfolds inside systems that were never built for them. Trauma does not just affect emotions or behavior. It reshapes how girls engage with the world—at school, at home, with peers, and within themselves. It disrupts routines, distorts identity, and chips away at the quiet sense of safety needed to grow. And too often, the environments meant to support them respond with punishment instead of care. From school policies and juvenile justice to the invisible pressure of social media, these forces shape not just what girls do each day, but who they believe they are becoming.

For occupational therapists, understanding these systems is essential. Healing does not happen in isolation. It happens through engagement, through relationships, and through the reclamation of meaningful roles in environments that finally feel safe enough to stay. This means therapists must look beyond the referral reason and begin with contextual inquiry, asking not only what the student is doing, but what they are navigating. For girls like Nyla, occupational therapy may begin with modifying the sensory and emotional demands of the school day: identifying classrooms where overstimulation is high, helping create regulation routines during long commutes, or collaborating with staff to reduce disciplinary exposure that reinforces shame. It may involve helping the student co-develop a predictable morning prep checklist that matches their living context, using visuals or text reminders tailored to unstable routines. It might also include facilitating restorative roles at school—opportunities for leadership, creative expression, or peer mentorship that allow the student to be seen for her strengths, not just her struggles.

Additionally, therapists can support reengagement with valued occupations that have been lost or interrupted. For Nyla, this could mean reintroducing a journaling practice, helping her request flexible deadlines without stigma, or connecting her with a trusted adult mentor on campus. Occupational therapy in these cases is not about fixing behavior; it is about rebuilding participation by restoring agency, predictability, and the right to feel safe enough to show up fully. When therapists recognize the layers underneath the behavior and adapt the environment to fit the girl, rather than forcing the girl to fit the system, participation becomes possible again.

Disruption of Daily Routines and Role Development

In the life of an adolescent girl, routines are often where identity begins to take shape. Whether she's brushing her hair before school, texting a friend about a class presentation, or finding quiet in the rhythm of after-dinner chores, these ordinary moments offer stability, predictability, and connection. For many teens, they are the backdrop against which self-concept, motivation, and emotional regulation quietly develop. But trauma changes the way these moments are lived. It fractures rhythm, interrupts roles, and replaces familiarity with unpredictability.

Relational stress, particularly when chronic or unrecognized, can dismantle the ability to engage in daily activities. Girls may oversleep or struggle with insomnia. Meals are missed, avoided, or emotionally fraught. Homework is forgotten not out of carelessness, but because the brain is working overtime to manage internal chaos. A teen may withdraw from peers or become hyper-responsible at home, filling in emotional gaps she was never meant to hold.

Both the **Model of Human Occupation (MOHO)** and the **Person-Environment-Occupation (PEO) model** provide insight into how trauma affects these patterns. MOHO emphasizes that motivation, habits, and performance are shaped by the interaction of personal factors and the surrounding environment (Park et al., 2019). In the presence of trauma, volition may be diminished, routines become fragile, and the ability to act with purpose may erode. A girl may begin to define herself by roles that reflect her environment's demands, such as caretaker, achiever, and avoidant student, rather than roles aligned with her emerging identity.

Through the PEO model, we understand how trauma shifts the fit between a girl, her environment, and the occupations available to her. When the internal experience of stress and dysregulation clashes with a school system that demands compliance, or a home environment that lacks emotional safety, the result is often disengagement. Occupations that once brought comfort may now feel overwhelming or out of reach. The environment no longer supports participation, it magnifies the mismatch.

From an occupational therapy perspective, these shifts offer critical information. Trauma doesn't just change how a girl feels, it changes how she engages. Using models like MOHO and PEO helps therapists look beneath the surface of avoidance or perfectionism and begin rebuilding occupational patterns that honor safety, autonomy, and self-discovery.

Systems That Shape Trauma Exposure and Response

Trauma in adolescence rarely exists apart from the systems that surround it. Girls do not just experience harm in isolation. They experience it in schools, child welfare programs, legal systems, and other institutions that hold power over their daily lives. These systems have the potential to either amplify trauma or interrupt it. Too often, they do the former.

In school settings, trauma frequently shows up in the form of absences, emotional dysregulation, difficulty concentrating, or sudden withdrawal. But these signs are easily misunderstood. Instead of being seen as indicators of distress, they are labeled as defiance, laziness, or poor character. Discipline policies that favor control over connection, such as suspension, referral to law enforcement, or behavioral demerits, often retraumatize students who are already struggling. These consequences are not distributed equally. Girls of color, girls in foster care, and girls with disabilities are disproportionately punished for behaviors that reflect underlying trauma, not willful disobedience.

The child welfare and juvenile justice systems reflect similar patterns. Girls who run away from unsafe homes, resist control in group placements, or react to perceived threats with intensity are often met with surveillance and restraint rather than support and safety. Foster placements may change frequently, breaking down any fragile trust that has been built. Incarcerated girls, many of whom have endured sexual abuse, neglect, or early loss, are often isolated from meaningful roles and stripped of autonomy, further entrenching their disconnection from identity and community.

From an occupational therapy perspective, these institutional responses matter deeply. Systems shape the environments in which roles are learned, routines are developed, and self-worth is constructed. When those systems respond to survival behaviors with punishment or indifference, they disrupt not only the girl's regulation but her access to meaningful occupation. School becomes a source of shame. Authority figures feel unsafe. Future-oriented thinking becomes nearly impossible.

Occupational therapists working within or alongside these systems must approach their work as both clinicians and advocates. This means using trauma-informed reasoning to reinterpret behaviors, designing supportive routines within restrictive settings, and addressing the environmental conditions that inhibit occupational growth. It also means helping girls reclaim agency in spaces where it has been taken from them, by scaffolding participation in decision-making, co-creating routines that feel safe, and affirming their rights to be heard, seen, and understood.

Digital Environments and Adolescent Trauma

Adolescence now unfolds across both physical and digital landscapes. According to Pew Research Center data from 2024, over 95 percent of teens have access to a smartphone, and more than one in three reports being online "almost constantly." For adolescent girls, digital platforms are not just tools for communication. They are spaces where identity is explored, social hierarchies are negotiated, and emotional needs are often met or denied. Social media has become a powerful site of occupation, one that shapes how girls perceive themselves, connect with others, and regulate emotion.

For girls with trauma histories, digital spaces can serve both as escape and exposure. A single post can trigger shame, exclusion, or humiliation. An online friendship can offer safety or reinforce patterns of dependency and invalidation. The boundaries between self-expression, performance, and surveillance are often blurred, especially when peer validation feels essential to emotional stability. In this context, trauma responses do not disappear online. They adapt. They show up as hypervigilant self-monitoring, compulsive scrolling, withdrawal, or the curated projection of a self that feels more acceptable than real.

Cyberbullying and digital peer violence are particularly damaging because they often occur invisibly to adults. The intensity of these interactions, combined with the inability to escape them, can heighten emotional dysregulation, sleep disturbances, and social withdrawal. Girls may begin to monitor their every post, curate a version of themselves they believe will be accepted, or disappear entirely from digital spaces as a form of self-protection. Some girls rely on the stimulation of scrolling and posting to avoid emotional stillness. Their devices become tools not just for connection, but for dissociation.

Occupational therapy must begin to view digital engagement as a core area of adolescent occupation. It is not enough to ask how much screen time a teen is getting. Practitioners must explore what that time means, what it regulates, and what it costs. Digital routines, just like school or home routines, can either support recovery or deepen patterns of dysregulation and shame. Therapists can help girls reflect on their digital identities, develop intentional media boundaries, and reframe online participation as an extension of authentic self-expression rather than performance or survival.

When supported through a trauma-informed lens, digital environments can be transformed from spaces of reactivity into opportunities for agency. A girl might use journaling apps to process emotion, create visual mood boards to explore identity, or engage in online peer groups that foster safety and shared understanding. By integrating digital occupations into assessment and intervention, occupational therapists can meet girls where they are, both on and offline, and help them build regulation, resilience, and connection across the full spectrum of their daily lives.

Contextualizing Trauma in Marginalized Girls

For girls who live at the margins of society, whether due to race, socioeconomic status, disability, or gender identity, trauma is more likely to be layered, culturally mediated, and shaped by systemic forces that remain invisible in most trauma frameworks. It is more likely to be chronic, less likely to be validated, and more often filtered through systems that misinterpret survival as misconduct. These girls are not only exposed to higher rates of adversity, but they also face layers of structural inequity that shape how trauma is experienced, responded to, and remembered.

The daily realities of marginalized girls are shaped by forces that extend far beyond individual relationships. They must navigate racism in the classroom, gendered expectations in their homes, under-resourced communities, or institutions that see their distress as disruption. This convergence of interpersonal and systemic harm creates compounded trauma, or wounds that are layered, ongoing, and often overlooked (Pazderka et al., 2021). Without an understanding of these intersecting contexts, trauma-informed care risks reinforcing the very exclusions it aims to address.

Marginalized Girls and Compounded Trauma

Marginalized girls often live at the crossroads of multiple adversities. Rather than encountering trauma as a singular or isolated event, many experience it as an ongoing condition—woven into daily interactions, institutional encounters, and community environments. These experiences accumulate over time, forming what is often referred to as compounded trauma. Unlike acute trauma, which may have a clear beginning and end, compounded trauma emerges from repeated invalidation, chronic stress, and exposure to environments that reinforce fear or erode self-worth.

For a girl growing up in a low-income neighborhood, compounded trauma may include navigating food insecurity, witnessing community violence, and being perceived as disruptive by teachers who overlook her learning needs. A girl of color may experience frequent microaggressions, disciplinary targeting, or cultural invalidation in school systems that were not designed with her identity in mind. A girl with a disability may face exclusion from peer groups, limited access to resources, and heightened vulnerability to abuse or neglect.

These layers of harm rarely exist in silos. They intersect in ways that shape how trauma is processed and how resilience is cultivated. From an occupational perspective, compounded trauma often disrupts not only emotional regulation but also patterns of engagement. Girls may withdraw from meaningful activities, assume rigid caregiving roles, or internalize messages of inadequacy that limit identity exploration and goal-setting. Without intervention, the impact of compounded trauma can extend into emerging adulthood, affecting academic persistence, vocational identity, and relational health.

Inequity doesn't just shape what girls are exposed to, it shapes how they are perceived, how they are supported, and whether they are given the benefit of being understood. By the time a marginalized girl enters the therapy room, she may already have a history of being misread, mistrusted, or punished for behaviors rooted in survival. For occupational therapists, the work is not only to support regulation or skill-building, but to understand the social architecture surrounding her life. This means asking deeper questions—about safety, about power, about belonging—and recognizing how systems either constrict or expand what is possible. A trauma-informed approach for marginalized youth must be unapologetically contextual. It must restore access to meaningful roles, affirm the complexity of identity, and resist the quiet harm of neutrality in the face of injustice.

Racial and Socioeconomic Inequities in Trauma Exposure

According to the CDC's 2023 *Youth Risk Behavior Surveillance* data, Black and Latina girls are significantly more likely than their White peers to report experiences of physical violence, sexual coercion, and chronic stress related to economic instability. These disparities are not incidental. They are the result of structural conditions such as intergenerational poverty, under-resourced schools, community disinvestment, and systemic racism that heighten vulnerability while limiting access to safety, validation, and care.

For many girls growing up in communities shaped by these forces, trauma begins long before a clinical threshold is met. It begins in the silence of being overlooked, in the pressure to grow up too quickly, in the normalization of chaos. A missed meal, a crowded apartment, a punitive teacher, a police siren outside the window, these everyday experiences accumulate. Over time, they wire the nervous system for vigilance and mold identity around survival rather than possibility.

These conditions do not just increase exposure to trauma; they shape the meaning of it. A girl who internalizes these experiences without language, space, or reflection may see herself as the problem. Her grief becomes anger. Her exhaustion is labeled defiance. Her dissociation is read as apathy. And too often, her responses are pathologized rather than contextualized.

Occupational therapists must recognize that these inequities are not peripheral; they are central to how trauma lives in the body and is expressed through occupation. Engagement in school, social activity, or creative exploration can feel unsafe or irrelevant when basic needs go unmet or cultural identity is not affirmed. Building trust in such contexts requires more than trauma-informed intention; it requires critical consciousness, humility, and the ability to name the systems at play without making the client responsible for navigating them alone.

When therapists understand how racial and socioeconomic forces shape occupational opportunities, they can begin to tailor interventions that restore agency, not just function. This may include co-creating culturally meaningful routines, advocating within school systems, supporting family rituals of resilience, or simply offering a space where a girl's full experience is seen and believed. The role of the occupational therapist is not only to respond to trauma, but to reimagine what healing can mean in spaces where injustice has long shaped who feels seen, safe, and worthy of care.

LGBTQ+ Youth and Trauma Risk

In a 2023 national survey by The Trevor Project, 41 percent of LGBTQ+ youth reported seriously considering suicide in the past year. Rates were even higher among transgender and nonbinary teens. These numbers do not simply point to mental health disparities. They speak to the emotional cost of growing up in a world that often greets identity with silence, resistance, or outright harm.

For many LGBTQ+ girls and gender-expansive youth, trauma is not a singular event. It is layered into the places that should offer safety. It begins in the comments at the dinner table, the bathroom pass denied at school, the name that is mispronounced on purpose. It lives in the quiet realization that showing up fully may come with consequences. Adolescence becomes a careful performance, where every gesture is weighed and every word rehearsed. This lived reality reflects findings on the contextual nature of trauma among sexual minority survivors (Berke et al., 2023).

The occupational toll is profound. Participation in everyday roles such as student, artist, or athlete begins to feel dangerous. A girl may avoid the classroom where she has been outed, skip the party where she feels unseen, or abandon dreams that once felt within reach. These choices are not rooted in disinterest. They are adaptations. Each one is a quiet act of protection against environments that have proven unkind.

For occupational therapists, this demands more than inclusive language or passive acceptance. It calls for clinical practices grounded in advocacy, curiosity, and cultural humility. That means using tools that reflect the full range of human identity, building spaces where authenticity is not a liability, and honoring that safety may not be found in the systems that surround the child—but within the relationship you co-create.

Therapy should never require someone to make themselves smaller to be helped. LGBTQ+ youth deserve more than survival strategies. They deserve the freedom to imagine a life they can participate in fully, with joy, purpose, and pride. Occupational therapy, when practiced through a queer-affirming and trauma-responsive lens, can be one place where that future begins to take shape. A more detailed exploration of trauma, identity formation, and occupational disruption among LGBTQ+ populations can be found in Chapter 10: Gender and Sexual Minority Women.

Trauma-Informed Occupational Therapy with Adolescents

Adolescents are rarely referred to therapy for the real reason they are struggling. They are sent because they stop attending class, lash out at home, refuse to follow rules, or seem unable to manage their emotions. But beneath the behavior is almost always something else, something quieter, harder to name, and often ignored for far too long. For girls navigating trauma, participation is not just difficult. It can feel impossible. And yet, the work of healing does not begin with fixing behavior. It begins with restoring safety, choice, and a sense of self that trauma has disrupted.

Trauma-informed occupational therapy is not about doing more. It is about doing differently. It means recognizing that what looks like avoidance may be a nervous system protecting itself. That what appears unmotivated may be the residue of burnout. And that what is dismissed as overreacting may be a body doing its best to survive. For therapists working with teens, the goal is not compliance, it is reconnection. Reconnection to the body, to identity, to creativity, to others, and ultimately, to a life that feels worth engaging in again. Table 2.6 outlines the core principles of trauma-informed practice and how they are translated into occupational therapy with adolescents. These principles guide the strategies that follow, from building safety and co-regulation to supporting creative expression and digital engagement.

These principles provide a foundational lens for working with teens who have experienced trauma. In occupational therapy, they are not abstract ideals but daily practices—reflected in how we structure sessions, invite participation, respond to silence, and affirm identity. When applied consistently, these principles not only support regulation and engagement but also help rebuild a teenager's sense of safety, autonomy, and connection in a world where those experiences may have been disrupted or denied.

Creating Safety and Regulation Through Occupation

Before a teen can learn, explore, or take risks, she must first feel safe enough to show up. Safety is not just physical. It is emotional, relational, and sensory. It is built in the smallest details: the tone of voice used in a session, the predictability of a routine, the dignity offered in being asked rather than told. Occupational therapy creates opportunities for safety through structure and choice.

Table 2.6 Trauma-Informed Principles in Occupational Therapy with Adolescents

Core Principle	Application in Adolescent OT Practice
Safety	Establish emotionally and physically safe spaces through predictable routines, consistent scheduling, and sensory-informed environments. With teens, this also includes honoring social safety by creating space where they are not judged for how they dress, speak, or express themselves.
Trustworthiness and Transparency	Adolescents often carry distrust of adults or systems. Be clear about roles, limits of confidentiality, and what each session will involve. Offer consistency in language, follow-through, and expectations to reduce uncertainty and power imbalances.
Peer Support	Adolescents are highly peer oriented. Group-based interventions, co-regulation through shared activities, and peer modeling can normalize their experiences and reduce shame. Carefully scaffold peer spaces to ensure emotional safety and inclusion.
Collaboration and Mutuality	Adolescents are in a critical stage of identity development. Involve them as equal partners in goal setting, session planning, and therapeutic pacing. Invite feedback and respect resistance as meaningful communication, not opposition.
Empowerment, Voice, and Choice	Give adolescents choice in the types of activities used (e.g., journaling vs. movement), how goals are framed, and how their progress is defined. Validate emotional intensity as developmentally appropriate and support agency without demanding emotional vulnerability too soon.
Cultural, Historical, and Gender Issues	Acknowledge the impact of racism, sexism, heteronormativity, and cultural invisibility on occupational engagement. Use inclusive language, reflect diverse identities in materials and interventions, and challenge internalized narratives around worth, identity, or belonging.

A calm, co-created schedule can anchor a nervous system that is struggling to regulate. A quiet corner with weighted tools and soft lighting can signal that rest is allowed here. A single shared activity done side by side, with no pressure to talk, can begin to rebuild trust.

Regulation is not taught through instruction. It is modeled, scaffolded, and practiced. When a therapist moves slowly, breathes evenly, and remains present without judgment, the body of a traumatized teen begins to learn that not every space requires defense. With repetition, this sense of internal safety begins to extend into the occupations of daily life, such as getting ready for school, making breakfast, or riding the bus. These small wins become the foundation for deeper therapeutic work.

Activity-Based Approaches for Emotional Expression

Adolescents do not always have the words to explain what they are feeling. Even when they do, speaking may not feel safe. Trauma can steal language. It can turn emotion into something too large or too dangerous to touch directly. This is why occupational therapy must offer other forms of expression. Art, movement, rhythm, and creation are not distractions. They are pathways. They allow teens to say what cannot be said.

A paintbrush becomes a way to process grief. A clay project becomes a metaphor for control and change. A walk through a garden becomes a moment of stillness that does not demand anything more. These are not just coping tools. They are active expressions of emotion that help integrate experience and restore coherence between body and mind.

Therapists should not worry about the aesthetic value of what is created. The goal is not beauty. It is honesty. In activity-based work, process is everything. This is where adolescents learn that their feelings do not have to be hidden, and that their expressions will not be punished. In a world that often demands silence or perfection, the act of making something can feel revolutionary.

Use of Technology and Media in Trauma Recovery

For many adolescent girls, digital life is not separate from real life. It is where friendships form, identities take shape, and emotions are expressed. Screens are not just tools. They are mirrors, stages, and sometimes, safe places to disappear. For youth living with trauma, digital spaces may offer escape from environments that feel unsafe, or they may reinforce patterns of avoidance and disconnection. Either way, technology is a central part of the occupational landscape and cannot be ignored in therapy.

Trauma-informed care means meeting adolescents where they are, and for many, that place is online. Rather than viewing technology only as a problem to be managed, therapists can approach it as an opportunity for connection and healing. A teen might use a journaling app to name feelings that are too hard to speak aloud. A playlist can regulate mood. A digital collage or short video can become a powerful way to tell a story that has yet found words. These tools are not secondary. They are extensions of how teens move through the world.

Therapists can also support routine-building through technology. Visual reminders, calming apps, and audio prompts can help organize daily life when executive functioning is taxed by stress. Screen-based strategies should not replace real connection, but they can bridge the gap between overwhelm and action. When used intentionally, digital tools offer structure, creativity, and emotional safety.

Most importantly, therapists must remain curious about a teen's relationship with media. Rather than asking how to reduce screen time, it is often more helpful to ask what a particular space or activity offers. What does it soothe? What does it replace? What need does it meet? From there, therapy becomes less about restriction and more about reflection. It becomes a space where even digital habits are explored with compassion, and where technology is no longer the enemy of healing but a potential partner in it.

Case Vignettes and Reflections

Trauma rarely announces itself. It lingers in the unsaid, reshaping the way a teen moves through the world, how she enters a room, how she avoids eye contact, how she hesitates before raising her hand (Gillies et al., 2016). In occupational therapy, we often meet adolescents in the middle of that quiet recalibration. What looks like resistance is often a form of protection. What seems like disinterest may be a sign of exhaustion. The work is not to correct, but to interpret, to offer something steady enough for the nervous system to lean against. The stories that follow are not about breakthroughs. They are about what happens when we stop rushing toward outcomes and notice what is already unfolding. They are reminders that healing is less about what we offer, and more about how we offer it—and whether we are willing to stay, even in the silence.

Case Example 1: Aaliyah, Age 12—School-Based OT with Emerging Grief and Withdrawal

When Aaliyah stopped raising her hand in class, no one panicked. When she started putting her head down on the desk during math, most assumed it was fatigue. When she quietly pulled away from the art club she used to love, there were murmurs. Maybe she was just growing out of it. Grief in children rarely enters the room shouting. It drips in slowly and often goes unnoticed until it begins to pool.

Aaliyah was a sixth-grade student in a public Title I school, receiving occupational therapy through an Individualized Education Plan for Attention Deficit Hyperactivity Disorder (ADHD). Her sessions focused on executive functioning, emotional regulation, and classroom routines. For over a year, she had been progressing well. She was organizing her binder, following transitions, participating in morning check-ins. She was steady, if quiet. Until she was not.

Midway through the school year, her teacher flagged a change. Aaliyah had grown silent. She was no longer engaging with classmates. Her posture had folded in on itself. When asked a question, she often responded with a shrug or stared at the floor. The school counselor referred her back to OT for a check-in. What was once a student working toward independence was now a girl pulling away from the world.

During a routine visual sequencing activity, Aaliyah looked up, blinked hard, and said quietly, "My brother died in October. We don't talk about it." Her voice did not shake. She did not cry. But everything about her shifted. The family had not informed the school. There had been no plan for grief, no support team, no adjustment to her goals. The therapist met with the counselor that same day. Together, they reviewed Aaliyah's IEP and made space within it, not just for academics, but for loss.

The therapist revised Aaliyah's sessions with intention. She did not ask her to talk. Instead, she invited her to make. They began each session with a calming sensory routine such as deep pressure using a weighted lap pad, five minutes of quiet coloring, or a visual breathing exercise using simple tracing patterns. Aaliyah chose a soft seat near the window and returned to it each time. It became hers.

Next came visual journaling. Aaliyah used magazine clippings, watercolor pencils, and gel pens to build image collages with words she rarely spoke aloud. *Still. Float. Gone.* One day she labeled a page with, "I want to be here, but I'm tired." The therapist did not ask her to explain. She nodded and added her own word to the corner of the page: *Brave.*

As trust built, they introduced co-regulated activities with gentle structure, such as collaborative drawing games or passing a single shape back and forth, each taking turns to transform it into something new. These small, shared acts of creation allowed Aaliyah to stay present without pressure. They were nonverbal conversations—low demand, high connection.

The therapist also helped modify her classroom transitions. Together they created a pocket-sized visual cue card Aaliyah could carry, reminding her of her daily routine and offering built-in breaks. They carved out five minutes each morning for her to visit the art room before the school day began. No expectation. No audience. Just space.

Over the months that followed, Aaliyah began to re-engage. She sat up taller. She returned to art club—not to participate at first, but to clean the brushes. Later, she asked to stay after school to finish a painting. When the school counselor invited her to a small grief group, she nodded but said she was not ready. "Maybe next month," she said, placing her latest journal page in her folder. "I think I'm almost ready to hear other people's stories."

Occupational therapy, in Aaliyah's case, was not about task completion. This approach aligns with community-based interventions that emphasize healing through meaningful occupation and relational support (Mazzeo & Bendixen, 2023). It was not about asking her to talk through her grief. It was about letting her name it in her own way, through color, through routine, and through quiet. It was not an intervention. It was an invitation back to herself.

Case Example 2: Leilani, Age 16—Outpatient OT in a Trauma-Informed Youth Wellness Program

Leilani did not arrive with a diagnosis. She arrived with three plastic bags, a tight jaw, and a list of places she no longer belonged. At sixteen, she had already moved through more homes than birthdays she could remember. School was a blur of unfinished credits and new names. Adults, she had learned, asked questions they rarely waited to hear the answers to.

She was referred to outpatient occupational therapy through a trauma-informed youth wellness clinic, part of a public behavioral health program for foster youth. The case manager's note was brief: "hypervigilant, avoids eye contact, not attending school consistently." Beneath that was the real story—difficulty sleeping, constant stomach pain, days spent curled into herself, absent from the world but present enough to comply.

At intake, Leilani chose the chair closest to the door. Her hood stayed up. She did not speak unless spoken to, and even then, her answers were clipped and cautious. When asked why she agreed to OT, she shrugged. "As long as I don't have to talk the whole time," she said. "I'm not good at that."

So the therapist did not start with talking. Instead, they started with rhythm. Sessions began and ended the same way: a check-in using a color-coded feelings chart, a moment of quiet through clay or sketching, a menu of options for the middle such as collage, music, design. Leilani chose. Sometimes she drew. Sometimes she rearranged planner stickers into routines she said she probably wouldn't follow but liked to see. No one asked her why.

Each week, a little more of her showed up. She built a sensory box for the clinic's group room, testing each fabric swatch and choosing the scents herself. She made playlists for different moods and asked the therapist to listen to one while they cleaned up the markers. When grounding techniques were introduced, such as walking barefoot on textured mats, holding cold washcloths to her face, she declined. "Too much," she said. So, the therapist offered image boards instead. Leilani curated her feelings through color and texture, building what she called "moods I wish I could have."

By the third month, she brought in a poem. "It's not about me," she said, placing it on the table. The therapist read it while Leilani drew silently beside her. Weeks later, she stood at the front of the wellness circle and explained her sensory box to other teens in the group. She asked if she could help make more for kids who were new. "So, they know what to expect," she said.

What emerged was not a sudden shift. It was slow and deliberate. The product of consent, control, and careful co-creation. Leilani did not need therapy that asked her to talk. She needed therapy that gave her space to choose how to speak. In colors. In playlists. In poems. And eventually, in her own voice.

Occupational therapy, for Leilani, became more than an intervention. It became a place where silence was not punished, where choice was not performative, and where healing did not require explanation—only the right conditions to unfold.

Therapist Reflections on Clinical Decision-Making

Working with adolescents who have lived through trauma is not about pulling tools from a clinical toolbox. It is about learning how to be with someone who is still deciding whether the world is safe enough to return to. It requires listening with patience, pacing with care, and choosing presence over performance. In both Aaliyah's and Leilani's stories, the most pivotal moments in therapy did not come from what was done, but from how it was offered—and when.

With Aaliyah, it was easy to assume her academic and social withdrawal meant she was slipping backward. But the truth revealed itself quietly: it was not a loss of skill, but the weight of grief. Her brother had died, and no one had said the words aloud. She no longer needed checklists and timers—she needed space. Visual journaling replaced planning grids. A weighted lap pad, a quiet corner, and ten minutes of drawing became her bridge back to classroom life. These were not deviations from her IEP. They were its evolution—adapted for a girl trying to hold herself together in a place that had not noticed she was breaking.

Leilani never once asked for help. She agreed to try occupational therapy "as long as it's not talking." She had changed homes three times that year and learned long ago that silence was safer than sincerity. For her, therapy began with structure—what time we started, where she sat, what choices she had each day. It unfolded through co-created visuals, shared music, and art that did not ask her to explain. Only after trust began to form did her voice follow—not on command, but on her own terms.

In both cases, the work began not with goals, but with consent. Not with fixing, but with witnessing. Trauma-informed occupational therapy is not a path you walk for someone. It is a space you hold, a rhythm you match, a scaffold you build gently enough for someone else to begin again. When we allow the occupation itself to lead—whether it is painting, journaling, or sitting in silence—we stop trying to pull healing out of someone and start letting it rise.

Summary and Implications

Healing for adolescent girls does not begin with a treatment plan. It begins in the everyday moments when safety is rebuilt through consistency, when silence is allowed without demand, and when creativity becomes a bridge back to self. Trauma in adolescence is rarely isolated. It is layered and shaped by environment, by history, and by systems that are too often underprepared to respond. For occupational therapists, this means moving beyond symptom management to truly understand what the body and behavior are trying to say. It means recognizing trauma responses as protective, not pathological, and adapting our approach to meet teens with compassion, structure, and flexibility.

When we intervene early and contextually, we are not only addressing regulation or participation. We are helping to rewrite the story a teen carries about herself and her place in the world. That work cannot happen in isolation. It demands a network of responsive systems, including schools, families, healthcare providers, and communities, working in concert. Occupational therapy is uniquely positioned to bridge these spaces. Through meaningful occupation, we help girls reclaim agency, restore rhythm, and reconnect with who they are becoming. In doing so, we do more than treat trauma. We lay the foundation for future wellness, one relationship, one routine, and one quiet act of choice at a time.

References

American Occupational Therapy Association (AOTA). (2020). Occupational therapy practice framework: Domain and process (4th ed.). *American Journal of Occupational Therapy, 74*(Suppl. 2), 7412410010. https://doi.org/10.5014/ajot.2020.74S2001

Berke, D. S., Tuten, M. D., Smith, A. M., & Hotchkiss, M. (2023). A qualitative analysis of the context and characteristics of trauma exposure among sexual minority survivors: Implications for posttraumatic stress disorder assessment and clinical practice. *Psychological Trauma: Theory, Research, Practice, and Policy, 15*(4), 648–655. https://doi.org/10.1037/tra0001464

Boynton-Jarrett, R., & Harville, E. W. (2012). A prospective study of childhood social hardships and age at menarche. *Annals of Epidemiology, 22*(10), 731–737. https://doi.org/10.1016/j.annepidem.2012.08.005

CDC. (2023). *Youth Risk Behavior Surveillance System (YRBSS)*. Centers for Disease Control and Prevention, U.S. Department of Health and Human Services. www.cdc.gov/healthyyouth/data/yrbs/index.htm

Chango, J. M., McElhaney, K. B., Allen, J. P., Schad, M. M., & Marston, E. (2012). Occurs and depressive symptoms in late adolescence: Rejection sensitivity as a vulnerability. *Journal of Abnormal Child Psychology, 40*(3), 369–379. https://doi.org/10.1007/s10802-011-9570-y

Danzi, B. A., & La Greca, A. M. (2021). Treating children and adolescents with posttraumatic stress disorder: Moderators of treatment response. *Journal of Clinical Child and Adolescent Psychology: The Official Journal for the Society of Clinical Child and Adolescent Psychology, American Psychological Association, Division 53, 50*(4), 510–516. https://doi.org/10.1080/15374416.2020.1823849

Dowdy, R., Estes, J., McCarthy, C., Onders, J., Onders, M., & Suttner, A. (2022). The influence of occupational therapy on self-regulation in juvenile offenders. *Journal of Child & Adolescent Trauma, 16*(2), 221–232. https://doi.org/10.1007/s40653-022-00493-y

Eder-Moreau, E., Zhu, X., Fisch, C. T., Bergman, M., Neria, Y., & Helpman, L. (2022). Neurobiological alterations in females with PTSD: A systematic review. *Frontiers in Psychiatry, 13*, 862476. https://doi.org/10.3389/fpsyt.2022.862476

Fialkowski, A., Shaffer, K., Ball-Burack, M., Brooks, T. L., Trinh, N. T., Potter, J. E., & Peeler, K. R. (2022). Trauma-informed care for hospitalized adolescents. *Current Pediatrics Reports, 10*(2), 45–54. https://doi.org/10.1007/s40124-022-00262-3

Gillies, D., Maiocchi, L., Bhandari, A. P., Taylor, F., Gray, C., & O'Brien, L. (2016). Psychological therapies for children and adolescents exposed to trauma. *The Cochrane*

Database of Systematic Reviews, 10(10), CD012371. https://doi.org/10.1002/14651858.
CD012371

Khan, S. (2025). *Occupational therapy and women's health: A practitioner guide* (1st ed.). Routledge. https://doi.org/10.4324/9781003531678

Mazzeo, G., & Bendixen, R. (2023). Community-based interventions for childhood trauma: A scoping review. *OTJR: Occupation, Participation and Health, 43*(1), 14–23. https://doi.org/10.1177/15394492221091718

Miller, E. (2019). Trauma-informed approaches to adolescent relationship abuse and sexual violence prevention. *Pediatric Annals, 48*(7), e274–e279. https://doi. org/10.3928/19382359-20190617-01

Park, J., Gross, D. P., Rayani, F., Norris, C. M., Roberts, M. R., James, C., Guptill, C., & Esmail, S. (2019). Model of Human Occupation as a framework for implementation of motivational interviewing in occupational rehabilitation. *Work (Reading, Mass.), 62*(4), 629–641. https://doi.org/10.3233/WOR-192895

Pazderka, H., Brown, M. R. G., Agyapong, V. I. O., Greenshaw, A. J., McDonald-Harker, C. B., Noble, S., Mankowski, M., Lee, B., Drolet, J. L., Omeje, J., Brett-MacLean, P., Kitching, D. T., & Silverstone, P. H. (2021). Collective trauma and mental health in adolescents: A retrospective cohort study of the effects of retraumatization. *Frontiers in Psychiatry, 12*, 682041. https://doi.org/10.3389/fpsyt.2021.682041

Sahi, R. S., Eisenberger, N. I., & Silvers, J. A. (2023). Peer facilitation of emotion regulation in adolescence. *Developmental Cognitive Neuroscience, 62*, 101262. https://doi. org/10.1016/j.dcn.2023.101262

Chapter 3

Stress and Trauma in Young Adult Women

Chapter Objectives

Upon completion of this chapter, the reader will be able to:

1. Describe the neurodevelopmental changes of early adulthood and explain how trauma influences executive function, emotional regulation, and occupational performance in young women.
2. Identify patterns of occupational disruption in emerging adulthood, including disrupted routines, role overload, identity confusion, and loss of volition.
3. Distinguish between high-functioning trauma responses and genuine occupational wellness by evaluating internalized stress, somatic symptoms, and relational patterns.
4. Apply trauma-informed occupational therapy strategies that promote nervous system regulation, identity reformation, and sustainable role engagement during early adulthood.
5. Evaluate the impact of structural barriers, such as financial strain, systemic inequities, and relational trauma, on the health, identity, and participation of young adult women.

Mei Lin Zhang was nineteen when she began to feel like her body was no longer hers. At her university, she had always been the quiet one, the dependable one, the girl who never caused trouble. But after joining a sorority to feel a sense of belonging, she found herself being asked to do things that made her stomach twist, such as blindfolded games, unwanted physical closeness, whispered dares that brought back the cold panic of high school nights she had tried to forget. Her

DOI: 10.4324/9781003658559-3

heart would race, her hands trembled, and she found herself dissociating during the rituals, unsure if the sounds around her were real
or remembered. She started avoiding mirrors, skipping classes, and
losing time during the day. When people laughed, she flinched. When
they touched her shoulder, she froze. Mei Lin smiled when she was
supposed to, but inside she was unraveling, haunted by the past and
overwhelmed by the pressure to pretend nothing was wrong.

Young adulthood is often romanticized as a season of growth, discovery, and
independence. Yet epidemiological data tell a different story. In the United
States, more than 40 percent of people aged 18 to 29 experience a psychiatric
disorder each year, with rates of depression, anxiety, and psychological distress
rising sharply among young women. Between 2005 and 2017, the prevalence of
major depressive episodes in women aged 18 to 25 increased from 8.1 to 13.2
percent—a shift mirrored globally across college-aged populations (Matud et al.,
2020). Beneath the surface of curated narratives lies a more complex reality. For
many women, this stage is marked by invisible rupture, chronic stress, and the
reemergence of unresolved trauma (Schwartz et al., 2015).

As the prefrontal cortex continues to develop and executive functions solidify, young women are expected to make decisions that shape the course of their
lives. Yet the structures that once offered safety, such as predictable routines,
consistent adult oversight, and institutional scaffolding, begin to recede. What
remains is often an abrupt increase in autonomy without the internal regulation
skills fully in place to manage it. The familiar rhythms of childhood give way to
uncertainty, and just as external demands intensify, internal vulnerabilities rise to
the surface. Chronic stress during this stage can further disrupt executive functioning and emotional regulation, especially in women with trauma histories,
compounding feelings of disorganization or overwhelm (Fleming et al., 2024).
Trauma does not always arrive with spectacle. More often, it presents as exhaustion, as perfectionism disguised as ambition, as relationships that echo past harm.

For those carrying histories of adversity or navigating systemic inequities, this
stage can reactivate trauma in ways that are both subtle and profound. Academic
pressure, unstable housing, toxic relationships, and the erosion of family support are not isolated stressors. Together, they undermine identity formation and
disrupt participation in daily life. Habits dissolve. Motivation weakens. Roles
become blurred, excessive, or abandoned altogether. Without trauma-informed
support, the passage into adulthood does not simply challenge. It can fracture.

Yet this period also holds powerful potential. When met with attuned and
equitable care, young women can rebuild what has been lost, reclaim authorship of their stories, and step into adult life with renewed clarity and connection.

Early adulthood offers a second window for healing and a pivotal opportunity to lay the foundation for lasting wellness.

Developmental Tasks and Vulnerabilities of Young Adulthood

At 24, Leilani Brown was in her first year of graduate school, raising a two-year-old, and working part-time as a medical assistant. After a brief marriage that ended quietly a year earlier, she moved back into a small apartment near campus to rebuild. Her classmates saw her as competent and collected, but inside she felt like she was constantly bracing. In clinic, she sometimes forgot routine tasks and caught herself zoning out during patient intakes. At school, she struggled to track readings and often froze during in-class discussions, afraid of saying something out of place. At home, she kept her son on a strict schedule, not because it worked, but because any deviation spiked her anxiety. In her first occupational therapy session, she admitted she barely slept, avoided asking for help, and felt a constant pressure to prove she belonged. "I keep telling myself I'm fine," she said, "but I'm tired in a way that rest doesn't fix." For Leilani, the demands of early adulthood had collided with unprocessed trauma, pulling her into roles that exceeded the nervous system capacity she never had the chance to fully develop.

Emerging adulthood, spanning roughly from ages 18 to 29, is a period of profound neurobiological, psychological, and social reorganization. It is a life stage where the scaffolding of childhood has been removed, but the stability of mature adulthood has not yet been built. For young women, this transition is often navigated within environments that are simultaneously demanding and under-resourced, such as college campuses, entry-level workplaces, healthcare systems that are unprepared to address the nuance of developmental trauma.

This is the age when identity formation intensifies. Women are not just exploring who they are, but are asked to define their values, chart career paths, navigate intimate relationships, and often assume caregiving or financial responsibilities. These demands arrive while executive functions such as future planning, emotional regulation, and risk assessment are still maturing, as these capacities are governed by neural networks that remain in flux well into the late twenties. In occupational therapy terms, this is a phase where role acquisition can outpace role competence, and where volition may be compromised by both internalized trauma and external instability.

Importantly, this period is also when early adversity often reemerges—not necessarily in the form of flashbacks or diagnostic criteria, but through dysregulated sleep, persistent anxiety, chronic somatic complaints, or a gnawing sense of failure despite outward achievement. Many young women carry histories of attachment disruption, emotional neglect, or systemic marginalization that were never fully processed. These unintegrated experiences surface just as they are being asked to "get it together," perform, and prove themselves worthy of belonging in adult systems. Understanding the developmental pressures of early adulthood through a trauma-informed and occupational lens allows for a more compassionate, contextualized approach to care. Rather than pathologizing perceived dysfunction, we can begin to see it as an expected outcome of navigating adulthood while still healing from a childhood that offered little room for safety, rest, or self-definition.

Identity Consolidation, Autonomy, and Occupational Role Expansion

Forming an adult identity is often imagined as a straightforward passage marked by milestones like graduating, finding a job, or settling into a defined role. In reality, this process is far more complex, especially for young women navigating a world shaped by cultural expectations, intergenerational responsibilities, and unresolved trauma. Identity development during this life stage involves not just direction but coherence, not just ambition but integration. It is the work of assembling a self that feels whole amid competing demands and fragmented environments.

A large-scale study by Schwartz et al. (2015) of nearly 9,737 college-attending young adults found that identity profiles are strongly linked to psychological outcomes. Those in the synthesized group reported the highest levels of well-being and the lowest levels of anxiety, depression, and risky behaviors. In contrast, individuals who demonstrated both high synthesis and high confusion had the poorest mental health outcomes. This pattern suggests that clarity in identity provides psychological protection, while internal conflict may intensify vulnerability.

Occupationally, young adulthood is defined by rapid expansion. Women often juggle multiple roles across education, employment, caregiving, and partnership, frequently without adequate structural support. These roles are not just tasks but expressions of self. When they accumulate too quickly or emerge in environments lacking affirmation, identity formation may falter. Many young women are managing invisible responsibilities behind the scenes, such as translating bureaucracies for parents, raising siblings, carrying cultural or financial burdens, all while expected to perform as if unencumbered.

Autonomy during this stage is also shaped by earlier experiences. For those raised in enmeshed or unpredictable environments, independence may not feel liberating. It may instead provoke anxiety, self-doubt, or guilt. What appears as avoidance or perfectionism is often a survival strategy, a way to manage risk when the developmental scaffolding for self-trust was never fully built. In occupational terms, this may present as overdependence in some contexts and over-control in others, each a way to navigate relational uncertainty.

In clinical and therapeutic contexts, these patterns call for more than encouragement to choose a major or define a career path. They require space for narrative reconstruction, for exploring the difference between internal desire and external pressure, and for slowly practicing self-direction in settings where it is safe to be uncertain. Supporting identity formation during this period means helping young women become the authors of their own lives, not just the performers of socially sanctioned roles.

Neurological Maturation and Executive Function Shifts

In clinical conversations, maturity is often conflated with age. But neuroscience tells a different story. The prefrontal cortex, which governs executive functions like impulse control, working memory, and long-range planning, does not reach full structural maturity until the late twenties. This matters, profoundly, for therapeutic work with young women. Many are navigating their most pivotal life transitions while still developing the very neural capacities that support reflection, regulation, and future-oriented decision-making. They are being asked to commit, to perform, to self-direct, and to self-regulate at precisely the moment when their brains are least equipped to do so consistently. And when they struggle, the dominant narratives often frame them as careless, unmotivated, or emotionally unstable.

For therapists, the takeaway is critical. Executive-function difficulties in early adulthood are not necessarily signs of pathology. They are often developmentally expected, particularly in women who are navigating trauma histories or system-level adversity. The ability to inhibit a response, sustain attention, or organize time is not simply a behavioral choice. It is a capacity that emerges through maturation, co-regulation, and experiential safety.

A trauma-informed lens reveals how chronic early stress reshapes this developmental arc. Studies have shown that adverse experiences in childhood can lead to hyperactivation of the limbic system and weakened connections between the prefrontal cortex and subcortical structures like the amygdala. In practice, this creates a brain that reacts before it reflects. It may also mean that the nervous system prioritizes short-term safety over long-term strategy, which has major implications for therapy that emphasizes planning or behavioral accountability.

For example, what may appear as poor time management in a college student might stem not from disorganization but from a nervous system locked in freeze response, unable to initiate tasks. A young woman who chronically misses deadlines may not be irresponsible but may be experiencing dorsal vagal shutdown, where the body's default response to overwhelm is immobilization. Conversely, another client may exhibit overplanning and rigid scheduling, which may appear to reflect strong executive skills but are actually strategies to avoid emotional unpredictability or re-experiencing past chaos. Both patterns reflect adaptations to trauma, not deficits in motivation or intelligence.

Traditional executive-function support (e.g., planners, timers, to-do lists) can fall flat without regulation. Instead, therapeutic interventions should begin by restoring predictability and somatic safety. This might include rhythm-based activities, sensory modulation, or embedded rest routines. Once physiological stability is reclaimed, cognitive scaffolds such as visual schedules, micro-goal setting, or values clarification can be layered in.

Therapists should also be cautious about overemphasizing independence. Many young women have learned to equate asking for help with failure. Others mask executive dysfunction with perfectionism or people-pleasing, further delaying the development of authentic self-direction. Co-creating routines, modeling reflective decision-making, and normalizing cognitive overload can create the kind of relational environment where executive function can finally begin to thrive. This is not a deficit to fix. It is a system to support. When we recognize the brain as still growing and often still healing, we shift therapy from correction to cultivation. And that shift changes everything.

Risk of Reactivated or Unresolved Trauma From Childhood or Adolescence

Not all trauma announces itself. For many young women, the impact of earlier adversity resurfaces not as flashbacks or overt distress but as subtle patterns such as unexplained fatigue, difficulty sustaining relationships, avoidance of opportunity, or a relentless inner voice that questions their worth. These patterns often emerge during young adulthood, a life stage that mirrors many of the original conditions under which trauma was first experienced: dependency, transition, uncertainty, and exposure to new power dynamics.

This phenomenon is not coincidental. The neurobiological systems that encode trauma, particularly those involved in fear conditioning, memory, and emotional regulation, remain sensitive to cues of relational threat or loss of control. When a young woman enters a college dorm, a new workplace, or an intimate partnership, the nervous system may detect echoes of earlier environments where safety was compromised. Without conscious awareness, she may experience these transitions as dangerous, triggering physiological states of fight, flight, or freeze even in the absence of immediate threat.

One client described feeling a wave of panic every night in her dorm room, though she could not name why. Over time, she realized the silence and isolation reminded her of childhood evenings spent alone while caregivers were absent or intoxicated, nights when she learned to stay quiet and brace for the unknown.

Developmentally, this is a period when earlier traumas often move from background noise to foreground disruption. Many young women who appeared resilient during adolescence begin to experience symptoms of anxiety, depression, eating disorders, or chronic pain during early adulthood. In clinical settings, this can be misread as decompensation or new-onset illness. But in reality, it often reflects the nervous system no longer being able to contain what was once suppressed in order to survive.

The challenge for clinicians is to recognize these presentations not as regressions but as invitations, signs that the individual has reached a level of developmental readiness to process what could not be processed before. Rather than pathologizing emotional dysregulation, avoidance, or inconsistent performance, therapists can view these signs as indicators of a system reaching its threshold and asking for repair.

Therapeutic responses must therefore be paced and attuned. Cognitive strategies alone may be insufficient if the client's body does not feel safe. Interventions that center on co-regulation, body-based grounding, and trauma-sensitive narrative work are often more effective than premature exposure to traumatic memories or high-demand behavioral plans. Clinicians should also be attentive to the ways in which systems, including higher education, healthcare, and employment, can retraumatize or invalidate young women, especially those from marginalized backgrounds.

Crucially, clinicians must learn to distinguish between behaviors that signal trauma and those that reflect disengagement or noncompliance. This requires moving beyond surface-level presentation and asking what the behavior is *protecting against*.

Trauma-based responses often follow patterns—they are persistent, relationally charged, and sometimes disproportionate to context. A trauma-informed lens asks not "Why is she avoiding class?" but "What happens in her body when she enters that classroom?" A young woman who seems to lack motivation may be experiencing learned helplessness after repeated experiences of not being heard or validated. One who is chronically late may not be disorganized but may have executive-function challenges rooted in chronic survival mode. Students who seem withdrawn or emotionally unavailable may not be apathetic but rather dissociated or overwhelmed.

There are subtle clues. Trauma reactions often coexist with shame, vigilance, and high sensitivity to perceived failure or rejection. They tend to escalate under relational pressure or sudden change. In contrast, behavioral disengagement tends to be more situational, often tied to external incentives or conscious choices. One of the simplest ways to differentiate is to look at *capacity vs. willingness*: Does the student want to succeed but seem unable to follow through, despite effort? That suggests trauma. Do they express indifference and resist any relational connection, even when safety is offered? That may point to a different root cause.

Unresolved trauma is not always loud. It can look like disinterest, delay, or collapse. But once the nervous system begins to feel safe enough, these behaviors shift. And for many young women, young adulthood is the first time they are developmentally and relationally ready to begin that process of repair.

Common Trauma Pathways and Stressors in Young Adult Women

At 35, Jennifer Gamin was one of five partners at a high-powered law firm and the only woman in the room. Her name on the glass door had been hard-earned, with each degree, each late night, and each courtroom win fueled by a quiet urgency to never be displaced again. Jennifer had spent her childhood bouncing from one foster home to another, never staying long enough to unpack, never safe enough to let her guard down. School became her sanctuary, the only place where achievement translated to stability. She graduated at the top of her class, excelled in law school, and worked her way up with unshakable discipline. But now, even at the top, she lived with a fear that everything could be taken away. When deadlines piled up or mistakes happened, her body reacted as if her security was on the line, with a tight chest, racing thoughts, and sleepless nights. Praise felt fleeting. Support felt conditional. Beneath her polished exterior was a nervous system still wired for survival, shaped by a childhood where failure didn't just mean disappointment, it meant being sent away.

Trauma in early adulthood rarely looks like crisis. More often, it emerges through accumulation. It is the slow layering of stressors that go unacknowledged, the repetition of relational dynamics that were never safe, and the quiet collapse that comes from trying to hold it all together without being seen. For many young women, this life stage is marked not by a singular traumatic event, but by the convergence of pressure, instability, and invisible labor across multiple domains of life.

This period is particularly vulnerable because the systems designed to support development—education, employment, healthcare, family—are often inaccessible, unpredictable, or outright harmful. As young women take on new roles and expectations, they are frequently doing so without reliable safety nets. The stressors they face are not just logistical. They are relational, existential, and deeply embodied.

What follows are four of the most common pathways through which trauma is sustained, reactivated, or deepened in young adulthood. These are not isolated categories. They intersect, compound, and shape the way young women show up in daily life. Understanding these patterns allows clinicians, educators, and advocates to move beyond surface-level problem-solving and into more attuned, responsive care.

Pathway 1: Academic and Career Pressures

It is possible to look successful on paper while quietly unraveling. Many young women do exactly that. In lecture halls and office spaces, they meet expectations with precision, carry family hopes on their shoulders, and perform competence like it is a currency. What often goes unseen is the toll it takes to keep performing when the nervous system is strained, the self-doubt is chronic, and the systems they are navigating were never built with them in mind.

Academic stress among young adult women has surged in recent years, not only due to increased enrollment but because of how performance is internalized. A 2024 study published in Heliyon found that impostor phenomenon is significantly more prevalent among female first-year medical students than their male peers, with 84 percent of women meeting the threshold compared to just 16 percent of men. The study linked these experiences to emotional stress, anxiety, and physical exhaustion, conditions that often go unaddressed in high-performing academic environments.

Impostor phenomenon is not simply a mindset problem. It is often the residue of environments that fail to affirm competence and identity in tandem. In women with histories of developmental trauma, it may resurface during high-stakes academic transitions or in competitive fields that reward output over process. For these students, the pressure to achieve is not only external. It is cellular. It becomes tied to safety, survival, and a sense of conditional belonging.

Career transitions pose similar challenges. Burnout and self-doubt often emerge just as women are expected to advocate for themselves professionally, negotiate their worth, and perform without error. In women from marginalized backgrounds, these effects are often compounded by experiences of cultural isolation and systemic exclusion.

For example, Laura, a first-year law student, experienced insomnia and nausea after receiving minor constructive feedback. These symptoms were not about perfectionism, but rather about early trauma cues being retriggered. Clinically, these patterns do not always present as crisis. They show up in more subtle ways, such as a client who cannot tolerate rest, a student who spirals after receiving constructive feedback, or a young professional who overworks to the point of collapse. These are not motivational problems. They are survival adaptations. And when they are misinterpreted, young women are often told to work harder, when what they truly need is permission to slow down.

A trauma-informed approach to academic and career stress asks different questions. It does not begin with time-management strategies or impersonal study tips. It begins with understanding what achievement has come to mean for this particular woman, what it protects her from, and what it costs her. It recognizes that success without safety is not sustainable. That confidence cannot be summoned in environments where women are expected to constantly prove they belong.

Occupational therapy and mental health support in this context must help women differentiate between authentic ambition and over-functioning. These two patterns often appear similar on the surface—driven, high-achieving, committed—but are rooted in profoundly different internal experiences. When ambition is fueled by curiosity, values, and self-expression, it can be energizing and sustainable. When it is driven by fear, shame, or the need for approval, it becomes a form of over-functioning that ultimately depletes the nervous system and fractures the self. See Table 3.1 for a clinical framework to distinguish between these presentations in practice.

It is also essential to create space for grief, including the time lost to anxiety, the goals pursued to earn approval, and the parts of themselves they

Table 3.1 Differentiating Authentic Ambition and Over-Functioning in Young Adult Women

Dimension	Authentic Ambition	Over-Functioning
Motivation Source	Rooted in values, purpose, and self-directed growth	Driven by fear of failure, rejection, or inadequacy
Emotional Quality	Energizing, fulfilling, allows for balance and rest	Exhausting, anxiety-provoking, requires constant effort to maintain
Relationship to Self	Self-worth remains stable regardless of outcomes	Self-worth depends on achievement and external validation
Boundaries	Can say no, delegate, and tolerate rest without guilt	Difficulty slowing down, saying no, or stepping back
Response to Setbacks	Processes challenges with self-reflection and perspective	Experiences setbacks as personal failure or confirmation of inadequacy
Relational Pattern	Seeks collaboration and reciprocal support	Overextends, takes on others' needs, avoids vulnerability
Somatic Indicators	Body feels grounded, rested, and regulated	Body feels tense, fatigued, or disconnected; sleep and appetite may be disrupted
Trajectory	Sustainable and aligned with long-term goals	Leads to burnout, emotional collapse, or identity confusion

had to silence in order to succeed. Only then can new definitions of success emerge, ones that include rest, boundaries, joy, and work that aligns with who they truly are.

Understanding the difference between authentic ambition and over-functioning allows therapists to approach high-achieving clients with greater nuance. It challenges the assumption that outward success reflects internal stability and reframes productivity as a possible adaptation to relational or systemic threat. For many young women, the compulsion to perform does not emerge in isolation. It is often shaped by broader forces such as economic pressure, cultural expectations, racialized labor, or the absence of dependable safety nets. When achievement becomes the only reliable source of identity or security, rest feels dangerous, and slowing down becomes a risk rather than a right. To intervene meaningfully, clinicians must consider not only what the client is doing but what the doing protects her from, and at what cost.

Pathway 2: Financial and Housing Insecurity

No one talks about the nervous system cost of being broke. Not in clinical terms. Not in classroom discussions. And rarely in therapy. But for many young women, financial strain and unstable housing are not side challenges. They are the defining conditions under which everything else must be negotiated: identity, health, relationships, even belief in the future.

Economic insecurity is not a temporary inconvenience. It is a state of prolonged uncertainty that shapes how a person thinks, feels, and organizes their day. For young women carrying student debt, earning less than their male peers, or financially supporting parents or siblings, every decision has consequences. Do I buy groceries or pay for my next class? Do I miss work to make this appointment, or push my health aside again? These calculations happen silently, invisibly, every day. Over time, they rewire the nervous system for survival, not growth.

Recent data from the Hope Center in 2024 found that nearly half of college students report some form of housing insecurity, and more than one-third experience food insecurity. The numbers are highest among women of color, parenting students, and those who identify as LGBTQ. These numbers translate into stories like Sara, a college sophomore commuting 90 minutes daily because campus housing waitlists were full and shelters were unsafe. She attended class with a backpack full of essentials in case she couldn't go home that night. But statistics do not capture the lived texture of this experience. It is waking up in someone else's apartment and pretending you got enough sleep. It is staying in a job or relationship that feels unsafe because it pays rent. It is becoming an expert in appearing fine while quietly unraveling.

In therapy, this does not always show up as a story. It shows up as missed sessions, as chronic fatigue, as a client who cancels when the weather is bad because the bus route is not safe. It shows up as difficulty planning, not because of poor executive function, but because the future feels too far away to imagine. These are not signs of resistance. They are symptoms of economic trauma.

Occupational therapy and mental health providers must learn to see these signals for what they are. A woman who cannot stick to a morning routine may not need more structure. She may need a bed of her own. A client who is disengaged from goal setting may not lack insight. She may be protecting herself from hoping for something she cannot yet afford to reach. The problem is not always the plan. The problem is the context in which the plan was made.

Therapeutic care must begin with that recognition. It requires providers to ask not just what the goals are, but what stability those goals rest upon. It may mean helping a client access housing supports or rewriting goals to reflect adaptive routines that flex across unpredictable settings. It may also mean slowing down, listening for what is not said, and naming the grief of time lost to survival. In this work, progress cannot be measured only by consistency or performance. Sometimes, it is measured by the first moment a client says, out loud, that they want more.

Because healing is not only about getting out of crisis. It is about rebuilding the right to imagine, to rest, to dream again without fear.

Pathway 3: Relational Trauma Across Systems

In a 2023 national survey of college women, nearly one in four reported staying in a relationship that made them feel unsafe emotionally, yet only a fraction of them named it as abuse. When asked why, the most common answer was, "It didn't feel different from what I was used to."

This is the hidden cost of relational trauma across systems. It does not always begin with partners or intimate encounters. It often begins much earlier—with emotionally inconsistent caregivers, with childhood roles that required caregiving rather than receiving care, or with family systems where love had to be earned through perfection, silence, or sacrifice. These early dynamics do not disappear when girls grow up. They evolve. They take on new forms in romantic relationships, academic spaces, and caregiving roles, often without being recognized as trauma at all.

What clinicians see as "low self-esteem" or "poor boundaries" is often the residue of chronic emotional survival. A young woman who avoids conflict may have learned that speaking up ends in abandonment. Another who overextends in every role may not be trying to prove something—she may be trying to keep herself from being discarded. These behaviors are not simply relational habits. They are protective mechanisms, shaped in childhood and reinforced by every system that made care conditional.

Familial rupture is often the first trauma, but it rarely ends there. Many young women enter adulthood having already experienced parentification, estrangement, or emotional enmeshment. Parentification, which occurs when a child is tasked with adult emotional or caregiving roles, can leave long-term effects on identity development and boundary formation. Some have aged out of foster care or lived in homes where physical needs were met, but emotional safety was absent. These conditions are linked to long-term PTSD risk when early adversity follows a chronic or compounding trajectory (El-Khoury et al., 2021). Meanwhile, others carry invisible intergenerational burdens, such as translating medical systems for immigrant parents, becoming the emotional regulator for a depressed caregiver, or being expected to succeed not just for themselves, but for everyone who never had the chance.

These histories can distort how intimacy is interpreted. Gaslighting, emotional volatility, and conditional affection in adult relationships may not feel like violations. They may feel familiar. Women who have never known safe attachment may stay in toxic partnerships not out of weakness but out of recognition, because the nervous system does not fear what it already knows how to survive. This is why relational trauma so often repeats itself. It is not because women are failing to choose better. It is because their earliest wiring taught them that care always comes with cost.

And the systems surrounding them often reinforce this logic. A young woman experiencing emotional abuse in a dating relationship may hesitate to speak up if her insurance requires a parent's consent, or if she fears being disbelieved by a professor or counselor. Those who leave home due to safety concerns may find themselves excluded from financial aid, unsupported in housing searches, or left to explain why they are entirely on their own at twenty years old. Systemic abandonment compounds relational trauma. It sends the message that safety is not a right but a luxury.

Rebuilding Relational Safety Through Attuned Therapeutic Practice

What does this mean for therapists and allied health professionals? It means we must be trained to see patterns, not just problems. A young woman who becomes anxious when praised may be waiting for the moment it is taken back. One who dismisses her own needs may not be passive, she may have learned that desire is dangerous. In therapeutic spaces, relational safety must be created gradually, not assumed from the start. This includes consistency, transparency, and permission for the client to notice, name, and even test the boundaries of trust.

Healing relational trauma is not a linear process. It requires helping women build new internal maps of what care can look like: stable, mutual, responsive, and earned simply by showing up as oneself. This work must be relational in structure, not just in content. That means offering consistency, reflecting emotional experiences without judgment, and modeling boundaries that are both firm and kind. It requires honoring the grief that comes with realizing how long one has survived without that kind of care. And it requires, above all, refusing to treat relational harm as a side effect of poor choices. It is a symptom of earlier blueprints that made harm feel like home. See Table 3.2 for examples of therapeutic strategies that support this kind of relational repair.

These practices are not quick fixes. They are small, deliberate contradictions to what trauma has taught a client to expect. When used consistently, they create the

Table 3.2 Strategies for Supporting Relational Trauma Recovery in Therapy

Relational Need	Therapeutic Strategy	Example in Practice
Rebuilding trust in connection	Offer consistency in scheduling, tone, and presence. Narrate ruptures and repairs openly.	"I noticed we had to reschedule last week. I want to make sure we reconnect here today—your time matters."
Expanding emotional range and expression	Name emotional patterns with compassion. Reflect nonverbal cues and validate ambivalence.	"You smiled just now, but your eyes looked heavy. It's okay to feel two things at once."
Repairing boundary confusion	Model and uphold healthy limits in session. Invite conversation when boundaries are tested.	"I'm going to hold our time to 50 minutes, and if we need to revisit something next week, we will. Your thoughts are still important even if we pause for now."
Countering internalized blame	Gently reframe self-criticism as an adaptive strategy. Avoid pathologizing survival behaviors.	"It makes sense that you learned to keep quiet as a child. That wasn't weakness—it was protection."
Introducing new models of care	Use language that reflects mutuality. Explore examples of safe relationships in real life or fiction.	"Who in your life now, or even in a book or movie, treats people in a way that feels safe to you?"
Making space for grief and longing	Validate loss without rushing resolution. Allow space for the mourning of unmet needs.	"It's okay to feel angry that no one protected you. That anger is part of the healing."
Supporting secure attachment experiences	Stay emotionally present during rupture. Encourage reflective practices over compliance.	"I noticed you seemed hesitant today. That's okay. We don't have to perform here—we can just explore what's coming up."

conditions for new relational learning, not just intellectually, but somatically. The goal is not to teach clients how to behave in relationships. It is to help them re-experience what it feels like to be seen, respected, and protected without earning it through perfection or silence. This is the essence of relational repair—not the absence of rupture, but the presence of repair that follows. Over time, these moments become internalized as new templates for safety, not just in the therapy room, but in life.

Occupational Disruption in Emerging Adulthood

Occupational science is the study of how humans engage in meaningful activities, or occupations, and how those activities both shape and are shaped by health, identity, culture, and context. It is a science rooted in the belief that what we do matters, not only to our physical well-being, but to our sense of self, purpose, and belonging. From this lens, participation is not simply about functioning. It is about being seen, being valued, and having access to a life that reflects one's desires and dignity.

For young women in emerging adulthood, that access is often compromised. What may appear as lack of motivation or inconsistency is frequently a deeper form of occupational disruption. These women are not failing to organize their lives. They are navigating bodies and nervous systems shaped by relational trauma, institutional exclusion, and cultural narratives that equate their worth with performance or care for others. The result is not just fatigue. It is disconnection from agency, identity, and meaning.

Occupational science challenges us to look beyond behavior and ask better questions: What roles is this person expected to perform? What occupations have they had to give up or never had access to? Who benefits from their over-functioning or their silence? These questions are essential in emerging adulthood, a life stage characterized by major transitions in education, employment, intimacy, and autonomy. For women with trauma histories or systemic barriers, these transitions often become inflection points where participation fractures.

Research supports this. A large study published in *Healthcare (Basel)* by Bouloukaki et al. (2023) assessed sleep quality and fatigue in over 900 university students before and during exam periods and found a marked deterioration in both domains. During the exam period, students' sleep quality scores worsened significantly, and fatigue levels rose in tandem. Notably, female students reported significantly higher fatigue scores than male students, even after controlling for other factors such as age, smoking, and physical activity. Increases in fatigue were also associated with depressive symptoms, chronic illness, and decreased exercise, factors disproportionately affecting women navigating both academic and emotional burdens. While these findings are often interpreted as temporary stress responses, they reveal deeper disruptions in occupational balance and self-regulation. For many women in emerging adulthood, exam periods do not simply reflect academic pressure, they mirror broader patterns of overextension and under-recovery that erode participation across roles and routines.

Occupational disruption in emerging adulthood is not abstract. It is lived in the granular details of daily life, when routines dissolve, when motivation slips away, and when roles become too heavy to carry. Disruption often reveals itself first in the erosion of daily rhythms, the loss of access to rest and leisure, and the collapse of productivity under the weight of invisible strain. For Jordan, a first-generation student, missing a single assignment felt like letting down her entire family. What appeared as procrastination was actually paralyzing guilt and the fear of being seen as undeserving. Each of these breakdowns offers insight into how trauma and systemic burden shape not just what young women do, but how they experience themselves through doing.

Impact on Routines

Stability in emerging adulthood often hinges on consistent routines—morning rituals, structured study schedules, and regular physical activity. These patterns do more than organize time; they regulate the nervous system, foster predictability, and anchor identity. However, for many young women, these routines begin to deteriorate under the weight of academic pressures and emotional stressors. Sleep becomes erratic, meals are skipped, and leisure activities are abandoned. These changes are not mere lapses in discipline but indicators of deeper occupational disruptions shaped by how trauma alters one's engagement with internal and external sensory environments (Harricharan et al., 2021).

A recent study examining the relationship between physical activity, fatigue, and sleep quality among university students during exam periods found that decreased physical activity levels were associated with increased fatigue and poorer sleep quality. This correlation was particularly pronounced among female students, highlighting the gendered impact of academic stress on occupational balance.

From an occupational therapy perspective, routines are foundational structures that support emotional regulation, cognitive clarity, and role integration. When these routines fracture, so does the individual's ability to participate meaningfully across domains (AOTA, 2020). For women who have internalized productivity as a measure of self-worth, the breakdown of structure often feels like personal failure rather than a response to overwhelming circumstances.

Interventions should focus on reframing rest and leisure as essential components of occupational health. Reestablishing daily rhythms might begin with small, manageable actions—consistent sleep schedules, scheduled breaks for physical activity, or reintroducing creative pursuits. These steps are not trivial; they are critical strategies for restoring occupational balance and promoting overall well-being.

Disrupted Volition, Motivation, and Identity Exploration

When routines begin to deteriorate, volition is often the next to weaken. Not all at once, but gradually and quietly. What used to feel energizing becomes overwhelming. What once sparked curiosity now feels like an obligation. For many young women in emerging adulthood, the disruption of motivation is not a sign of apathy. It is a nervous system protecting itself from a world that demands too much without offering enough safety or support in return.

Volition, as defined in occupational science, refers to the capacity to choose and initiate actions that are personally meaningful and identity-reinforcing (Skorikov & Vondracek, 2011). It is shaped by one's values, interests, sense of efficacy, and internalized expectations. When volition is intact, a person moves through the world with agency. But when it is compromised by trauma, chronic stress, or repeated invalidation, agency is replaced by hesitation, self-doubt, or emotional disengagement.

In clinical practice, this often shows up as a young woman who keeps changing majors not because she is lost, but because she has never been invited to explore who she is without someone else's agenda. Or the new graduate who procrastinates on job applications not because she lacks ambition, but because her nervous system has equated visibility with vulnerability. These are not failures of character. They are expressions of disrupted occupational identity (Fleming et al., 2024).

The developmental task of emerging adulthood is to build a self-directed life. But for many women, this process is constantly interrupted by cultural and familial expectations, survival demands, or unprocessed relational trauma, all of which contribute to disproportionate risks for affective dysregulation and identity fragmentation during this life stage. Their identities are shaped more by accommodation than authenticity. They pursue what is expected, not what is aligned. Over time, this gap between doing and being creates a kind of occupational dissonance, where action no longer reflects self-hood and motivation becomes harder and harder to access.

A 2023 study published in *Frontiers in Psychology* found that trauma-exposed college students reported significantly lower levels of intrinsic motivation, and a higher incidence of identity diffusion compared to their peers. Researchers noted that this population demonstrated more externalized goal orientation and described difficulty imagining a future that reflected their true preferences and values. These findings align with what we see clinically: when safety is uncertain and worth is externally defined, choice is no longer empowering. It is paralyzing.

Restoring volition begins with reducing performance-based pressure and increasing opportunities for self-authorship. For some clients, this may look like exploring what brings energy rather than what earns approval. For others, it may mean tolerating the discomfort of trying something new without a guarantee of success. Identity development is not a cognitive exercise. It is lived, practiced, and felt in action. In therapy, it must be reclaimed not through motivational techniques alone, but through co-regulation, permission to pause, and the space to explore desire without judgment.

Emerging adulthood presents a critical developmental window in which individuals can begin to reorient their actions based on internal values rather than external expectations. This process of self-authorship is particularly salient for young women whose prior experiences may have prioritized compliance, performance, or relational caretaking over autonomous decision-making. Within this context, even a subtle expression of authentic interest is not merely a sign of psychological progress. It represents a reengagement with volition, a reclaiming of identity, and a foundational step toward long-term occupational well-being.

Role Overload and Collapse

Praise often follows young women who appear dependable, organized, and consistently available. These traits are culturally reinforced and professionally rewarded—but rarely interrogated. What is less visible is the cost of sustaining this kind of constancy. For many women in emerging adulthood, adult life does not begin with one defining moment. It begins with the gradual accumulation of roles: student, employee, caretaker, advocate, partner. Some are pursued intentionally. Others are assumed by default or necessity. Over time, even those who seem the most competent may begin to fracture under the cumulative weight of these expectations.

In occupational science, role overload refers to the experience of managing too many roles with too few resources. But in practice, it is more than a scheduling problem. It is a nervous system problem. It is an identity problem. And it is often a gendered problem, exacerbated by unspoken expectations around performance, perfectionism, and emotional labor. Young women are not only managing tasks, they are managing the feelings, needs, and stability of those around them, often at the expense of their own regulation and well-being.

Clinically, this may show up as cognitive fatigue, anxiety, executive dysfunction, or the quiet erosion of self-confidence. A client might say, "I feel like I am failing everyone," or "I do not know who I am outside of what I do for other people." These are not merely signs of stress. They are indicators that occupational roles have outpaced the woman's capacity to participate meaningfully, and without loss.

A 2024 review published in *Global Advances in Integrative Medicine and Health* examined well-being among self-identified women working in healthcare professions across 26 countries. The review found that women consistently reported significantly higher levels of stress and burnout than their male counterparts, with direct correlations to role strain, psychological distress, and challenges with work–life integration. While this study focused on professional women, its findings are deeply relevant to the broader experience of role overload in emerging adulthood—especially for young women navigating multiple high-stakes roles without adequate support. When occupational demands outpace regulation and recovery, the result is not only exhaustion but the erosion of identity, motivation, and long-term well-being.

Role overload is often invisible. Many women meet expectations and exceed them, performing competence while quietly losing access to joy, rest, and volition. What appears as resilience can sometimes be survival. What looks like strength is often depletion, masked by performance. In high-achieving academic environments, impostor feelings and perfectionistic striving can obscure inner struggle (Wrench et al., 2024). Research shows that these emotional burdens often correlate with heightened depression, anxiety, and maladaptive coping among college-aged women, even when external performance appears intact (Mahmoud, 2012). Emotional creativity and achievement motivation, while often praised, can also interact with trauma symptoms and exacerbate psychological distress in university students (Bulathwatta & Lakshika, 2023).

Intervening in these patterns requires more than teaching task prioritization or self-care routines. It requires helping women reevaluate what roles are sustainable, and which ones have been assumed out of fear, habit, or unresolved obligation. It involves acknowledging grief for the identities neglected in service of others, for the boundaries never modeled, and for the costs of being over-relied upon. Occupational therapy must support not just functioning but freedom—the freedom to choose, to decline, to rest, and to redefine what success and selfhood can look like on their own terms.

To prevent role overload from progressing into collapse, assessment must go beyond time management or symptom tracking. Therapists should explore both the quantity and emotional weight of roles, as well as the client's perceived satisfaction, autonomy, and alignment with those roles. Tools such as the *Role Checklist* can help identify role patterns across time, while the *Canadian Occupational Performance Measure* can illuminate discrepancies between what a woman is doing and what actually matters to her. Assessing satisfaction, not just performance, reveals where misalignment may be eroding volition. Narrative-based inquiry and values clarification tools can further uncover roles assumed from survival rather than choice. Research suggests that many women, particularly those with histories of maltreatment, may display adaptive but draining role performance shaped by autonomic dysregulation and chronic stress adaptation (Toth & Cicchetti, 2013; Chaaya et al., 2025). Intervention begins with recognition, naming the overload, validating the toll, and co-creating strategies to either redistribute, redefine, or release roles that are no longer sustainable. When women are supported in reclaiming authorship of their roles, the result is not less ambition but more intentional participation.

Trauma-Informed Occupational Therapy in Early Adulthood

> Every morning, Talia Davis opened her laptop to a maze of tabs, including unfinished job applications, shopping carts she never checked out, and email drafts she could not bring herself to send. She made to-do lists at night but rarely looked at them the next day. She would start laundry, then forget it in the machine. Meals were skipped or microwaved without hunger. In class, she took notes meticulously but often missed the next assignment deadline. In therapy, she said, "I feel like I am constantly circling but never moving forward." Her time was full but without flow, marked by long periods of drifting followed by bursts of anxious urgency. What appeared as disorganization was a nervous system caught between demand and depletion.

Trauma-informed care is not a technique. It is a stance, one that recognizes how lived experiences of adversity shape the way a person thinks, moves, copes, and connects. In early adulthood, trauma does not simply linger in memory. It shows up in decision paralysis, in fragmented routines, in the exhaustion that follows brief periods of functioning. For young women especially, trauma-informed care must be grounded in more than empathy. It must be grounded in precision, particularly as research shows the cumulative toll of trauma on female reproductive and neuroendocrine health across the lifespan (Hillcoat et al., 2023). This stage of life demands that they construct an identity, pursue independence, navigate institutions, and show up in roles that often ask more than they are resourced to give.

Occupational therapy in this context becomes both a clinical practice and a relational act, particularly within women's health, where trauma-informed strategies must attend to gendered patterns of stress, identity development, and occupational disruption (Khan, 2025). It asks not only what is not working, but what has been survived. It asks what was once adaptive that no longer serves, and what has never felt safe enough to begin. Trauma-informed occupational therapy in early adulthood must move beyond symptom reduction or behavior shaping. It must engage with the systems, both internal and external, that have shaped the client's ability to participate in daily life. It must support the slow rebuilding of routines, roles, and identities not defined by past harm but by present agency.

For young adult women, a trauma-informed approach does more than validate lived experience. It reorients the therapeutic lens toward context. Rather than asking why someone is disorganized or unmotivated, it asks what that behavior is protecting them from. Rather than pushing for independence, it examines what dependencies were necessary for survival. Trauma-informed care helps therapists recognize that emotional regulation, executive function, and role performance are not fixed traits but flexible outcomes, shaped by relational safety, nervous system stability, and access to support. Research has shown that trauma, particularly among women facing housing insecurity or other social disadvantages, can significantly affect independent living skills, highlighting the need for occupational therapy that addresses both psychosocial and functional barriers to participation (Davis & Kutter, 1998; Moledina et al., 2021). In this way, trauma-informed care becomes a tool for clinical discernment, helping to distinguish what is willful from what is wired, and what is resistance from what is protection.

What follows are entry points. They are not protocols or solutions, but invitations to design therapy through collaboration, co-regulation, and structural humility. In the work of early adulthood, the goal is not to fix, but to re-anchor. To meet instability with scaffolding. And to hold space for the kind of healing that makes sustainable participation possible.

Rebuilding Routines and Anchoring Structure

Routines are often mistaken for mundane habits, but in occupational science, they are far more than that. Routines scaffold our sense of time, safety, and identity. For individuals with trauma histories, particularly young women navigating early adulthood, the absence of routine is not just disorganization. It is an occupational expression of disrupted neurobiology. The ability to sustain even basic patterns of self-care or productivity is deeply tied to nervous system regulation, cognitive bandwidth, and perceived safety in one's environment.

What makes trauma-informed care distinct is its refusal to pathologize these breakdowns. Instead, it interprets them as meaningful data. A woman who cannot maintain a consistent sleep schedule may not lack discipline. She may be living in a state of hypervigilance that makes rest physiologically unsafe. A student who starts and stops multiple projects may be navigating an over-coupled sense of urgency and shame. Rebuilding structure in this context is not about imposing order. It is about cultivating safety through rhythm.

Visual tools like co-created weekly planners or energy–mood maps help externalize overwhelm. Rather than assigning a premade template, therapists can design flexible visual aids with the client that reflect her cognitive load, emotional cycles, and capacity across the week. One client used a circle-based visual, not a list, because linear formats triggered memories of punitive school settings. Sasha preferred sticky notes to planners, as one smudge in her notebook would send her spiraling into shame. Together, we built a visual schedule with imperfection baked in. Another client marked time not by hours, but by "low brain," "medium brain," and "bright brain" segments, helping her attune to when she could realistically engage.

Scaffolding through instability is also key. Rebuilding routines may begin with anchoring just one daily touchpoint—brushing teeth to music, lighting a candle before studying, or sending a two-word check-in text to a support person. When co-regulated and customized, these micro-routines become somatic cues of predictability, stability, and emerging autonomy.

Role Navigation and Identity Repair

There is a hidden occupational cost to surviving trauma during girlhood. Many women enter adulthood with roles they never chose but learned to perform flawlessly: the helper, the fixer, the overachiever, the emotional container. These roles often ensured proximity to care or protection in earlier environments, but in early adulthood, they become constraining. What looks like capability can mask a profound disconnection from self-authorship.

Identity repair in occupational therapy begins not with surface-level goal setting, but with curiosity: What roles have you inherited, and which ones have you never had space to try on? Narrative interventions help externalize identity as a process rather than a fixed trait. In doing so, therapists must consider the sociocultural context that shapes occupational identity. Iwama et al. (2009) describe the therapeutic value of culturally responsive models like the Kawa model, which center the client's cultural narrative in clinical reasoning. Role mapping, both visually and verbally, allows clients to categorize their current roles, trace their origins, and explore the ones they long for but feel unqualified to claim.

One client described herself as a "therapist in every friendship," a role she had unconsciously adopted since adolescence. Through structured reflection and values clarification, she realized that what she most desired was reciprocity and vulnerability, roles that had been unavailable in her earlier relationships. Together, we explored what it would mean to step out of hyper-responsibility and into shared emotional labor. Another client used collage to represent the identities she was shedding and the ones she was growing into, offering a nonverbal path toward integration.

Repair is not about discarding the past but about facilitating a therapeutic process in which identity can be re-examined with intentionality and choice. From an occupational therapy perspective, this means helping clients distinguish between roles that reflect self-determined values and those that emerged in response to trauma, social conditioning, or survival imperatives. Therapists can support this process by incorporating structured interventions such as guided role exploration, values clarification, and narrative reframing. When women are supported in identifying how performance-based roles have shaped their occupational identity, they can begin to reclaim a sense of authorship. This shift holds significant implications for clinical practice: identity becomes a domain of intervention, not only in the psychosocial sense, but as a foundation for sustainable participation, improved volitional engagement, and long-term well-being.

Addressing Injustice and Systemic Barriers

Trauma-informed care is incomplete without a systems lens. For many young adult women, trauma does not occur in isolation. It is compounded by the social structures that fail to protect, include, or affirm them. Research shows that trauma-related symptoms among sexual minority women are often exacerbated by low social support, sexual assault, and minority stress, further complicating participation in daily life (van Stolk-Cooke et al., 2023). The cumulative impact of racism, ableism, classism, heterosexism, and gender-based violence is not peripheral to clinical care. It directly shapes occupational participation. Whether it manifests as withdrawal from academic programs, underemployment, medical mistrust, or resignation from caregiving roles, systemic injustice often limits not only what women can do, but what they believe is available to them.

Occupational therapists have a critical role in identifying and addressing these barriers. Advocacy in educational and workplace settings may involve supporting a woman through the process of requesting accommodations, navigating hostile learning environments, or documenting discrimination under the Americans with Disabilities Act. For students impacted by harassment or sexual violence, therapists may assist in understanding Title Nine rights, gathering documentation, and providing emotional support across the process. These moments require not only logistical guidance but attuned presence. The goal is not simply access—it is protection of dignity and power.

Anti-oppressive practice also requires reflection on the therapy space itself. Are we unintentionally reinforcing dominant cultural norms around independence, self-regulation, or emotional restraint? Are we pathologizing resistance or honoring it as a response to unsafe conditions? Therapy, in this context, becomes an act of justice when it centers voice, context, and collaborative power. See Table 3.3 for key clinical strategies that support trauma-informed advocacy and systems navigation.

Trauma recovery is not just about restoring the nervous system. It is also about challenging the environments that created harm in the first place. Effective occupational therapy goes beyond improving individual function. It asks

Table 3.3 Clinical Strategies for Addressing Systemic Barriers

Strategy	Application in Practice	Clinical Benefit	Example in Practice
Environmental and occupational mapping	Identify institutional, cultural, or physical barriers limiting participation	Highlights systemic obstacles affecting function	Mapping a college campus with a student to identify unsafe locations or inaccessible services

(Continued)

Table 3.3 (Continued)

Strategy	Application in Practice	Clinical Benefit	Example in Practice
Role-play and scripting for advocacy	Prepare clients for difficult conversations with professors, employers, or administrators	Builds confidence and communication skills	Practicing a script for requesting deadline flexibility after trauma disclosure in a graduate program
Culturally informed contextual interviews	Explore the sociopolitical factors shaping identity, safety, and performance	Brings invisible labor and trauma responses into the open	Asking about responsibilities like translating for family or managing cultural stigma around mental health
Rights education and systems literacy	Teach frameworks like ADA and Title Nine in client-centered language	Supports informed decision-making and self-advocacy	Reviewing Title Nine protections with a student pursuing action after campus sexual harassment
Resource linkage and referrals	Connect to peer support, legal aid, or culturally responsive services	Promotes continuity of care and broader community connection	Referring a queer client to a trauma-informed LGBTQ resource center that offers legal and housing support

what systems made participation feel unsafe, and what can be done to change them. When therapists support clients in understanding their rights, practicing difficult conversations, and navigating unjust systems, they are not simply offering tools. They are helping clients reclaim voice, power, and agency. For young women who have faced marginalization, this support can shift the difference between quiet survival and confident self-advocacy. Healing is not only what happens within the body. It is also what becomes possible when the world begins to respond with safety, dignity, and respect.

Emotional and Sensory Regulation

The body keeps score, but it also keeps rhythm. For young women shaped by trauma, regulation is not a skill they were born knowing. It is a capacity that must be rebuilt, moment by moment, through safety, rhythm, and relationship. What we often label as emotional dysregulation is not a flaw in personality or effort.

It reflects the imprint of a body whose early neurobiological development was shaped by instability and threat, which interferes with the maturation of emotional regulation systems (Edgelow et al., 2020).

Occupational therapists are uniquely positioned to help rewrite that narrative, not through conversation alone, but through the body's own language: movement, repetition, sensation, presence. Occupational therapists restore regulation not by demanding composure but by creating conditions where composure becomes possible. A steady hand in a shared task. A breath that slows. The quiet click of puzzle pieces returning to their place. These are not small things. They are the architecture of healing. Mindfulness-based practices have been shown to induce neurobiological changes that support regulation and healing, reinforcing the value of embodied routines in therapy (Calderone et al., 2024)

Emerging neuroscience confirms what many survivors already know in their bones. The capacity to regulate emotion does not come from logic. It comes from embodied safety (Kearney & Lanius, 2022), where the reintegration of somatic awareness is a central component of trauma recovery. The vagus nerve, the core of the parasympathetic nervous system, is not activated by instruction. It responds to experience—the sound of a calm voice, the softness of light, the cadence of breathing. Regulation begins not with what we teach but with how we show up.

But knowing *what* to do is not the same as knowing *when* to do it.

Regulation strategies are most effective when they are timed with intention. At the start of a session, consider using gentle sensory input or co-regulated movement to help clients transition from external stressors into the therapeutic space. This may look like shared breathing while setting up materials, stretching together, or walking while talking. These practices cue the nervous system that the environment is safe and allow the session to begin from a more regulated baseline.

During moments of escalation, when a client begins to shift into fight, flight, or freeze, grounding strategies should take priority. Use activities that are structured, rhythmic, and sensory-rich: sorting colored beads, kneading clay, or matching socks from a laundry basket. Avoid abstract questions or verbal processing during this window. Instead, anchor the client in sensation and task completion to reestablish regulation.

In mid-session dips, those quiet moments when a client's energy suddenly drops or they appear checked out, activation strategies may help. Offer short bursts of vestibular or tactile input, such as gentle rocking in a chair, textured fidget tools, or dynamic standing tasks. Invite choice, but keep demands low. The goal is not productivity; it is reconnection.

At the end of a session, downshift intentionally. Clients who have been in high arousal or intense emotional states should not leave abruptly. Build in 5 to 10 minutes of sensory regulation to close the session, such as deep breathing while folding a blanket, hand massage with lotion, or selecting and listening to music together. This closing rhythm helps encode safety into the session and supports smoother transitions back into daily life.

Therapists should also assess what state the client is bringing in, considering not just their behavior, but their body. Are they collapsed or on edge? Is their speech rapid, flat, or delayed? Regulation must begin at the level of the nervous system before it can emerge in the language of goals or performance. Every session is a chance to become a co-regulator. Every shared moment is an opportunity to restore rhythm. To support regulation is not to fix distress. It is to say, I can be with you in it. And sometimes, that is enough to shift the entire nervous system toward healing.

Case Vignettes and Clinical Reflections

Trauma in young adulthood often hides in plain sight. It wears the face of the high-achieving student, the overextended employee, the friend who remembers everyone's birthday but forgets to eat. In occupational therapy, we often meet young women at the moment when the scaffolding begins to crack, not yet in crisis, but in quiet depletion. Their routines are intact, their calendars full, their smiles rehearsed. But the nervous system tells another story.

What looks like motivation may be hypervigilance. What sounds like confidence may be masking collapse. The work of therapy in this stage is not to push harder. It is to pause longer. To recognize that many young women are navigating adult expectations with bodies still learning how to feel safe. The stories that follow are not about dramatic turning points. They are about subtle shifts, moments when therapy becomes less about what we do, and more about how we help someone remember who they are underneath what they perform.

Case Example 1: Nia, Age 21—University Student with Perfectionism and Panic

Nia was the kind of student who looked like she had it all together. Dean's list every semester. Student government. A competitive research internship. But behind the color-coded planner was a nervous system operating in chronic overdrive. She was referred to campus-based occupational therapy after a panic attack during a lab class. Her intake revealed multiple indicators of sympathetic nervous system hyperarousal: persistent insomnia, poor appetite awareness, somatic tension, and a deeply internalized fear of underperformance which research shows can heighten vulnerability to compulsive coping behaviors and emotional dysregulation (Conti et al., 2023). Although her presenting concern was framed as "test anxiety," it became clear that her occupational performance challenges were rooted in trauma-adapted perfectionism and disconnection from basic regulatory routines.

The OT prioritized rapport-building and nervous system stabilization as the first phase of intervention. Rather than beginning with goal-setting or verbal cognitive strategies, the therapist used observational assessment to gather baseline data. Nia gripped her pen tightly, apologized excessively, and hesitated before sitting still. These subtle cues shaped the direction of care.

Intervention Phase 1: Regulation and Body-Based Anchoring

Each session began with a brief **sensory-based entry routine**—a structured sequence that paired proprioceptive input with movement: walking the perimeter of the room with weighted textbooks, followed by slow, patterned tracing on textured paper, then a seated breath reset. These activities supported **interoceptive awareness** and promoted parasympathetic activation, creating a somatic foundation for occupational engagement.

Intervention Phase 2: Occupational Mapping and Routinization

Rather than focus on generalized "time management," the therapist facilitated a **weekly occupational mapping activity** using visual–spatial planning tools. Together, they co-designed a calendar system that prioritized nervous system–friendly color codes:

* Blue: cognitive demand (classes, studying)
* Yellow: physiological need (meals, hydration, sleep routines)
* Green: recovery occupations (leisure, stillness, low-demand sensory input)

This visual planning tool functioned not only as an organizational aid but as a **cognitive reframing strategy**, helping Nia externalize her internal pressure and see rest as a scheduled necessity rather than a sign of laziness. The therapist embedded **values-based planning** by encouraging Nia to identify what brought her a sense of connection or joy, even if it was small—music breaks, walking to class without headphones, organizing her notes at a local cafe.

Intervention Phase 3: Identity Integration and Autonomy

Midway through therapy, Nia disclosed that she "felt less like a student and more like a performance." In response, the therapist used **motivational interviewing—a collaborative, client-centered approach designed to strengthen personal motivation and commitment to change by exploring and resolving ambivalence.** Through this lens, they explored occupational identity and internalized narratives around productivity and worth. Together, they drafted short-term, trauma-informed goals centered not on GPA or deliverables, but on nervous system restoration and sustainable engagement. Goals included:

* Initiate one non-academic occupation per day (e.g., reading, art, cooking)
* Complete three full meals per day with sensory support (e.g., grounding scent, music)
* Practice one nervous system down-regulation routine before bed 5x/week

Over time, Nia began to tolerate blank space in her calendar without panic. Her appetite returned. She began sleeping in two-hour blocks, then three. This gradual improvement in sleep is particularly notable given research indicating that poor sleep quality is linked to diminished resilience in young women, with gender-specific vulnerabilities tied to both biological and psychosocial factors (Bouloukaki et al., 2023). When asked how her week had gone, she paused and said, "I did less, but I felt more like myself." That moment marked a shift—not the elimination of anxiety, but the reclamation of self. Occupational therapy, in Nia's case, was not about managing tasks. It was about reestablishing internal safety, reframing performance-based identity, and supporting the nervous system as the true starting point for meaningful participation.

Case Example 2: Priya, Age 27—First-Generation Professional with Burnout and Role Overload

Priya, a 27-year-old public health coordinator, arrived to occupational therapy with a well-managed appearance and a barely contained nervous system. She was referred by her primary care physician for persistent fatigue, a decline in daily functioning, gastrointestinal discomfort, and "non-cardiac chest tightness." Despite a full medical workup, her symptoms persisted. "I feel like I'm failing everyone, and there's no off switch," she said in her first session. Her tone was calm. Her body was not.

As a first-generation college graduate supporting both her nuclear and extended family, Priya had internalized the belief that rest was irresponsible. She described feeling like a "machine," unable to delegate or disconnect without guilt. Her days were packed with professional tasks, domestic caregiving, and family advocacy—an invisible triad that yielded no room for her own care. The occupational therapist identified occupational imbalance, intergenerational over-functioning, and trauma-adapted hyper-independence as key drivers of her occupational disruption. The initial focus was on nervous system stabilization and externalization of cognitive and emotional load.

Intervention Phase 1: Role Externalization and Energy Mapping

To help Priya name the weight she was carrying, the therapist introduced a role-mapping exercise, drawing from the Model of Human Occupation. Together, they charted her formal and informal roles, breaking each into sub-occupations. A visual energy cost map was then created, color-coded by perceived physical, cognitive, and emotional exertion. The result was staggering: every hour of her week was filled, and nearly all roles were coded red (high effort). This mapping became a shared tool, not only for intervention planning but for validating the legitimacy of her exhaustion.

Intervention Phase 2: Boundary Rituals and Task Recovery

Priya resisted the idea of canceling responsibilities, so the therapist began with occupational reframing, not removal. They co-designed transition rituals between roles, using sensory grounding and environmental cues to signal closure and rest. Examples included:

- Ending workdays with a lavender hand massage and a guided playlist
- Using a visual "shutdown" checklist for her laptop workspace
- Creating a personalized "permission card" to visibly affirm when enough had been done

These routines introduced micro-boundaries that helped her body differentiate between urgency and recovery, even when external demands remained constant.

Intervention Phase 3: Restorative Occupations and Identity Work

Once physiological symptoms began to stabilize, the therapist facilitated a values clarification and identity reauthoring process using visual journaling and narrative prompts. Priya was asked: "What parts of your identity exist beyond being useful to others?" Her voice shook when she said, "I don't know." That became the goal.

They established short-term, trauma-informed goals, including:

- Engage in one personally meaningful leisure occupation per week without multitasking
- Decline or reschedule at least one non-essential task per week, using a co-created script
- Track sleep and digestion using a body awareness log, with weekly reflection

When Priya began attending weekly community yoga sessions, not as exercise, but as time "no one else could claim," the therapist noted the shift. Her planner still held many roles, but she had begun to color-code for herself.

The turning point came when she said, "I took a nap this weekend. Not because I was sick. Just because I was tired." It was the first time she had allowed herself to feel fatigue without shame.

Occupational therapy, in Priya's case, was not about teaching self-care. It was about undoing the narratives that framed self-preservation as failure. Through sensory regulation, narrative work, and the reconstruction of boundaries, Priya reclaimed her right to rest, an important occupation, not as a reward for doing enough, but as a non-negotiable part of being whole.

Therapist Reflections on Clinical Decision-Making

Working with young adult women often requires unlearning what we've been taught about motivation, performance, and readiness. Both Nia and Priya entered therapy with outward markers of competence—high-achieving, articulate, deeply responsible. But their bodies told a different story. What they needed was not more support to push through. They needed permission to slow down, fall apart, and reconstruct themselves from a place of safety, not survival.

Respecting autonomy meant relinquishing the urge to correct or reframe prematurely. In both cases, the therapist did not lead with behavioral interventions. Instead, she co-created conditions that allowed each client to surface in their own time. For Nia, this meant waiting through long silences and choosing regulation before goal setting. For Priya, it meant affirming that delegation and stillness were not failures of character, but unfamiliar forms of self-preservation.

Pacing was essential. When trauma is disguised as productivity, slowing down can feel intolerable. The therapist recognized this and approached change not as a sharp pivot, but as a gentle recalibration—one boundary at a time, one moment of rest, one routine infused with sensory intention. Each decision was deliberate—small enough to avoid activating shame, meaningful enough to shift the body's internal rhythm.

Co-regulation served as the true starting point of both interventions. The therapist's own nervous system became a stabilizing force—through presence, voice, rhythm, and attunement. Before asking the client to reflect, plan, or prioritize, the therapist modeled calm, consistency, and neutrality. These were not soft skills. They were clinical interventions in their own right, foundational for restoring trust in relational safety.

Identity affirmation was threaded throughout. Trauma, particularly in early adulthood, can fracture a young woman's sense of self. When achievement becomes the only accepted version of worth, rest feels dangerous, and slowness feels like failure. Therapy became a space to explore: Who am I outside of my usefulness? What do I want, beyond what I've been praised for? These questions were not answered quickly. But they were asked—again and again—until the client's own voice began to rise.

In both cases, progress was not measured by task completion or symptom reduction. It was marked by softness returning to the body, by moments of self-directed pause, by the quiet reclamation of time, space, and worth. Trauma-informed occupational therapy, in this context, was not a treatment plan. It was a collaboration. A steady rhythm offered in a world that had only ever demanded performance.

Summary and Implications

In early adulthood, trauma often reveals itself not in acute crises, but in persistent patterns of overextension, emotional suppression, and somatic distress that remain largely invisible to the systems surrounding young women. This life stage, characterized by emerging independence, role negotiation, and identity formation, is especially vulnerable to the effects of unresolved developmental and relational trauma. Yet because the behaviors that arise from chronic dys-regulation often mimic socially desirable traits like ambition, responsibility, and adaptability, the underlying strain on the nervous system frequently goes unrecognized. What appears as high performance may in fact reflect a body bracing for failure, a mind conditioned to equate rest with danger, and a self-worth tethered to utility. From a neuroendocrine standpoint, this can lead to a sustained state of sympathetic dominance, disrupted circadian and hormonal rhythms, and increased risk for long-term mental and physical health complications.

For occupational therapists, this calls for a reframing of both assessment and intervention. Trauma-informed care in young adult women must begin with attunement to physiological signals of distress—sleep disturbance, appetite changes, pain syndromes, and sensory overwhelm—not as isolated symptoms, but as embodied narratives. Interventions that prioritize sensory regulation, co-regulated routines, values-based occupational mapping, and narrative reframing offer not just temporary relief but foundational recalibration. Therapeutic goals must move beyond productivity benchmarks to include restoration of rhythm, discernment of authentic occupational identity, and the capacity to say no without shame. Importantly, the therapist's role is not to motivate or instruct, but to pace alongside—to serve as a regulated presence that models safety, flexibility, and self-compassion in a world that often demands constant output.

References

American Occupational Therapy Association (AOTA). (2020). Occupational therapy practice framework: Domain and process (4th ed.). *American Journal of Occupational Therapy, 74*(Suppl. 2), 7412410010. https://doi.org/10.5014/ajot.2020.74S2001

Bouloukaki, I., Tsiligianni, I., Stathakis, G., Fanaridis, M., Koloi, A., Bakiri, E., Moudatsaki, M., Pouladaki, E., & Schiza, S. (2023). Sleep quality and fatigue during exam periods in university students: Prevalence and associated factors. *Healthcare (Basel, Switzerland), 11*(17), 2389. https://doi.org/10.3390/healthcare11172389

Bulathwatta, A., & Lakshika, R. (2023). Role of emotional creativity and achievement motivation on trauma symptoms among university students. *Frontiers in Psychology, 14*, Article 1203226. https://doi.org/10.3389/fpsyg.2023.1203226

Calderone, A., Latella, D., Impellizzeri, F., de Pasquale, P., Famà, F., Quartarone, A., & Calabrò, R. S. (2024). Neurobiological changes induced by mindfulness and meditation: A systematic review. *Biomedicines, 12*(11), 2613. https://doi.org/10.3390/biomedicines12112613

Chaaya, R., Sfeir, M., Khoury, S. E., Malhab, S. B., & Khoury-Malhame, M. E. (2025). Adaptive versus maladaptive coping strategies: insight from Lebanese young adults navigating multiple crises. *BMC public health, 25*(1), 1464. https://doi.org/10.1186/s12889-025-22608-4

Conti, L., Fantasia, S., Violi, M., Dell'Oste, V., Pedrinelli, V., & Carmassi, C. (2023). Emotional dysregulation and post-traumatic stress symptoms: Which interaction in adolescents and young adults? A systematic review. *Brain Sciences, 13*(12), 1730. https://doi.org/10.3390/brainsci13121730

Davis, J., & Kutter, C. J. (1998). Independent living skills and posttraumatic stress disorder in women who are homeless: Implications for future practice. *American Journal of Occupational Therapy, 52*(1), 39–44. https://doi.org/10.5014/ajot.52.1.39

Edgelow, M., Harrison, L., Miceli, M., & Cramm, H. (2020). Occupational therapy return to work interventions for persons with trauma and stress-related mental health conditions: A scoping review. *Work (Reading, Mass.)*, *65*(4), 821–836. https://doi.org/10.3233/WOR-203134

El-Khoury, F., Rieckmann, A., Bengtsson, J., Melchior, M., & Rod, N. H. (2021). Childhood adversity trajectories and PTSD in young adulthood: A nationwide Danish register-based cohort study of more than one million individuals. *Journal of Psychiatric Research*, *136*, 274–280. https://doi.org/10.1016/j.jpsychires.2021.02.034

Fleming, L. L., Harnett, N. G., & Ressler, K. J. (2024). Sensory alterations in posttraumatic stress disorder. *Current Opinion in Neurobiology*, *84*, 102821. https://doi.org/10.1016/j.conb.2023.102821

Harricharan, S., McKinnon, M. C., & Lanius, R. A. (2021). How processing of sensory information from the internal and external worlds shape the perception and engagement with the world in the aftermath of trauma: Implications for PTSD. *Frontiers in Neuroscience*, *15*, 625490. https://doi.org/10.3389/fnins.2021.625490

Hillcoat, A., Prakash, J., Martin, L., Zhang, Y., Rosa, G., Tiemeier, H., Torres, N., Mustieles, V., Adams, C. D., & Messerlian, C. (2023). Trauma and female reproductive health across the lifecourse: motivating a research agenda for the future of women's health. *Human reproduction* (Oxford, England), *38*(8), 1429–1444. https://doi.org/10.1093/humrep/dead087

Iwama, M., Thomson, N. A., & Macdonald, R. M. (2009). The Kawa model: The power of culturally responsive occupational therapy. *Disability and Rehabilitation*, *31*(14), 1125–1135. https://doi.org/10.1080/09638280902773711

Kearney, B. E., & Lanius, R. A. (2022). The brain-body disconnect: A somatic sensory basis for trauma-related disorders. *Frontiers in Neuroscience*, *16*, 1015749. https://doi.org/10.3389/fnins.2022.1015749

Khan, S. (2025). *Occupational therapy and women's health: A practitioner guide* (1st ed.). Routledge.

Mahmoud, J. S. R. (2012). The relationship among young adult college students' depression, anxiety, stress, demographics, life satisfaction, and coping styles. *Issues in Mental Health Nursing*, *33*(3), 149–156. https://doi.org/10.3109/01612840.2011.632708

Matud, M. P., Díaz, A., Bethencourt, J. M., & Ibáñez, I. (2020). Stress and psychological distress in emerging adulthood: A gender analysis. *Journal of Clinical Medicine*, *9*(9), 2859. https://doi.org/10.3390/jcm9092859

Moledina, A., Magwood, O., Agbata, E., Hung, J. H., Saad, A., Thavorn, K., & Pottie, K. (2021). A comprehensive review of prioritised interventions to improve the health and wellbeing of persons with lived experience of homelessness. *Campbell Systematic Reviews*, *17*(2), e1154. https://doi.org/10.1002/cl2.1154

Schwartz, S. J., Hardy, S. A., Zamboanga, B. L., Meca, A., Waterman, A. S., Picariello, S., Luyckx, K., Crocetti, E., Kim, S. Y., Brittian, A. S., Roberts, S. E., Whitbourne, S. K., Ritchie, R. A., Brown, E. J., & Forthun, L. F. (2015). Identity in young adulthood: Links with mental health and risky behavior. *Journal of Applied Developmental Psychology*, *36*, 39–52. https://doi.org/10.1016/j.appdev.2014.10.001

Skorikov, V. B., & Vondracek, F. W. (2011). Occupational identity. In S. J. Schwartz, K. Luyckx, & V. L. Vignoles (Eds.), *Handbook of identity theory and research* (pp. 693–714). Springer Science + Business Media. https://doi.org/10.1007/978-1-4419-7988-9_29

Toth, S. L., & Cicchetti, D. (2013). A developmental psychopathology perspective on child maltreatment. *Child Maltreatment*, *18*(3), 135–139.

van Stolk-Cooke, K., Price, M., Dyar, C., Zimmerman, L., & Kaysen, D. (2023). Associations of past-year overall trauma, sexual assault and PTSD with social support for young adult sexual minority women. *European Journal of Psychotraumatology*, *15*(1), 2287911. https://doi.org/10.1080/20008066.2023.2287911

Wrench, A., Padilla, M., O'Malley, C., & Levy, A. (2024). Impostor phenomenon: Prevalence among 1st year medical students and strategies for mitigation. *Heliyon*, *10*(8), e29478. https://doi.org/10.1016/j.heliyon.2024.e29478

Chapter 4

Trauma Associated with Perinatal Events

<hr />

Chapter Objectives

Upon completion of this chapter, the reader will be able to:

1. Describe the neurobiological changes that occur during pregnancy and postpartum, and explain how these shifts influence maternal identity, nervous system regulation, and daily occupational engagement.
2. Identify trauma responses in the perinatal period, including physical, emotional, and behavioral symptoms that may reflect unresolved trauma, and distinguish these from normative postpartum experiences.
3. Analyze the occupational impact of perinatal trauma, including birth trauma, pregnancy loss, medical complications, and structural inequities, with attention to roles, routines, and maternal self-perception.
4. Apply trauma-informed occupational therapy strategies that support regulation, agency, and identity restoration through co-regulation, sensory input, narrative processing, and choice-based care.
5. Evaluate the importance of culturally responsive care and structural advocacy in perinatal occupational therapy, and articulate how systemic inequities influence trauma recovery and engagement in care.

Juliette Campbell was 23 when she gave birth to her first child. While her pregnancy had been medically uneventful, the delivery quickly became life-threatening. Following an extended labor, she experienced a severe postpartum hemorrhage and required emergency surgical intervention. Her infant, born with respiratory distress, was immediately admitted to the neonatal intensive care unit, where he remained for over three weeks. In the days that followed, Juliette

DOI: 10.4324/9781003658559-4

reported feeling disoriented, emotionally detached, and hypervigilant. She described being physically present but mentally elsewhere, unable to rest, and overwhelmed by the sound of monitors and alarms.

Occupational therapy was initiated to support regulation, reengagement, and identity restoration. Early sessions focused on body-based grounding strategies to increase present-moment orientation, including sensory-based self-contact, paced breathing, and environmental orientation cues. As she stabilized, the therapist integrated structured co-occupations that promoted maternal agency, such as collaborative caregiving routines, sensory cocreation activities, and narrative tools to help Juliette process her birth experience within a safe and validating space. Her perceived stress levels, measured using the Impact of Events Scale, showed a clinically meaningful reduction over the course of treatment. However, in follow-up sessions several weeks later, Juliette expressed persistent fears of separation. Even brief periods away from her baby induced acute anxiety. She declined social invitations, postponed her return to school, and described an ongoing sense of unease that others might not care for her infant as attentively as she could.

This residual trauma response reflected the nervous system's ongoing need for safety, consistency, and control. Occupational therapy shifted focus to support graded exposure to separation, co-developing safety scripts, and expanding Juliette's window of tolerance for participation outside the NICU environment. The work was not about independence for its own sake. It was about helping her reestablish a felt sense of safety in her body, her environment, and her evolving role as a mother.

The United States remains one of the most dangerous high-income countries in which to give birth. In 2023, 669 maternal deaths were recorded, representing a rate of 18.6 deaths per 100,000 live births. But these numbers only scratch the surface of a deeper crisis. According to the CDC (2024), Black women are still dying at more than three times the rate of White women, with a staggering maternal mortality rate of 50.3 deaths per 100,000 live births. These disparities persist regardless of education, income, or access to prenatal care. Behind these statistics is another layer that is often hidden from view: trauma.

Recent data from the CDC and maternal health task forces reveal that mental health conditions, including suicide, substance use, and trauma-related disorders, are now among the leading causes of pregnancy-related deaths in the United States. These deaths are often preventable. They are not the result of individual failure, but of systemic neglect, fragmented care, and a healthcare system that too often fails to listen, to adapt, or to make space for women's lived experiences.

The perinatal period marks a profound transformation across neurological, relational, and occupational domains. It is a time of heightened physiological vulnerability and significant identity reorganization. For women who experience birth trauma, pregnancy loss, emergency medical interventions, or mistreatment in obstetric care, this transition is often accompanied by fear, disconnection, and a disruption of self. These experiences are not isolated. They are frequently overlooked, minimized, or rendered invisible within clinical spaces. Yet their impact is enduring, shaping not only physical health but also the continuity of daily routines, the performance of maternal roles, and a woman's felt sense of safety, agency, and orientation to the world around her.

Reproductive Transitions as Neurobiological and Occupational Events

Pregnancy initiates a neurological transformation that is as significant as it is invisible. Unlike the visible expansion of the belly or the shift in gait, the maternal brain reshapes itself quietly reorganizing structure, sensitivity, and function in preparation for caregiving, attunement, and protection. These changes are not incidental. They are biologically orchestrated, hormonally mediated, and designed to recalibrate how a woman interprets sensory input, evaluates social cues, and responds to threat or connection.

Hormones such as estrogen, progesterone, cortisol, and oxytocin act as chemical architects in this process, influencing neural pathways responsible for emotion regulation, memory, executive function, and stress response. What neuroscience reveals is that these brain changes are not just short-term adaptations, they persist into the postpartum period, often for months or even years. For some women, especially those with trauma histories or high-stress exposures, the postpartum brain remains in a state of heightened vigilance or dysregulation, influencing how they bond, rest, or engage in everyday roles (Caglayan et al., 2023). See Table 4.1 for an overview of key neurobiological changes that occur during the perinatal period.

Understanding these neurological shifts is foundational to effective perinatal care. These are not temporary side effects of pregnancy, nor are they signs of decline. They reflect adaptive neuroplasticity, with changes that prepare a woman to detect subtle emotional cues, respond rapidly to distress, and remain attuned to the rhythms of another life. But when compounded by trauma, chronic stress, or lack of postpartum support, these same adaptations can contribute to dysregulation, identity disruption, and occupational disengagement. For clinicians, and particularly for occupational therapists, recognizing these brain-based

Table 4.1 Neurobiological Brain Changes in Pregnancy and Postpartum

Brain Region/System	Neurobiological Change	Onset and Duration
Gray Matter (Social Cognition Areas)	Reduction in volume to enhance maternal attunement and social cognition	Begins in 2nd trimester, persists up to 2 years postpartum
Amygdala	Increased reactivity to emotional and social stimuli	Increases during late pregnancy, heightened postpartum for approximately 6 months
Prefrontal Cortex	Temporary inefficiencies in executive function (planning, decision-making)	Altered function in 3rd trimester, stabilizes by approximately 1 year postpartum
Hippocampus	Reduced volume and function (linked to cortisol and sleep deprivation)	Changes in late pregnancy, gradual recovery by 6 to 12 months postpartum
Oxytocin System	Upregulation of oxytocin receptors; supports bonding and trust	Heightened during labor and early postpartum, effects depend on safety and bonding context
HPA Axis (Stress Response System)	Elevated baseline cortisol levels; increased stress sensitivity	Activated early in pregnancy, may remain dysregulated up to 1 year postpartum in trauma
Default Mode Network	Reorganization to prioritize social and relational processing	Shift begins in 3rd trimester, can last into second postpartum year

changes is essential to interpreting behavior, structuring intervention, and pacing care in ways that honor the body's unfolding biology.

Trauma and the Dysregulated Perinatal Nervous System

Nadira Adel had made it through the pregnancy without major complications, but she never quite felt at ease. She flinched when strangers touched her belly. She avoided looking too far ahead. At night, her thoughts raced: "What if something goes wrong?", "What if they don't believe me?" After delivery, she found herself scanning her baby for signs of distress, checking her breathing over and over. Even the sound of the baby monitor made her chest tighten. She couldn't explain why simple tasks felt so hard. Her body ached. Her sleep was shallow. Her partner kept saying, "The hard part's over now," but Nadira wasn't so sure. She didn't feel calm. She felt alert. Like she was still waiting for something to go wrong.

The maternal nervous system does not begin at zero when pregnancy starts. It carries forward the imprint of everything that came before, including early attachment experiences, chronic stress exposure, systemic racism, relational trauma, and medical mistrust (Ahmad et al., 2022). For many women, pregnancy unfolds within a body already conditioned to scan for danger and override discomfort. In this context, the biological transitions of the perinatal period may amplify, rather than soothe, the body's sense of threat.

During pregnancy, the HPA axis becomes increasingly active. This is a normative process, intended to support fetal development and maternal vigilance. But when baseline stress levels are already elevated, this upregulation can tip into hyperactivation. Cortisol remains chronically high. Rest becomes elusive. Somatic symptoms such as headaches, joint pain, gastrointestinal issues, and chest tightness may surface—not as primary medical concerns, but as the nervous system's language of overload.

Trauma also interferes with the oxytocin system. Oxytocin is often described as the hormone of bonding and trust, but its effects are context-dependent. In safe, relationally attuned environments, oxytocin promotes warmth, closeness, and caregiving behaviors. But in the aftermath of trauma, oxytocin signaling may be blunted or paradoxically dysregulating, triggering discomfort instead of calm. For some women, physical touch, skin-to-skin contact, or even eye contact with their newborn may evoke sensations of vulnerability or danger. These responses are not signs of detachment. They are signs of a nervous system that has not yet reestablished safety.

Occupational therapists supporting women during the perinatal period must learn to read beyond behavior. Disengagement from infant care may reflect sensory overload, emotional exhaustion, or trauma-related dysregulation rather than disinterest or detachment. A rigid adherence to routines may be an effort to create predictability in an environment that feels volatile. These patterns are not signs of failure but protective adaptations shaped by the nervous system's ongoing search for safety. Trauma-informed care in this context requires attunement, pacing, and coregulation, not correction. To support clinical insight, therapists may incorporate assessments such as the *Mother-to-Infant Bonding Scale (MIBS)*, the *Postpartum Bonding Questionnaire (PBQ)*, or the *Perinatal PTSD Questionnaire (PPQ)* to better understand the emotional and relational landscape. These tools help identify when a mother's behaviors reflect typical adjustment and when they may indicate unresolved trauma or compromised attachment. The therapeutic goal is not to compel participation through expectation, but to cultivate the relational and sensory safety that makes engagement possible. See

Table 4.2 Differentiating Normative Versus Trauma-Related Perinatal Responses and Occupational Therapy Strategies

Observed Behavior/ Symptom	Normative Pregnancy/ Postpartum Response	Possible Trauma-Related Indicator	Occupational Therapy Interpretation and Strategy
Difficulty sleeping	Common in third trimester and early postpartum due to hormonal shifts and newborn care demands	Persistent insomnia beyond 6 weeks postpartum with racing thoughts or physiological arousal	Introduce nervous system down-regulation strategies such as breath pacing, weighted items, or guided body scans
Hyper-focus on infant care tasks	Can reflect adaptive learning and bonding, especially in new mothers	Compulsive over-functioning linked to hyperarousal or fear of failure	Use co-regulated routines and emphasize safety over perfection in infant care
Emotional numbness or flat affect	Temporary emotional withdrawal during postpartum adjustment	Emotional numbing as a protective dissociative response	Provide low-demand, sensory-rich occupations to rebuild presence and emotional connection
Avoidance of physical closeness with infant	May occur in early postpartum if mother is physically uncomfortable or fatigued	Avoidance rooted in prior trauma, discomfort with touch, or unresolved birth trauma	Respect boundaries while offering options for safe touch or parallel engagement
Excessive worry or scanning for danger	Mild vigilance is common, especially in new mothers	Chronic hypervigilance or exaggerated fear of harm, especially without identifiable cause	Normalize fear but work on grounding strategies and safety cues within daily routines

(Continued)

Table 4.2 (Continued)

Observed Behavior/ Symptom	Normative Pregnancy/ Postpartum Response	Possible Trauma-Related Indicator	Occupational Therapy Interpretation and Strategy
Rigidity with routines or caregiving schedules	Can reflect attempts to create structure during a time of major change	Rigid control as a trauma response to unpredictability or past loss	Introduce flexible routines with visual anchors and stress-reducing transitions
Disinterest in self-care or hygiene	Reduced priority for self-care is common in early postpartum	Rigid control as a trauma response to unpredictability or past loss	Introduce flexible routines with visual anchors and stress-reducing transitions
Strong startle response or emotional lability	Can reflect hormonal fluctuations and sleep deprivation	Intensified reactivity due to nervous system sensitization	Support emotional literacy through body-based regulation and graded emotional exposure

Table 4.2 for examples of how to differentiate between typical perinatal experiences and signs that may signal deeper disruption.

Understanding how trauma presents in the perinatal period requires more than checklists or structured assessments. It calls for therapeutic presence and the ability to interpret what is felt but not always said. Behaviors such as emotional withdrawal, compulsive routine-following, or hesitation with physical closeness are often misread as disinterest, inflexibility, or failure to bond. In reality, they may reflect a nervous system working to protect itself. A woman who appears distant may be internally overwhelmed. A mother who fixates on feeding or sleep schedules may be creating a sense of order in a world that has felt unpredictable. Occupational therapy offers a space where these patterns can be understood without judgment and gently shifted through relational safety, choice, and small moments of co-regulated rhythm. Healing begins through consistency, through attention to what feels tolerable, and through occupations that help women feel both competent and connected.

Occupation as Identity and Restoration in the Perinatal Period

Identity is not something we hold. It is something we do. During the perinatal period, what a woman does, hour by hour and day by day, changes in ways that

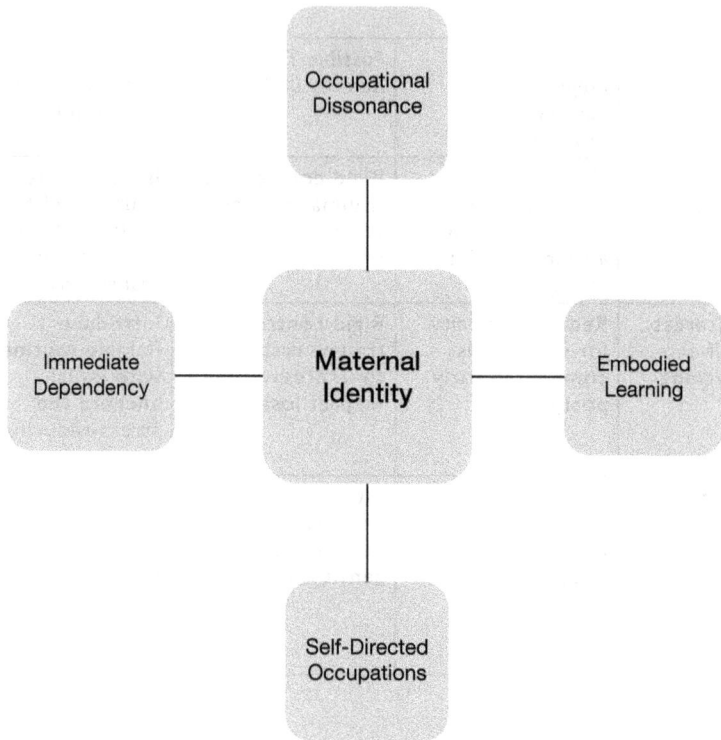

Figure 4.1 Core domains influencing maternal identity in the perinatal period.

redefine how she understands herself. This stage does not simply introduce new responsibilities. It reshapes the meaning of occupation. Every action becomes shared. Every decision, from when to eat to how to move, is filtered through the presence of another life. As illustrated in Figure 4.1, maternal identity in the perinatal period is shaped by multiple interconnected domains that influence how a mother experiences and navigates her daily life.

Immediate dependency is a defining aspect of early motherhood. A woman's daily activities are no longer fully her own. Caring for an infant becomes central. Yet this dependency is unidirectional. It does not offer reciprocity or pause. She may begin to feel unseen within the very routines she upholds. She may give without acknowledgment, function without feedback, and slowly lose sight of herself within the tasks she performs.

This stage is also characterized by **embodied learning**. The mother's body becomes a site of knowing but also of discomfort, fatigue, and new physical demands. There is no rehearsal for most postpartum tasks. They are learned through repetition, touch, and motion. Activities such as holding, feeding, and calming an infant are physical acts of learning, often accompanied by uncertainty and exhaustion. The learning is immediate and constant. It happens through the body, not the intellect.

For many women, this period brings a quiet yet persistent experience of **occupational dissonance**. The daily activities she performs may be essential, but they may feel disconnected from who she was before. A woman who once created art, led meetings, or traveled freely may now spend her days tracking feedings and organizing nap schedules. These new tasks may carry deep purpose but not necessarily personal fulfillment. When occupations feel misaligned with internal identity, the result can be disengagement or emotional blunting. This is not a failure of maternal instinct. It is a natural response to loss of self-direction.

Rebuilding identity during this period requires attention to **self-directed occupations**, those rooted in personal choice rather than obligation. Small actions such as journaling, preparing a favorite meal, or taking a walk alone serve as vital affirmations that she still exists outside of her caregiving role. These activities are not indulgent. They are essential. They remind her of who she is beyond what she provides. See Table 4.3 for clinical strategies aligned with four core domains of occupational identity in the perinatal period.

These four domains offer a practical lens for identifying where identity is strained and where it can be gently rebuilt. The goal is not to resolve all tension, but to restore a sense of ownership in daily life. When therapists understand that identity is actively shaped through engagement, they can offer interventions that move beyond function alone. A woman's capacity to feel like herself again often begins in the smallest choices—what she wears, how she moves, what she reclaims as hers. By protecting space for self-directed action within the context

Table 4.3 Clinical Applications: Supporting Identity Through Occupation

Focus Area	Clinical Insight	Suggested Occupational Therapy Strategies
Immediate dependency	Acknowledge how constant caregiving has impacted privacy, choice, and autonomy	Ask open questions about what feels missing or lost; validate the emotional toll of full-time responsibility
Embodied learning	Recognize that new occupations are learned through physical trial and repetition	Offer sensory-based tools and language that support body awareness, comfort, and task mastery
Occupational dissonance	Identify disconnect between current roles and personal meaning or satisfaction	Help the client explore what feels misaligned and why; support reflection without judgment
Self-directed occupations	Reinforce that personal choice within daily life is a form of identity protection	Create time-bound goals around personally meaningful activities; document emotional and functional responses

of caregiving, therapy becomes a means of restoring not only participation, but presence.

Pathways to Trauma in the Perinatal Period

Trauma during the perinatal period is more prevalent than often recognized. Studies estimate that up to one in three women experience their birth as traumatic, with factors including perceived threat to life, loss of control, and lack of informed consent. These events are not limited to high-risk deliveries or major medical complications. They also occur in seemingly routine clinical interactions where women feel ignored, coerced, or denied agency. In addition to birth-related trauma, many women face medical complications, emergency procedures, infant separation, and poorly supported postpartum recovery. Others endure pregnancy loss, stillbirth, or the psychological distress of neonatal intensive care.

Systemic inequities further compound these risks. Racism, obstetric violence, and structural barriers disproportionately affect women of color, low-income women, and those with intersecting vulnerabilities. Still others experience forms of trauma that remain largely invisible—subtle acts of dismissal, minimization, or moral judgment that leave no formal record but erode safety and trust in care. These pathways are not mutually exclusive. They often intersect and accumulate, shaping how women engage in daily life and how they reconstruct identity after trauma. Recognizing the complexity of these experiences is essential to providing responsive, trauma-informed care.

Birth Trauma: Lack of Consent, Emergency Procedures, Loss of Agency

Birth trauma is not defined by a specific outcome but by the perception of threat, violation, or helplessness during the birthing process. A healthy baby and a physically intact parent do not guarantee a psychologically safe experience. Birth can become traumatic when a woman feels her body is no longer her own—when decisions are made without her input, when procedures are performed without clear explanation, or when she is spoken about rather than spoken to. Emergency interventions, though medically necessary, can leave women disoriented, frightened, or disconnected from the experience entirely. Even in non-emergent settings, rushed timelines, dismissive tones, and a lack of consent can turn what should be an empowering moment into one marked by powerlessness and fear.

The implications extend well beyond the delivery room. Women who experience birth trauma may struggle with bonding, breastfeeding, or returning to daily activities. They may avoid medical care or experience physiological symptoms when triggered by clinical settings. Occupational engagement often narrows as trauma restricts energy, safety, and choice. Occupational therapy in this context must recognize that physical recovery is not enough. Restoring a sense of control, voice, and trust becomes the primary therapeutic focus. This includes creating environments where women can express what went wrong, reestablish personal agency, and reengage in life beyond the identity of patient or survivor. See Table 4.4 for strategies used by occupational therapists for addressing trauma-related responses in the labor and early postpartum period.

Occupational therapists working in perinatal care must be prepared to address the functional impact of birth trauma even when the trauma itself is not explicitly named. Many women will not use the language of trauma but will describe feeling overwhelmed, disconnected, or unable to resume everyday roles. These are

Table 4.4 Occupational therapy strategies for addressing trauma-related responses in the labor and early postpartum period.

Observed Concern	Potential Trauma-Related Mechanism	Occupational Therapy Strategy
Expressed fear or panic during routine postpartum exams (e.g., pelvic checks, blood pressure assessments)	Procedural trauma; perceived loss of control or violation during labor	Use anticipatory co-planning before any hands-on activities; support client in scripting boundaries or consent phrases (e.g., "pause," "explain first")
Avoidance of infant care tasks such as diapering, bathing, or feeding	Somatic flashbacks linked to emergency procedures, surgical pain, or feeling helpless	Grade reintroduction to caregiving tasks through parallel engagement; encourage safe touch and pacing without performance pressure
Intense reactivity to sounds, alarms, or crying	Auditory triggers associated with birth setting or NICU experience	Introduce noise-mapping and auditory modulation strategies; create calming soundscapes or use noise-canceling tools during caregiving routines
Inability to recall parts of labor or detachment when recounting birth	Dissociation during traumatic delivery; shutdown as nervous system defense	Support trauma-informed birth processing using visual timelines, guided drawing, or occupational storytelling to gently reconstruct memory

(Continued)

Table 4.4 (Continued)

Observed Concern	Potential Trauma-Related Mechanism	Occupational Therapy Strategy
Sleep disruption unrelated to infant schedule	Heightened startle reflex or hypervigilance; nervous system does not perceive safety	Facilitate sleep-supportive routines using sensory-based wind-down plans (weighted items, tactile comfort strategies, nighttime occupational rituals)
Refusal to return to birthing hospital or avoidant behavior in healthcare settings	Medical avoidance due to distrust or retraumatization	Collaborate on exposure mapping and environmental adaptations for future visits; rehearse advocacy scripts and plan co-attendance if needed

not just emotional responses. They are occupational disruptions rooted in nervous system survival strategies. By recognizing patterns of avoidance, reactivity, or disengagement, therapists can begin to gently rebuild participation through relational safety, consent-based practice, and activities that restore choice and control.

Postpartum Complications: Medical Trauma, NICU, Physical Recovery

The postpartum period is often framed as a time of healing, but for many women, it becomes a continuation of medical crisis. Complications such as hemorrhage, infection, severe tearing, emergency surgeries, or unanticipated readmissions can trigger trauma responses long after delivery. These events are often fast-moving and poorly explained, leaving women confused and afraid. The experience of being treated as a patient rather than a person, being monitored, medicated, and immobilized, can strip away any sense of mastery over one's body. In some cases, physical trauma is compounded by separation from the infant or by care teams who minimize discomfort or urgency. Even when complications are well-managed clinically, they may still result in psychological wounds that are slow to heal.

When infants require intensive medical care, the maternal recovery process becomes even more complex. The NICU environment is characterized by uncertainty, loss of routine, and restricted maternal roles (Kaliush et al., 2023). Women may be discharged before their infants, or find themselves navigating rigid visiting protocols, unfamiliar equipment, and constant alarms. Their own emotional and physical needs often go unacknowledged in the presence of a critically ill newborn. This can lead to guilt, numbness, or hypervigilance, making it difficult to engage in basic tasks of self-care or bonding. From an occupational perspective, recovery is not only about healing tissue or reducing pain. It is about helping women reintegrate into their lives in ways that honor what they have been through and make space for new patterns of care, both for their infants and for themselves. See Table 4.5 for occupational therapy strategies that address common challenges following postpartum complications and NICU-related trauma.

Table 4.5 Occupational Therapy Strategies for Postpartum Complications and NICU-Related Trauma

Observed Concern	Trauma-Related Factors	Specific Occupational Therapy Strategies
Avoidance of showering, toileting, or dressing due to pain or fear of re-injury	Surgical recovery (e.g., C-section, perineal tear), fear of pain, low body trust	Create visual self-care sequences with adaptive pacing; use tactile desensitization techniques and safe movement practice in bathroom settings
Reluctance to eat, sleep, or rest despite physical exhaustion	Hypervigilance, guilt about "not doing enough," disrupted circadian regulation in NICU	Introduce caregiver rest schedules; use external prompts for meals and hydration; integrate brief restorative occupations that support regulation
Emotional disconnection or lack of responsiveness during infant visits	Disrupted bonding due to medical separation or procedural fear	Facilitate gentle, non-demanding co-occupations such as singing, hand-holding, or cloth scent exchange between mother and baby
Over-monitoring of vital signs, alarms, or care team activities	Anxiety related to unpredictability or fear of loss	Co-create visual schedules of NICU rounds; introduce grounding tools (e.g., worry stones, fidget bands); normalize uncertainty through reflective discussion

(Continued)

Table 4.5 (Continued)

Observed Concern	Trauma-Related Factors	Specific Occupational Therapy Strategies
Disinterest in future planning or postpartum transitions	Grief, loss of perceived birth experience, or overwhelmed executive function	Break down postpartum planning into single-decision frameworks; use environmental cues and external organizers to simplify transitions
Avoidance of medical facilities or staff	Trauma triggers related to prior hospitalization or provider interaction	Develop a care map with sensory-based coping supports (e.g., essential oil, stress object); rehearse provider communication and advocacy scripts

Postpartum trauma often occurs in tandem with survival. Unlike other trauma experiences that may result in withdrawal from activity or setting, women recovering from medical complications and NICU stays are often expected to resume caregiving roles immediately. They are praised for their strength even as their bodies and nervous systems remain in crisis. This can lead to an internal split between performance and reality, where a woman appears highly functional but privately struggles with pain, fear, or emotional numbing. Occupational therapy must account for this mismatch by observing not only what the woman is doing, but how she is doing it. High participation does not always signal high integration. Supporting true recovery means creating space for rest, refusal, and rehabilitation, even when the external environment demands resilience.

Pregnancy Loss and Disenfranchised Grief

Pregnancy loss is often treated as a private event, but its impact can be pervasive and long-lasting. Whether it occurs in the first trimester or after a full-term labor, the disruption extends beyond physical recovery. For many women, the loss is compounded by the absence of public acknowledgment, rituals, or community validation. Terms like miscarriage and stillbirth carry clinical precision but rarely capture the emotional weight of the experience. In the case of termination for medical reasons (TFMR), grief may also be layered with isolation, silence, and moral complexity. Without space to process the emotional and occupational fallout, women may internalize a sense of failure, detachment, or shame that affects not only their mental health but their engagement in daily life.

Occupational disruption after loss is often subtle but deeply embedded in routine. Formerly joyful tasks like organizing a nursery, attending medical appointments, or engaging with peers may now provoke avoidance, sadness, or withdrawal. Loss of role identity, particularly for women who had begun to see themselves as mothers, can create an identity void that is difficult to articulate (Boss, 2016). Grief may surface during unrelated tasks or at unpredictable times (Khosravi, 2021). From a therapeutic perspective, supporting women after pregnancy loss requires more than emotional validation. It involves helping them navigate an altered occupational landscape by redefining goals, reclaiming routine, and creating rituals that allow them to carry their grief forward without becoming consumed by it. See Table 4.6 for occupational therapy adaptations that support clients experiencing grief after pregnancy loss or medically indicated termination.

Table 4.6 Occupational Therapy Modifications Following Pregnancy Loss or TFMR

Observed Concern	Underlying Grief Response	Therapeutic Reframe	Relevant Evidence or Theory
Disengagement from previously anticipated roles (e.g., parenting, planning)	Identity disruption, loss of expected future	Pause forward-looking goals. Use narrative-based sessions to explore role loss, reorient values, and reintroduce routine-based on emotional tolerance	Boss (2016): Ambiguous Loss; Neimeyer (2001): Constructivist Grief Therapy
Avoidance of healthcare settings or baby-related stimuli	Exposure to grief triggers or reactivation of loss	Modify setting (e.g., offer virtual sessions), remove infant-related prompts (e.g., waiting room posters); introduce sensory-grounding kits for hospital navigation	Briere and Scott (2012): Trauma exposure therapy adapted for grief
Emotional volatility or guilt interfering with daily task initiation	Internalized blame or shame, disenfranchised grief	Normalize grief as non-linear; redefine productivity and support restorative occupations	Doka (1989): Disenfranchised Grief

(Continued)

Table 4.6 (Continued)

Observed Concern	Underlying Grief Response	Therapeutic Reframe	Relevant Evidence or Theory
Client declines structured scheduling or goal tracking	Emotional overload or fear of re-engagement	Use flexible, narrative-rich interventions (e.g., art journaling, reflective walks, photo curation of memory)	Khosravi (2021): Tasks of Mourning
Overcompensation through excessive activity or volunteering	Avoidance of emotional processing	Use pacing and activity journaling to distinguish purposeful engagement from emotional numbing; introduce symbolic occupations or ritual	Stroebe and Schut (1999): Dual Process Model of Grief

Many clients navigating pregnancy loss are not looking to return to a baseline. They are attempting to reorient themselves in a world that no longer looks the same. Occupational therapy can serve as both a witness and a guide in this process. By focusing on what feels manageable, meaningful, and emotionally tolerable, therapists can help women reclaim small moments of agency and rebuild connection to self, not by bypassing grief, but by honoring it within the fabric of everyday life.

Structural and Invisible Trauma

Trauma in the perinatal period does not always occur through a single event. For many women, especially those from historically marginalized communities, trauma emerges through repeated exposure to systemic inequities and everyday acts of dismissal. Structural trauma includes practices and policies that devalue or endanger women through discrimination, neglect, or coercion. This includes obstetric racism, delayed pain management, forced sterilization, restricted access to respectful care, and the overmedicalization or criminalization of women of color, disabled women, and those in poverty. These harms are often embedded within standard protocols, making them difficult to name yet deeply damaging in their cumulative impact.

Alongside structural trauma, women frequently experience invisible trauma, subtle forms of invalidation that are often excused as routine. These may include being talked over during delivery, having pain minimized, or having emotional distress dismissed as hormonal. While less overt than procedural harm, these experiences can erode a woman's sense of safety, dignity, and autonomy. They may contribute to mistrust in healthcare, avoidance of future care, or reduced engagement in postpartum support. Occupational therapists must be alert to these invisible patterns. A woman's withdrawal from care or emotional flatness in clinical sessions may be protective, not passive. Trust-building becomes the intervention itself. See Table 4.7 for strategies that align occupational therapy with the needs of clients affected by structural and invisible trauma in perinatal care. See Table 4.7 for ways occupational therapists can identify and explore structural and invisible trauma through therapeutic inquiry and clinical observation.

Table 4.7 Common client presentations that may signal structural or invisible trauma in the perinatal period.

Observed Presentation	Potential Trauma Category	Occupational Therapy Approach to Further Explore
Client appears overly agreeable or avoids expressing preferences	Invisible trauma (minimization, prior dismissal of voice)	Ask, "Has there ever been a time in healthcare when you felt like your preferences were not heard?" or "How do you usually like to be involved in decisions about your care?"
Withdrawal or lack of affect when discussing delivery experience	Structural trauma (systemic neglect, coercion, obstetric violence)	Use gentle occupational storytelling: "Some births are hard to talk about. Would it help to draw or map out what you remember?"
Declines follow-up appointments despite physical symptoms	Structural trauma (distrust, racial bias, provider harm)	Reflective questioning: "Is there anything about returning to the clinic that feels uncomfortable or stressful?"
Refuses body-based care (e.g., guided movement, sensory processing)	Invisible trauma (internalized shame, medicalization of body)	Offer permission-based frameworks: "What feels okay today in terms of movement or body-based activities?"
Focused on meeting goals but avoids discussing emotions	Coping strategy to maintain control after trauma	Normalize emotional labor: "Sometimes getting through the day means pushing feelings aside. Do you want space for that here, or would you prefer to focus just on tasks today?"

Occupational therapists are uniquely positioned to notice what often goes unseen. When a woman minimizes her needs, withdraws during care, or avoids certain environments, it may not be due to disinterest or disengagement—it may be a reflection of past harm. Structural and invisible trauma are not always disclosed, but they leave traces in how someone moves, interacts, and participates. Recognizing these patterns is not just about observation. It is about knowing when not to push, when to ask differently, and when to offer safety without conditions. In this way, the therapeutic relationship becomes a counter-narrative to systems that have silenced, rushed, or overlooked her. This is where the real work begins—not with fixing, but with creating the conditions for healing to unfold.

Trauma-Informed Assessment in Perinatal Care

Assessment in perinatal care often begins before a word is spoken. The way a woman enters the room, carries her body, or responds to physical proximity offers cues about safety, overwhelm, or exhaustion. For occupational therapists, the goal is not immediate data collection, but the creation of a space where emotional and physiological defenses can soften. Perinatal trauma does not always manifest through visible distress. It may appear as high-functioning behavior, perfectionism in caregiving, or polite detachment. These responses are not indicators of wellness. They are strategies for managing unpredictability and preserving control in a system that may have once felt unsafe (Briere & Scott, 2012). Standardized tools often miss this nuance, focusing on what a client can do rather than what she is protecting herself from (Biggs et al., 2021). A trauma-informed approach to assessment asks how she engages with the roles and routines that have shaped her identity—especially those that were disrupted, medicalized, or never chosen in the first place. Table 4.8 outlines trauma-informed assessment strategies specific to perinatal occupational therapy, with attention to nervous system cues, occupational identity, role shifts, and relational dynamics.

Effective assessment in perinatal occupational therapy is not about covering every domain—it is about recognizing when a woman's nervous system is protecting her from re-entering one. A client who declines help with dressing after a cesarean may not be resisting care, but may be avoiding the site of a traumatic scar that no one has acknowledged. Another may appear attentive and engaged while reporting feeding routines, yet grip her chair tightly and shift posture when asked how her body feels. In NICU follow-up, a woman might freeze when asked about her discharge experience, eyes glazing over—not out of disinterest, but because memory recall triggers physiological threat. In outpatient rehab, a mother may insist she is "fine," despite bracing her abdomen with every movement, unable to tolerate pelvic activation due to unprocessed procedural trauma.

These are not clinical anomalies, they are patterns. Trauma does not always announce itself, but it often reveals itself through what the body does and does

Table 4.8 Trauma-informed assessment strategies in perinatal occupational therapy

Assessment Focus	What to Observe or Ask	Trauma-Informed Strategy
Nervous system regulation	Does the client appear hypervigilant, fatigued, frozen, or over-activated? Are there shifts in breath, posture, or voice tone when certain topics arise?	Begin with grounding or centering (e.g., breath pacing, warm drink, gentle weighted input); delay formal assessments if the client appears dysregulated
Relationship to daily roles	How does the client speak about feeding, sleeping, or bonding? Do they avoid or overemphasize competence in caregiving roles?	Ask, "What parts of your day feel manageable?" or "What feels most demanding even if it seems small?"
Birth, NICU, or postpartum medical experience	How does the client describe or avoid aspects of labor, cesarean recovery, or separation from baby? Is there confusion, gaps in memory, or avoidance of details?	Invite birth storytelling through drawing, timelines, or journaling; allow nonverbal processing or pacing across sessions
Scar sensitivity or body-based trauma (e.g., C-section, perineal tear)	Does the client avoid touching or discussing certain body areas? Is there visible tension or bracing during movement or palpation?	Frame all physical contact as optional; offer alternatives like mirror work, guided body mapping, or scar desensitization led by client
Vital signs and physiological cues	Are heart rate, blood pressure, or respiratory patterns elevated in safe settings? Does client experience dizziness, faintness, or freeze states under observation?	Consider trauma-sensitive monitoring (e.g., allow client to self-track); debrief after physiological spikes to build interoceptive awareness
Lactation, chest binding, or feeding experiences	How does the client describe their relationship with feeding or body exposure? Are there emotions linked to success, failure, or pressure?	Use gender-affirming, nonjudgmental language ("Would you like to talk about feeding, lactation, or chest care?"); allow grief or frustration without problem-solving

(Continued)

Table 4.8 (Continued)

Assessment Focus	What to Observe or Ask	Trauma-Informed Strategy
Pelvic engagement, posture, or core stability	Is the client hesitant to engage in movement requiring core activation or pelvic awareness? Do they report discomfort but avoid specifics?	Use body-neutral prompts like "How does this movement feel?" or "Let's notice what changes when we shift position." Always offer consent and choice for pelvic-related assessments
Trust and relational safety	Does the client express needs, ask questions, or assert preferences? Or do they defer, stay silent, or over-accommodate?	Provide structure for shared decision-making: "Here's what I was thinking for today—what feels okay to you, and what would you rather skip or change?"

not do. The most relevant data may not come from intake forms or goal sheets, but from silence, tension, or avoidance. A trauma-informed therapist learns to slow down in these moments, not to fill the space, but to make it safer. When assessment is reframed as a process of relational attunement rather than checklist completion, women begin to show us not just what they can do, but what they are protecting. From this foundation, therapy can begin, not with interventions, but with the conditions that make them possible.

Creating a Safe Therapeutic Space

Eliza Miller, a thirty-two-year-old woman, had been admitted to the inpatient psychiatric unit following a diagnosis of postpartum psychosis. She appeared disoriented at times, alternated between long silences and bursts of pressured speech, and frequently turned her head as if responding to sounds others could not hear. She was hypervigilant about her surroundings, had difficulty maintaining sleep, and expressed confusion about whether her baby was safe, despite reassurance from staff. Her occupational therapist began each session with quiet consistency, sitting beside her rather than across from her, and inviting her to choose a familiar object to hold—often a soft blanket or a small photo of her newborn. Sessions started with a brief grounding routine: both placing their feet on the floor, holding a warm cup of tea, and taking three slow breaths while focusing on a steady point in the room. Once Eliza's breathing slowed and her gaze steadied, the therapist gently introduced daily care activities as invitations. The room's lighting was softened, noise was minimized, and Eliza always had the choice to pause or decline. During hygiene tasks, she was offered privacy and structure—clear steps, minimal language, and the presence of a support person nearby. These small, attuned actions helped Eliza gradually feel less fragmented, more anchored in her body, and safer in the therapeutic space—laying the groundwork for functional engagement and recovery.

In perinatal occupational therapy, creating safety requires more than a calm tone or a warm room. It requires the ongoing negotiation of pace, presence, and power. Women recovering from trauma may enter a session hyper-alert, scanning for judgment, or disconnected from their own physical sensations. Their ability to engage is not just shaped by the activity, but by how the activity is introduced, whether they feel they can opt out, and whether their boundaries are honored without hesitation or consequence. A therapeutic space is safe not because nothing difficult happens there, but because the client knows she will not be pushed past her capacity.

Consent is not a one-time question. It is a posture. Whether the task is movement-based, narrative, or sensory, the invitation must always be accompanied by permission to decline. For women whose trauma occurred in clinical settings, regaining trust begins when they experience control in the therapeutic environment. This might mean offering choices about the order of tasks, the positioning of chairs, or even how a session begins and ends. Small adaptations like offering weighted items, allowing breaks, or narrating transitions aloud can create powerful shifts in how the nervous system perceives threat. Building body awareness can also be done gradually through grounding routines or mirrored movement—approaches that support reconnection without requiring exposure. The therapist's job is not to activate emotion, but to build capacity for presence. In doing so, safety becomes something the client does not just expect but begins to feel.

A trauma-sensitive environment is less about décor and more about dynamics. It is shaped through intentional, often subtle choices that communicate safety without needing words. Placing chairs side by side rather than face to face reduces the intensity of eye contact, which can feel confrontational or overwhelming for clients in a heightened state of vigilance. This positioning supports parallel processing and shared focus, particularly helpful when engaging in emotionally charged discussions. Asking before adjusting a pillow, touching a client's arm, or repositioning equipment respects body autonomy and reinforces that the client is in control of her physical space, something often lost during medical procedures or birth trauma. Allowing clients to keep personal items within reach (like a water bottle, photo, or baby blanket) helps anchor them to familiarity and supports sensory regulation through self-chosen comfort objects.

For women who have experienced bodily violation, coercion, or emotional dismissal, these micro-interactions can determine whether a space feels regulating or retraumatizing. Narrating actions clearly ("I'm going to move this chair closer—does that feel okay to you?"), offering opt-outs routinely ("Would you like to skip this part today?"), and maintaining consistency in scheduling and tone help reduce unpredictability, a core trigger for many trauma responses. Lighting that can be adjusted allows women to control the sensory load of the room, while surfaces that are soft but functional (like supportive cushions or textured mats) provide grounding without overstimulation. Having sensory tools—like weighted lap pads, fidget items, or calming scents—available without requiring justification honors individual coping strategies without labeling them as clinical needs. Even the way silence is held, without rushing to fill it, shows respect for the client's internal timing and emotional pacing.

Safety is not a static feature of a room. It is a dynamic process of attunement, where the environment flexes to the nervous system of the person within it. When space, structure, and interaction are shaped around a woman's cues, rather than requiring her to mask, perform, or accommodate, therapy becomes less about fixing and more about facilitating the conditions for restoration.

Nervous System Regulation Strategies: Co-Regulation, Sensory Modulation, and Breathwork

In the perinatal period, trauma is often layered onto an already sensitive nervous system. Hormonal shifts, disrupted sleep, feeding demands, surgical recovery, and chronic pain are common experiences. But when trauma is present, these physical changes intersect with a persistent sense of danger. A woman who felt powerless during labor, was separated from her infant, or dismissed in postpartum care may live in a heightened state of physiological threat. She may brace during diapering, flinch at routine checks, or freeze when asked about her delivery. These are not mental reactions. They are embodied responses to unresolved harm. The role of occupational therapy is not to teach coping in isolation, but to facilitate experiences of safety through intentional engagement.

Co-regulation often becomes the first entry point. A therapist's voice, pacing, and presence can help guide the nervous system toward balance. In NICU follow-up, for example, a mother who appears flat during play may not be disengaged but frozen. Matching her rhythm through mirrored play, soft tone, or shared silence can restore connection. Sensory modulation may include using a warm compress before movement, offering grounding objects during intake, or adjusting lights and sound to reduce overwhelm. Breathwork, often misapplied as a direct intervention, can be introduced indirectly for trauma survivors—through humming, rocking, or singing with a baby. These co-occupational strategies invite regulation without triggering control-based breathing patterns that may feel unsafe.

The goal is not to push the nervous system into calm. It is to offer repeated experiences where the body begins to expect safety again. These moments may be brief, such as a softened shoulder, a slower exhale, an easier reach, but over time, they build capacity. In perinatal occupational therapy, nervous system regulation is not a step before intervention. It is the intervention. It is what allows participation to feel possible, sustainable, and safe.

The goal is not to force calm but to create repeated opportunities for the body to sense safety. A relaxed shoulder, a fuller breath, or a fluid motion becomes the evidence that healing is underway. In perinatal occupational therapy, nervous system regulation is not a precursor to treatment. It is the treatment. It is what makes participation feel not only possible, but safe enough to stay.

Restoring Maternal Occupations

Three weeks after giving birth, Pia Agarwal told her midwife she felt like she had disappeared. She could change diapers in the dark, nurse while standing, and smile politely when her mother-in-law asked how she was doing. But when left alone, she stared at the wall or folded baby clothes she didn't remember buying. Her body hurt constantly, but she kept brushing it off as normal. She avoided photos with her baby and felt a wave of nausea anytime someone said, "You must be so happy." In occupational therapy, she described herself as functional but floating. "It's like I'm doing everything a mom should do," she said, "but none of it feels like mine." Her sleep was shallow and restless. Movement felt like dragging. She no longer listened to music. Bonding felt like a performance. What looked like survival was, in fact, depletion layered with shame.

Postpartum recovery is not simply a return to baseline, it is a neurobiological recalibration. The maternal brain, reshaped by the hormonal tides of pregnancy, must now sustain caregiving, healing, and identity reorganization while operating under chronic physiological load. Sleep, movement, emotional attunement—these are not soft concepts. They are biological imperatives that, when disrupted, destabilize health at the most cellular level.

Restoration in this phase is often mistaken for endurance. But healing does not occur through perseverance alone. It begins with safety, physiological, emotional, and environmental. For women navigating trauma or chronic stress, basic functions like sleep, movement, and connection are not automatic. They are interrupted processes that require intentional support. Occupational therapy becomes essential here, not as a set of surface-level strategies, but as a clinical pathway back to coherence. Through structured, relational, and sensory-informed care, therapists help re-establish stability across disrupted systems, making it possible for women to reconnect with themselves, their roles, and the world around them (Khan, 2025; Precin, 2011). See Table 4.9 for common patterns of occupational disruption during the postpartum period and corresponding trauma-informed strategies for clinical use.

While Table 4.9 outlines common disruptions and their neurobiological underpinnings, restoring maternal occupations requires a deeply client-centered

Table 4.9 Maternal Occupational Focus and Trauma-Informed Clinical Strategies

Maternal Occupational Focus	Common Disruptions	Neurobiological Factors	OT Strategies for Restoration
Sleep and Rest	Insomnia, light sleep, intrusive thoughts, early waking	Cortisol elevation, HPA axis hyperactivity, hypervigilance	Establish circadian anchors (light exposure, wind-down routines), use sensory grounding (weighted items, breath pacing), normalize fragmented sleep cycles
Physical Mobility	Pelvic pain, fatigue, avoidance of movement, poor posture	Musculoskeletal strain, cesarean or perineal trauma, inflammatory load	Functional movement training, body mechanics during infant care, gradual re-engagement in self-paced mobility tasks
Leisure Engagement	Loss of interest, guilt during rest, absence of pleasure	Dopamine suppression, anhedonia, trauma-linked emotional blunting	Introduce micro-occupations for joy, co-regulated creative tasks, frame leisure as recovery not indulgence
Maternal Bonding	Emotional numbness, difficulty connecting, fear of failure	Dysregulated oxytocin system, attachment disruption, relational trauma	Parallel play with infant, safe touch desensitization, narrative reframing of caregiving moments

approach. Therapeutic strategies should not begin with assumptions or generic protocols, but with listening—understanding what rest, movement, leisure, and connection mean to that individual woman in her current context. For sleep hygiene, for example, some mothers may find comfort in silence and darkness, while others feel safer with soft background noise or a dim light on. Breathwork may be grounding for one person and triggering for another.

Rather than offering prescriptive checklists, occupational therapists are called to collaborate by exploring through dialogue, observation, and trial which sensory and behavioral cues best support regulation. Physical mobility strategies must similarly be tailored. A woman recovering from cesarean delivery with a toddler at home has different movement demands than a first-time mother navigating pelvic floor pain. Functional retraining, then, is not a one-size-fits-all process. It requires co-creating routines that respect pain thresholds, energy reserves, caregiving tasks, and personal goals. Research by Ryan and Deci consistently shows that when therapeutic strategies are closely aligned with a person's values, preferences, and lived context, not only is adherence more likely, but the interventions themselves are more effective (Ryan & Deci, 2020). Client-centered care is not just ethical, it is evidence-based.

This personalized lens extends to leisure and maternal bonding as well. While leisure is often viewed as a luxury in early postpartum care, it can serve as a lifeline when framed within a woman's existing interests and available capacity. For one mother, leisure might mean journaling for five minutes in the morning with a warm cup of tea. For another, it might be laughing through a favorite podcast while doing dishes. Therapists should explore not only what used to bring joy, but what feels accessible and safe now. Similarly, maternal bonding strategies must account for trauma history, sensory preferences, cultural norms, and evolving attachment. Eye contact, touch, and skin-to-skin contact are powerful but may not feel tolerable to all women, especially in the wake of obstetric violence or relational trauma. Co-regulated occupations—such as synchronized walking, infant massage with the mother's guidance, or simply being present during tummy time—can be adapted to support safety and choice. When therapeutic experiences are rooted in autonomy and attunement, women are more likely to engage meaningfully and are more likely to heal. The role of occupational therapy is not to dictate the path forward, but to walk alongside, co-constructing occupations that rebuild not only function, but agency and trust.

Culturally Responsive Care and Structural Advocacy

A 2024 study published in the *Journal of Midwifery and Women's Health* found that Black women in the United States are significantly more likely to be mistreated during childbirth. This includes being yelled at, ignored, or threatened, especially when compared to their White counterparts. These negative care experiences are not isolated moments; they are linked to increased rates of postpartum depression, posttraumatic stress, and disengagement from essential postpartum services (Spurlock & Pickler, 2024). Culturally responsive care is not a courtesy. It is a clinical imperative. For trauma-informed occupational therapy to be truly effective, it must extend beyond individual healing to address the systemic, relational, and cultural forces that either scaffold recovery or deepen harm.

Occupational therapists are uniquely positioned to act as both clinicians and advocates within this space. Culturally responsive care begins with the recognition that trauma does not occur in a vacuum—it is shaped by legacies of racism, sexism, colonialism, and ableism that are often embedded in the healthcare system itself. These structural forces impact not only the delivery of care but also the very meaning of safety, autonomy, and connection for each client. For some postpartum women, healing might be supported through ancestral practices, intergenerational caregiving, or spiritual rituals that do not fit into conventional Western models (Miljkovitch et al., 2022). Others may require harm-reduction strategies when navigating healthcare systems that have historically silenced or violated them. The role of the occupational therapist is not to standardize these experiences, but to honor them by collaborating in creating care plans that reflect the client's worldview, values, and definitions of healing (Khan, 2025).

This means adjusting therapeutic goals and interventions to fit, not fix. It means understanding how a mother's decision not to breastfeed may be rooted in previous bodily autonomy violations. It means recognizing how racial micro-aggressions in a NICU may lead to withdrawal from early bonding routines. It means knowing that eye contact, direct touch, or certain posture cues may be culturally dissonant or even dysregulating depending on trauma history. When providers fail to account for these realities, interventions, however well-intended, can feel alienating or unsafe. But when therapists center client preferences, language, and lived experience, outcomes improve. Women are more likely to participate in therapy, more likely to report emotional gains, and more likely to build sustainable routines for recovery.

Culturally responsive care also requires structural action. Therapists must speak up in team meetings, challenge discharge plans that ignore social determinants, and advocate for interpreter services, longer perinatal follow-ups, and flexible scheduling. Clinical notes and documentation can capture more than just function; they can highlight barriers rooted in inequity. At the institutional level, departments must invest in training that addresses implicit bias, racial trauma, and health disparities, treating them not as add-ons but as foundational competencies. Supervisors must cultivate environments where humility, self-reflection, and continuous learning are not optional, but expected.

Above all, therapists must do the work of looking inward. Cultural responsiveness is not achieved by completing a module or mastering the right terminology. It is a dynamic, relational process that requires listening deeply, apologizing when harm occurs, and building relationships that are accountable to the people most impacted by injustice. As one mother in the study said, "I didn't need a perfect provider. I needed someone who made me feel like I mattered." That is what culturally responsive care delivers: not perfection, but presence. Not saviorism, but solidarity. Not scripts, but space to co-author what healing looks like.

For occupational therapists, this co-authorship begins with curiosity, not only about the client, but also about the self. Cultural humility requires more than knowledge; it demands reflection, attunement, and a willingness to confront the ways in which power and privilege show up in practice. Table 4.10 outlines a guide designed to support occupational therapists in translating cultural

Table 4.10 Prompts and Reflective Questions to Support Culturally Responsive, Trauma-Informed Practice

Focus Area	Reflective or Clinical Questions	Purpose
Building Trust	"How does this client define safety? Have I asked?" "Am I showing up consistently in tone, timing, and follow-through?"	Foster relational consistency and emotional predictability
Understanding Cultural Context	"What cultural beliefs, roles, or responsibilities shape how this client approaches healing?" "Do I know who this client considers part of their support system?"	Tailor interventions to lived experience and family/community structures
Respecting Autonomy	"Am I giving the client real choices—not just multiple options I created?" "Have I asked what *they* want to work on today?"	Avoid paternalism; reinforce agency and control
Language and Communication	"Am I using jargon-free, culturally affirming language?" "Do I need an interpreter or cultural broker present?"	Support accessibility and honor linguistic identity
Checking Bias and Power	"Am I making assumptions about motivation, parenting, or compliance?" "How do my own identities influence this interaction?"	Increase awareness of implicit bias and structural influence
Repair and Responsiveness	"If rupture occurred in care, have I acknowledged and addressed it?" "What might this client need to feel heard again?"	Promote trust repair and accountability when harm occurs

responsiveness into clinical behavior. These questions and prompts can be used during client interactions, team meetings, and personal reflection to deepen therapeutic alignment with each client's unique sociocultural context.

Culturally responsive care requires occupational therapists to recognize the impact of systemic racism, discrimination, and historical harm on maternal health experiences. When women of color express concern, question their care, or disengage from services, these behaviors must be understood within the context of prior medical trauma and ongoing inequity—not as noncompliance. Therapists have a responsibility to ensure that care is accessible, relevant, and affirming. This includes advocating for inclusive policies, equitable resource allocation, and the dismantling of barriers that prevent full participation in care. It also means speaking up in clinical spaces where bias, dismissal, or cultural erasure occur. Trauma-informed practice is incomplete without an active commitment to justice. Therapists must not only support individual healing but also contribute to structural change within the systems where they work.

Case Vignettes and Reflections

The following vignettes illustrate how trauma-informed, culturally responsive occupational therapy can support maternal recovery through individualized care. These cases reflect common yet often overlooked challenges in the postpartum and perinatal periods, including birth trauma, grief, identity disruption, and the complexity of bonding. Each clinical reflection explores therapeutic reasoning, pacing, and the nuances of when to lead and when to listen. These are not prescriptive formulas, but dynamic processes shaped by empathy, flexibility, and deep respect for each woman's lived experience.

Case Example 1: Maya, Age 32—Postpartum PTSD After Emergency Cesarean and NICU Stay

Maya, a 32-year-old first-time mother, was referred to occupational therapy three months postpartum following an emergency cesarean and an eight-day NICU stay for her infant son. Although her physical recovery had progressed without complication, Maya exhibited significant emotional distress. She reported chronic sleep disturbances, hypervigilance, and panic episodes triggered by hospital imagery or reminders of her son's birth. Despite her infant's stable health, she described feeling detached and numb during daily caregiving: "I'm doing everything I'm supposed to, but it feels mechanical—like there's a wall between me and my own life."

Maya also struggled with self-blame and feelings of failure, particularly around her perceived inability to bond with her son. She avoided baby photos, declined support group invitations, and resisted well-meaning advice from family. During initial sessions, she appeared guarded but cooperative, downplaying her symptoms with phrases like "I know I'm lucky" and "other people have had it worse." The therapist recognized signs of sympathetic nervous system activation and prioritized therapeutic pacing and regulation.

Initial intervention focused on co-regulated engagement and somatic stabilization. This included sensory-based grounding strategies tailored to Maya's preferences, such as deep pressure tools, rhythmic rocking, and breathwork embedded into caregiving tasks. As trust developed, the therapist gently introduced narrative strategies to help Maya process her disrupted postpartum experience. Visual mapping exercises helped Maya plot key emotional events during her birth and postpartum period on a large sheet of paper, creating a tangible, externalized version of her story. Timeline reconstruction involved collaboratively sequencing events, such as hospital admissions, procedures, and early caregiving moments, to help Maya reframe fragmented or overwhelming memories into a more coherent narrative. The therapeutic plan did not center on "bonding" as an outcome but instead emphasized restoring agency, redefining maternal identity, and creating safe, functional routines rooted in Maya's values.

As Maya's emotional regulation improved and her nervous system became more responsive to safety cues, the therapeutic focus expanded to include the reengagement of maternal roles through occupation-based interventions that supported identity, volition, and relational attunement. The therapist used graded exposure to support Maya's reconnection with her infant—not through performance-based expectations of bonding, but through accessible, emotionally manageable occupations that fostered shared experience.

Maya began with structured sensory-motor routines that emphasized rhythm and co-occupation, such as infant massage using guided scripts, singing familiar lullabies while walking outdoors, and participating in infant bathing rituals using predictable sequences and sensory input tailored to both her and her baby's regulation profiles. These sessions also included reflective pauses, where Maya was invited to notice her own internal state without judgment, cultivating interoceptive awareness and reinforcing that emotional presence could coexist with caregiving.

As Maya's capacity for relational engagement grew, the therapist layered in narrative identity work that centered maternal strengths. This included values-based journaling, where Maya identified qualities she hoped to embody as a parent, and photo sequencing activities that allowed her to select and annotate images from her early postpartum journey—reclaiming her story on her terms. The therapist also introduced symbolic co-creation, such as collaboratively crafting a "resilience mobile" for the nursery using small objects that represented strength, survival, and connection. These objects became visual anchors for Maya during moments of dysregulation.

Importantly, the therapist collaborated with Maya to build community supports that felt safe and empowering. Rather than large parent groups, the therapist facilitated a soft introduction to peer connection through parallel participation in a small, therapist-led sensory play group. Maya was able to observe, participate gradually, and eventually share experiences in a way that felt authentic rather than performative.

These interventions were not focused on returning Maya to a pre-trauma version of motherhood. They were designed to help her redefine maternal identity on her own terms, honoring the reality of what she had endured while supporting her capacity to experience joy, agency, and relational presence again.

Case Example 2: Ana, Age 29—Pregnancy After Stillbirth and Identity Reconstruction

Ana entered therapy at 22 weeks pregnant, carrying the invisible weight of a prior full-term stillbirth that had occurred just one year earlier. Her voice was steady but guarded during intake. She described feeling grateful for the new pregnancy, but also overwhelmingly fearful, numb, and detached from any sense of hope. "It's like I'm holding my breath through this whole experience," she said. Despite having supportive family and access to medical care, Ana found herself withdrawing from occupations she had once loved—photography, yoga, weekend gatherings with friends. She had declined a baby shower, delayed setting up a nursery, and avoided talking about the future with her partner, afraid that even acknowledging excitement might "jinx" the pregnancy.

Initial sessions focused on creating a therapeutic environment where avoidance and ambivalence were not pathologized but honored as understandable adaptive responses. Instead of framing engagement in prenatal activities as the ultimate therapeutic goal, the therapist worked to normalize Ana's protective strategies while gently widening her window of tolerance for emotional connection. Interventions centered around grounding practices, interoceptive awareness, and revisiting occupations that fostered emotional regulation rather than immediate attachment to the pregnancy itself. Ana reengaged in nature photography with a specific focus on tracking seasonal transitions, which became a metaphorical space to explore the coexistence of endings and beginnings. Short, open-ended journal prompts such as "What does safety feel like today?" or "How do I want to mother this moment?" helped her reconnect with a sense of agency without pressure to perform optimism.

As Ana's comfort with therapy deepened, the occupational therapist incorporated physical therapeutic strategies to support bodily connection and preparation. Gentle prenatal yoga-based movements were reintroduced, not as fitness goals but as somatic reconnection tools. Seated pelvic tilts, diaphragmatic breathing in supported positions, and guided body scans helped Ana notice areas of bracing or disconnection. Scar mobilization techniques and positional education were offered with sensitivity to her previous delivery experience, supporting both pelvic health and trust in her body's evolving capacity. These physical interventions were always nested within relational safety—offered as invitations rather than tasks.

Psychosocially, the therapist supported Ana in reframing avoidance through a lens of nervous system protection. Identity-based interventions included value-mapping sessions, where Ana articulated the qualities she associated with herself as a mother, a partner, and a grieving person. These values were then used to guide decision-making, such as setting boundaries with extended family, selecting sensory elements for her birth environment, or choosing how and when to share updates with others.

The concept of dual occupancy, holding space for grief and hope simultaneously, was central to their work. Ana was invited to design rituals that honored both children: a small bracelet she wore daily as a tactile reminder of connection, letters she wrote and sealed for each baby, and a playlist that included both lullabies and songs of mourning. Preparatory discussions with her partner emphasized creating emotional safety over logistical preparation, allowing them to approach birth planning not from fear of recurrence, but from a place of shared intention.

As the pregnancy progressed, Ana described a subtle shift. She was still afraid, but she was no longer ruled by that fear. She could envision moments of connection, imagine future experiences, and allow herself small acts of joy without feeling betrayal toward her grief. Therapy did not eliminate anxiety. It gave her a set of embodied, relational, and reflective tools to move through it. She learned to mother both the child she lost and the one she was preparing to meet—without silencing either love or needing to resolve one in order to welcome the other.

Therapist Reflections on Clinical Decision Making

Both cases illustrate that trauma in the perinatal period is not defined by a single catastrophic event but by the accumulation of experiences that disrupt agency, safety, and occupational coherence. In Maya's case, a traditional emphasis on maternal–infant bonding would have risked retraumatization by demanding emotional connection her nervous system was not yet prepared to access. The therapeutic process instead centered on restoring physiological regulation, scaffolding agency in caregiving, and gradually reintroducing relational engagement through graded exposure. Strategies such as sensory-based stabilization, visual mapping, and narrative sequencing were essential not only for processing traumatic memories but also for externalizing and reframing her lived experience in a safe and embodied way.

In Ana's case, trauma resurfaced not in the aftermath of birth, but in anticipation of it. Pregnancy following stillbirth required a therapeutic approach that honored avoidance and ambivalence as valid protective responses. Rather than directing engagement toward immediate attachment, therapy focused on restoring connection to self, supporting bodily trust, and helping Ana cultivate dual emotional occupancy, grieving the child she lost while making space for hope in the pregnancy she carried. Physical therapeutic strategies such as somatic grounding, scar mobilization, and guided breath supported reconnection with her body, while identity-based interventions created space for her to reclaim meaning in motherhood on her own terms.

Importantly, recovery was not measured by outward emotional expressions or participation in normative rituals. It was reflected in both clients' increasing capacity to remain present, make value-aligned choices, and engage in occupational roles without overwhelming distress.

Occupational therapy in the perinatal period must resist imposing linear timelines or standardized expectations (Lynch et al., 2023). Healing is layered, relational, and deeply individual. It begins with listening, builds through safety, and unfolds through participation that is flexible, intentional, and rooted in dignity.

Summary and Implications

The perinatal period is marked by profound neurological, relational, and occupational change—made more complex when trauma is present. Trauma during this time often stems not only from medical events but also from loss of agency, birth-related violations, pregnancy loss, and systemic inequities that disrupt maternal roles and daily routines. Changes in brain function during pregnancy and postpartum affect emotion regulation, executive functioning, and social engagement (Peterson & Tom, 2021). When layered with trauma, these shifts can result in physiological hyperarousal, emotional withdrawal, and difficulty connecting to caregiving roles. These responses are not signs of failure but adaptations to overwhelming or invalidating environments.

Occupational therapists are uniquely positioned to support healing during this window of vulnerability and transformation. Trauma-informed care must go beyond symptom screening to include attuned presence, validation, and the restoration of safety through occupation (Isobel, 2023). By addressing both neurobiological changes and contextual barriers, therapists can help rebuild agency, restore occupational identity, and lay the foundation for long-term resilience. Though rooted in the perinatal phase, unresolved trauma may continue to shape health and participation well beyond postpartum, reinforcing the need for care models that honor complexity, continuity, and choice.

References

Ahmad, S. I., Rudd, K. L., LeWinn, K. Z., Mason, W. A., Murphy, L., Juarez, P. D., Karr, C. J., Sathyanarayana, S., Tylavsky, F. A., & Bush, N. R. (2022). Maternal childhood trauma and prenatal stressors are associated with child behavioral health. *Journal of Developmental Origins of Health and Disease*, *13*(4), 483–493. https://doi.org/10.1017/S2040174421000581

Biggs, C., Tehrani, N., & Billings, J. (2021). Brief trauma therapy for occupational trauma-related PTSD/CPTSD in UK police. *Occupational Medicine (Oxford, England)*, *71*(4–5), 180–188. https://doi.org/10.1093/occmed/kqab075

Boss, P. (2016). The context and process of theory development: The story of ambiguous loss. *Journal of Family Theory & Review*, *8*(3), 269–286. https://doi.org/10.1111/jftr.12152

Briere, J., & Scott, C. (2012). *Principles of trauma therapy: A guide to symptoms, evaluation, and treatment* (2nd ed.). Sage Publications.

Caglayan, I. S., Uzun Cicek, A., Yilmaz, Y., & Sahin, A. E. (2023). The role of childhood trauma on prenatal attachment: A cross-sectional study. *The Journal of Nervous and Mental Disease*, *211*(4), 281–288. https://doi.org/10.1097/NMD.0000000000001610

Doka, K. J. (1989). Disenfranchised grief. In K. J. Doka (Ed.), *Disenfranchised grief: Recognizing hidden sorrow* (pp. 3–11). Lexington Books/D. C. Heath and Com.

Isobel, S. (2023). Trauma and the perinatal period: A review of the theory and practice of trauma-sensitive interactions for nurses and midwives. *Nursing Open*, *10*(12), 7585–7595. https://doi.org/10.1002/nop2.2017

Kaliush, P. R., Kerig, P. K., Raby, K. L., Maylott, S. E., Neff, D., Speck, B., Molina, N. C., Pappal, A. E., Parameswaran, U. D., Conradt, E., & Crowell, S. E. (2023). Examining implications of the developmental timing of maternal trauma for prenatal and newborn outcomes. *Infant Behavior & Development*, *72*, 101861. https://doi.org/10.1016/j.infbeh.2023.101861

Khan, S. (2025). *Occupational therapy and women's health: A practitioner guide*. Routledge.

Khosravi, M. (2021). Worden's task-based approach for supporting people bereaved by COVID-19. *Current Psychology (New Brunswick, N.J.)*, *40*(11), 5735–5736. https://doi.org/10.1007/s12144-020-01292-0

Lynch, A., Ashcraft, R., & Tekell, L. (Eds.). (2023). *Trauma, occupation, and participation: Foundations and population considerations in occupational therapy*. AOTA Press.

Miljkovitch, R., Danner-Touati, C., Gery, I., Bernier, A., Sirparanta, A., & Deborde, A. S. (2022). The role of multiple attachments in intergenerational transmission of child sexual abuse among male victims. *Child abuse & neglect*, *128*, 104864. https://doi.org/10.1016/j.chiabu.2020.104864

Neimeyer, R. A. (2001). The language of loss: Grief therapy as a process of meaning reconstruction. In R. A. Neimeyer (Ed.), *Meaning reconstruction & the experience of loss* (pp. 261–292). American Psychological Association. https://doi.org/10.1037/10397-014

Peterson, A., & Tom, S. E. (2021). A life course perspective on female sex-specific risk factors for later life cognition. *Current Neurology and Neuroscience Reports*, *21*(9), 46. https://doi.org/10.1007/s11910-021-01133-y

Precin, P. (2011). Occupation as therapy for trauma recovery: A case study. *Work (Reading, Mass.)*, *38*(1), 77–81. https://doi.org/10.3233/WOR-2011-1106

Ryan, R. M., & Deci, E. L. (2000). Self-determination theory and the facilitation of intrinsic motivation, social development, and well-being. *American Psychologist*, *55*(1), 68–78. https://doi.org/10.1037/0003-066X.55.1.68

Spurlock, E. J., & Pickler, R. H. (2024). Birth experience among Black women in the United States: A qualitative meta-synthesis. *Journal of Midwifery & Women's Health*, *69*(5), 697–717. https://doi.org/10.1111/jmwh.13628

Chapter 5

Navigating Trauma and Occupational Transitions Across Midlife and Aging

Chapter Objectives

Upon completion of this chapter, the reader will be able to:

1. Describe how neurobiological, hormonal, and cognitive changes in midlife and older adulthood interact with trauma histories to influence occupational participation.
2. Identify key life transitions such as menopause, caregiving, widowhood, and chronic illness as potential trauma reactivators that disrupt routines, roles, and identity.
3. Apply trauma-informed occupational therapy strategies that support nervous system regulation, rebuild occupational identity, and promote participation across evolving life stages.
4. Evaluate the impact of sociocultural factors such as ageism, racism, and gender bias on women's access to equitable and trauma-responsive care in later life.
5. Design occupation-based interventions that support grief integration, identity reconstruction, and meaningful engagement in midlife and older adulthood.

By the time she turned 53, Orlina Baker had become an expert at minimizing herself. A dedicated hospital administrator, mother of two adult children, and caregiver to her aging father, she rarely missed a meeting or a meal prep, yet could not remember the last time she felt present in her own body. After a medically indicated hysterectomy, her doctor told her recovery would be routine, but nothing about her inner life felt normal. She cried in her car after work without knowing

DOI: 10.4324/9781003658559-5

why, skipped yoga without meaning to, and sometimes stared at her own reflection unsure of who was looking back. Her sleep was shallow. Her mind raced. She began forgetting tasks she had performed effortlessly for years. "I am not broken," she told her occupational therapist, "but I feel scattered. Like I keep doing and doing, and none of it feels like mine anymore."

What Orlina was experiencing was not simply a reaction to surgery. It was the collision of neuroendocrine shifts, accumulated stress, and a quiet but persistent loss of agency. The abrupt hormonal decline following hysterectomy can trigger changes in brain regions responsible for memory, mood regulation, and identity processing. For women with trauma histories or longstanding caregiving roles, these shifts can resurface unprocessed grief, amplify cognitive fog, and destabilize routines that once grounded their lives. When such transitions go unacknowledged, women like Orlina are left to navigate a crisis of self in silence, misunderstood by systems that treat healing as purely physical and aging as purely inevitable.

By the time a woman reaches the second half of her life, she has often lived through a complex accumulation of transitions across physical, emotional, relational, and occupational domains. These trauma-related symptoms often intensify during major health transitions such as menopause, caregiving responsibilities, chronic illness, or bereavement. A recent study published in *Menopause* found that trauma-related symptoms, including PTSD, are not isolated to early life but continue to evolve across adulthood, often intensifying during major health transitions such as menopause, caregiving responsibilities, and chronic illness onset.

Yet the impact of trauma at midlife often remains invisible, buried under cultural expectations of resilience, productivity, and caregiving. In one qualitative study, midlife women recovering from serious health events described the experience not only as a medical battle but as "a shattering of identity," where previous roles as professionals, caregivers, and partners no longer felt accessible. Health care often focuses on disease management, while the occupational consequences of trauma such as withdrawal, disconnection, emotional numbing, and disrupted routines go unrecognized.

For women with histories of relational, systemic, or medical trauma, midlife can become a second critical window: a period where healing can deepen or where unaddressed wounds can resurface, magnified by hormonal, cognitive, and occupational changes. Trauma-informed occupational therapy has an essential role in scaffolding recovery, identity rebuilding, and future-oriented occupational engagement during this often-overlooked stage of development. As women continue into later adulthood, new patterns of trauma exposure and occupational disruption emerge—shaped by widowhood, displacement, physical decline, and systemic neglect.

Neurobiological and Occupational Shifts in the Second Half of Life

In June 2017, Rachel Weiss, a counselor from Perth, Scotland, hosted the first Menopause Café at a local coffee shop. Inspired by the Death Café movement, Weiss aimed to create a space where individuals could openly discuss menopause over tea and cake. The event attracted women in their 40s and 50s who shared experiences of memory lapses, mood swings, and a sense of identity shift—symptoms they had often faced in isolation. The success of this gathering led to the establishment of Menopause Cafés worldwide, providing support and breaking the silence surrounding midlife transitions.

These shared narratives highlight the profound neurobiological transformations occurring during midlife. Declining estrogen levels impact brain regions responsible for memory, emotion regulation, and executive function. For many women, especially those with prior trauma, these changes can exacerbate feelings of disconnection and cognitive challenges, affecting daily life and occupational roles. See Table 5.1 for neurobiological changes during menopause and potential occupational impacts.

Hormonal Changes and Brain Health

Estrogen plays a vital role in supporting neuroplasticity, emotional resilience, and cognitive regulation across the lifespan. During menopause, estrogen levels decline sharply, influencing the hippocampus, amygdala, and prefrontal cortex—regions essential for memory, executive functioning, and emotional processing. These shifts often manifest as forgetfulness, slowed information processing, emotional volatility, and sleep disturbances.

For women with a trauma history, the neurobiological shifts of midlife may amplify existing vulnerabilities. Research suggests that early trauma sensitizes the HPA axis, making the brain more reactive to hormonal changes later in life (Lee & Lee, 2022). As estrogen's regulatory support diminishes, women with trauma exposure may experience intensified cognitive fog, executive dysfunction, and mood lability, further disrupting their engagement in daily occupations.

Understanding these neurobiological changes is critical for occupational therapists working with women in midlife. When cognitive fog, emotional variability, or physical fatigue disrupt daily roles, they are often misinterpreted as personal shortcomings rather than recognized as biologically mediated shifts. A trauma-informed, neurobiological lens allows therapy to focus not only on

Table 5.1 Neurobiological Changes During Menopause and Potential Occupational Impacts

Neurobiological Change	Description	Potential Occupational Impact
Estrogen decline	Reduction in estrogen affecting hippocampus, amygdala, and prefrontal cortex	Memory difficulties, reduced emotional regulation, decreased cognitive flexibility during multitasking
Disrupted thermoregulation	Fluctuations in hypothalamic set point causing hot flashes, night sweats	Sleep disruption leading to daytime fatigue, decreased concentration, irritability during work or caregiving
Decreased synaptic plasticity	Reduced ability for neurons to form new connections and adapt	Slower learning of new tasks, increased frustration with changing routines or technology demands
Changes in autonomic regulation	Increased sympathetic nervous system activation, decreased parasympathetic tone	Heightened stress response, difficulty managing complex tasks under pressure, social withdrawal
Altered cortisol regulation	Dysregulation of HPA axis, leading to elevated cortisol	Emotional lability, anxiety, impaired sustained attention and decision making, avoidance of challenging occupations
Sleep fragmentation	Reduced deep sleep and increased awakenings throughout the night	Cognitive fog, emotional reactivity, reduced occupational stamina across the day (Thurston et al., 2019)

symptom management but also on sustaining meaningful occupational engagement. As internal changes unfold, they often collide with external pressures related to work, caregiving, and evolving family roles, creating fertile ground for role strain and identity disruption.

Estrogen plays a vital role in supporting brain health across the lifespan. It enhances synaptic plasticity, promotes blood flow to key regions such as the hippocampus and prefrontal cortex, and modulates neurotransmitters involved in mood and executive functioning. As estrogen levels decline during menopause, these protective mechanisms weaken, often leading to difficulties with memory, attention, emotional regulation, and cognitive flexibility (Saadedine et al., 2024 [2002]). For women with a history of trauma, the effects of hormonal changes may be even more pronounced. Chronic trauma exposure sensitizes the brain's stress systems, and when layered onto the hormonal volatility of menopause, it can amplify cognitive fog, emotional lability, and executive dysfunction. Rather than isolated symptoms, these experiences often reflect a convergence of neuroendocrine shifts and unresolved trauma, significantly impacting daily occupational performance and emotional well-being.

For women with a trauma history, the cognitive symptoms of menopause often emerge earlier, more severely, or with greater disruption to daily life. Trauma exposure primes the HPA axis to remain in a heightened state of alert, disrupting the body's ability to regulate stress, memory, and executive function. When the additional strain of hormonal decline is layered onto this foundation, symptoms such as brain fog, emotional lability, and difficulty planning or organizing tasks can intensify. These cognitive challenges are not solely biological nor solely psychological; they are the result of a cumulative burden on the nervous system that demands a trauma-informed lens to accurately interpret and address.

Occupational Identity, Role Strain, and Resilience in the Second Half of Life

Midlife often ushers in a complex reorganization of occupational roles, challenging long-standing identities and routines that once anchored a woman's daily life. A recent study published in *The American Psychologist* emphasized that midlife represents a unique convergence of transitions and shifting demands, distinct from earlier and later phases of life (Infurna et al., 2020). Career trajectories may shift due to ageism, caregiving demands, health changes, or personal choice. Women who previously defined themselves through professional accomplishment may encounter new barriers to engagement, while others find that sustaining former levels of productivity becomes increasingly difficult due to cognitive and emotional changes associated with menopause and cumulative trauma exposure.

At the same time, caregiving responsibilities often expand in midlife rather than diminish. Many women find themselves managing the emotional and medical needs of aging parents while continuing to support adolescent or adult children. This "sandwich generation" dynamic compresses occupational roles, often leading to feelings of exhaustion, role overload, and invisibility. Sleep disturbances, mood volatility, and cognitive fog linked to hormonal changes further strain the ability to meet these overlapping demands, disrupting routines that once provided stability and predictability.

These cumulative pressures can lead to occupational identity disruption, a loss of coherence between how a woman perceives herself and the roles she is able to enact (Håkansson et al., 2005). Women who once anchored their sense of purpose in caregiving, professional excellence, or community leadership may experience grief as familiar capacities shift or diminish. For those with histories of trauma, the destabilization of roles may trigger earlier patterns of hypervigilance, withdrawal, or internalized blame, increasing the risk of occupational disengagement and emotional distress.

Yet midlife also offers profound opportunities for resilience and redefinition. Many women use this period of transition to realign their occupational identities with evolving values and emerging possibilities. Creative occupations, advocacy work, entrepreneurship, mentorship, and health promotion activities often become new avenues for meaning making. Rather than restoring old roles, women in midlife often engage in the courageous work of building new ones—roles that are more authentic, more sustainable, and more deeply rooted in self-determined priorities.

Trauma-informed occupational therapy can support this process by validating grief over occupational losses, scaffolding the exploration of emerging identities, and helping women construct routines and roles that honor both their histories and their current realities. Therapy must move beyond simply restoring "function" to supporting meaning, agency, and relational coherence in the face of evolving life demands. By doing so, occupational therapy can play a transformative role in promoting resilience during one of the most complex and powerful periods of adult development.

Trauma Pathways Across the Second Half of Life

At 57, Vanessa Hall had begun to treat her car like a waiting room. Most mornings, she sat in the driver's seat outside her workplace, staring at the building, hands still on the steering wheel, willing herself to go inside. After twenty years at the same nonprofit, her job now felt hollow, the rhythm unfamiliar. A missed promotion had left her questioning not just her competence but her place. Her divorce had fractured more than her home, it impacted her community, her routines, and her sense of continuity. One child had stopped returning calls. The other texted occasionally, mostly about money.

When she was diagnosed with an autoimmune disorder, she told the doctor, "That sounds about right," and never picked up the medication. Her occupational therapist asked how she was managing. Vanessa shrugged. "I refill the dog's water bowl. I pay the bills. I keep the plants alive. I guess that means I'm functioning." She laughed, but it didn't reach her eyes. "I'm not unraveling, I'm just . . . ghosting my own life." Even the mirror had become too much. "I look at myself and don't recognize the woman staring back. She seems tired of being resilient."

Trauma in the second half of life rarely stems from isolated catastrophic events. Instead, it emerges from the layering of relational rupture, medical disruption, systemic inequity, and identity loss that accumulate across decades. These trauma pathways may manifest differently in midlife and older adulthood, but they share common roots in cumulative stress, societal invisibility, and the gradual erosion of coherence between identity and occupation.

In midlife, trauma often takes shape through the convergence of caregiving demands, health vulnerabilities, shifting family dynamics, and the growing disconnect between cultural expectations and lived experience. Divorce, chronic illness, financial instability, caregiving for aging parents, and systemic discrimination rarely occur in isolation. Instead, they compound upon earlier experiences of relational, developmental, or structural trauma. As women navigate these overlapping stressors, new patterns of hypervigilance, emotional withdrawal, somatic distress, and occupational disengagement frequently emerge. Understanding these midlife-specific trauma pathways is critical for designing interventions that address not only individual symptoms but also the broader occupational and systemic landscapes shaping women's health and identity during this pivotal life stage.

Accumulated Relational Trauma

Midlife often brings relational changes that do not occur in isolation but instead interact with earlier patterns of trauma, creating new emotional fractures that disrupt occupational life. Divorce during this period frequently carries heavier occupational consequences than it might have earlier in adulthood, unraveling routines built around partnership, shared caregiving, financial interdependence, and family stability. Women facing divorce in midlife are often tasked with reconstructing their daily lives while grieving the loss of relational identity, home structures, and envisioned futures. For those with prior trauma, these ruptures can intensify patterns of hypervigilance, emotional detachment, or internalized blame, complicating reentry into new social, community, or occupational roles.

Caregiving for aging parents adds another layer of relational and occupational complexity. Many women step into caregiving roles that demand significant emotional, financial, and logistical labor, often without adequate support. When earlier relationships with parents were marked by neglect, abuse, or emotional distance, caregiving can resurface unresolved grief, anger, or confusion about boundaries. These dynamics frequently lead to compassion fatigue, emotional exhaustion, or role overload. At the same time, the experience of an empty nest—often idealized as a period of freedom—can bring unexpected grief and identity disruption, particularly for women whose occupational roles were closely tied to motherhood. The sudden absence of caregiving responsibilities may leave women grappling with disconnection and purposelessness, especially when layered atop other midlife stressors. Without trauma-informed support, these relational transitions can reinforce patterns of withdrawal, survival-based coping, and occupational disengagement that complicate recovery and resilience.

Medical Trauma and Chronic Health Conditions

Midlife and older adulthood often bring increased engagement with the healthcare system, whether through chronic disease management, surgical interventions, or preventive screenings. Yet these encounters are not experienced uniformly. For many women, the onset or progression of conditions such as cancer, autoimmune disease, or cardiovascular illness becomes a defining inflection point. It alters not only biological health but also occupational identity, daily structure, and one's felt relationship with the body (Fakhry et al., 2021). Medical interventions that are clinically necessary may simultaneously act as traumatic experiences, especially when they involve loss of bodily control, prolonged recovery, or interactions with providers that feel dismissive or dehumanizing. For women with histories of relational or systemic trauma, the clinical setting itself may echo earlier experiences of helplessness or violation, reinforcing patterns of hypervigilance, avoidance, or emotional numbing.

These trauma-shaped experiences influence how women engage in health-related occupations in both visible and hidden ways. Some may avoid medical appointments altogether, delay follow-up care, or disengage from rehabilitation because of anxiety, distrust, or dissociative symptoms that are misunderstood as noncompliance. Others may perform health routines mechanically, such as medication management or exercise programs, without emotional presence or internalized benefit. Occupational disruption in this context often extends beyond the condition itself, encompassing a fractured sense of safety, autonomy, and body trust.

For women in midlife and beyond, chronic illness may also be accompanied by grief over changes in function, shifting roles, or the inability to maintain previously valued identities such as caregiver, professional, or partner. Feelings of shame or inadequacy may arise when productivity is reduced or when energy must be redirected toward self-care. Without trauma-informed care, occupational therapy may risk addressing tasks without fully supporting the emotional and relational terrain that shapes engagement. A trauma-informed approach in this context includes pacing interventions around emotional readiness, validating fear or frustration linked to health routines, and restoring agency through collaborative goal setting, choice-based care routines, and somatic awareness strategies that reconnect women to their bodies without retraumatization.

Systemic and Structural Trauma

The experience of trauma in midlife is not solely interpersonal or medical; it is fundamentally shaped by systemic and structural forces that govern access to care, economic security, and occupational opportunity. Ageism and sexism converge in midlife to render women increasingly invisible within healthcare systems, labor markets, and public discourse. Midlife women may find their symptoms minimized, their health concerns reframed as inevitable decline, or their professional contributions devalued in favor of younger counterparts (Verburgh et al., 2024). These experiences are not isolated indignities; they accumulate over time, forming chronic layers of structural trauma that shape emotional resilience, occupational engagement, and health outcomes.

For women from historically marginalized groups, including women of color, LGBTQ+ women, and women with disabilities, the impact of systemic inequities during midlife is often compounded. Racial disparities in healthcare access and quality, workplace discrimination, and financial vulnerabilities stemming from long-term economic exclusion intersect to create heightened occupational precarity. The stress of navigating biased systems while simultaneously managing the layered responsibilities of caregiving, health maintenance, and relational transitions can trigger survival-based adaptations such as emotional numbing, hypervigilance, and occupational withdrawal. Trauma-informed occupational therapy must move beyond addressing individual symptoms to confront these structural dimensions, advocating not only for therapeutic adaptation but also for systemic change that restores occupational justice and equity across the lifespan. See Table 5.2 for an overview of common midlife stressors, associated trauma pathways, and the occupational disruptions that often result.

In older adulthood, trauma may reemerge through loss of autonomy, institutional displacement, widowhood, or the erosion of previously meaningful roles. When trauma is left unaddressed, it may manifest as apathy, avoidance, or occupational disengagement. These responses are often misinterpreted as aging rather

Table 5.2 Common Midlife Stressors, Trauma Pathways, and Occupational Disruptions

Life Event	Trauma Pathway	Occupational Disruption
Divorce	Hypervigilance, mistrust in relationships, emotional withdrawal	Disruption of home routines, loss of caregiving roles, occupational isolation
Caregiving for aging parents	Compassion fatigue, emotional exhaustion, role overload	Decreased self-care, diminished leisure engagement, occupational imbalance
Empty nest transition	Identity loss, grief reactions, disconnection from social roles	Loss of parenting identity, reduced community participation, purposelessness
Chronic illness diagnosis (e.g., cancer, autoimmune disease)	Somatic hyperawareness, healthcare avoidance, loss of body trust	Decreased work performance, disruption of health management routine

(Continued)

Table 5.2 (Continued)

Life Event	Trauma Pathway	Occupational Disruption
Medical trauma (e.g., invasive procedures, dismissive care)	Dissociation, distrust of healthcare systems	Avoidance of medical care, disengagement from rehabilitation occupations
Financial instability	Chronic stress, executive dysfunction, restricted occupational access	Withdrawal from employment, disrupted educational and financial occupations
Experiences of ageism or sexism in healthcare	Emotional numbing, advocacy fatigue, distrust of providers	Decreased engagement in health maintenance, emotional disengagement from professional and social occupations
Racism or systemic inequities	Heightened stress responses, cumulative trauma burden	Fragmented occupational participation, avoidance of community and healthcare systems

than understood as unresolved disruption. Just as in midlife, these experiences call for nuanced, relational, and justice-driven occupational responses.

Trauma during midlife often disrupts the routines, roles, and relational patterns that once provided structure, identity, and meaning. These changes rarely occur in isolation; instead, they accumulate over time, intersecting with evolving health challenges, relational transitions, and systemic inequities. Without intentional support, the erosion of occupational coherence can deepen emotional distress, diminish agency, and restrict participation in meaningful life domains. Addressing midlife trauma requires interventions that not only target functional recovery but also restore occupational identity, rebuild relational safety, and create new avenues for engagement rooted in self-determined values and capacities.

Trauma and Occupational Disruption in Older Adulthood

At 82, Elise Walker had recently moved in with her daughter after a fall made living alone unsafe. She had spent over four decades in her own home, surrounded by routines that gave structure to her days: radio in the morning, crossword at lunch, a walk to the mailbox every afternoon. Now, in a well-meaning but unfamiliar environment, Elise found herself waiting for others to tell her when to eat, when to bathe, when to rest. She declined most suggestions in occupational therapy, saying "I'm not used to needing help," though her therapist noted she flinched during touch and startled easily when approached from behind.

Once known for her hospitality, Elise no longer cooked, played piano, or wore the jewelry she used to put on each morning. When asked why, she replied, "There's no one left to notice." Her routines had not only been disrupted, but they had also been erased, along with the roles that once anchored her identity. Underneath her quiet compliance was a nervous system shaped by earlier relational trauma and now reactivated by loss, dependency, and institutional rhythms she could not control.

While trauma in midlife is often framed through the lens of hormonal and role transitions, trauma in older adulthood is more frequently obscured masked by assumptions about aging, decline, or emotional detachment. Yet for many older women, trauma does not recede with time. It resurfaces. It evolves. And it often intersects with physical vulnerability, cognitive change, institutional systems, and the slow erasure of previously held roles (Cook & Simiola, 2018).

Older adulthood is a period marked by cumulative loss, including the loss of loved ones, homes, and roles once central to daily life. These losses are not isolated events. They reverberate through a woman's routines, relationships, and sense of purpose. When trauma is unacknowledged, it is often misread as apathy or confusion. When occupational disruption is overlooked, it becomes normalized as part of aging rather than recognized as a site of potential intervention. For many women, the experience of aging is not only shaped by biological changes but by earlier trauma that has been suppressed or dismissed, only to reemerge when resources for coping are most diminished.

Occupational therapy has an essential role in addressing trauma during this stage, not only through physical support or cognitive strategies but by restoring the conditions that allow older women to engage meaningfully with their lives. This includes honoring grief, challenging invisibility, and helping women navigate environments and expectations that often strip them of autonomy. When previous routines are disrupted by relocation or loss, therapists can support the reintroduction of structure through personalized morning rituals, meaningful music selections, or opportunities for self-expression in dressing or grooming. For women who no longer cook due to physical limitations or reduced social connection, therapists may adapt culinary occupations by incorporating seated preparation methods, accessible tools, or family storytelling through shared recipes.

When long-standing caregiving roles have ended, occupational identity can be reconstructed through life review projects, mentorship roles, or guided participation in community activities that affirm purpose. For those impacted by medical trauma or systemic distrust, therapists can facilitate advocacy coaching, prepare scripts for clinical interactions, and offer choice-based care routines that restore agency during health management. Even when cognitive decline is present, participation can be supported through visual cues, sensory anchors, and simplified co-occupations that reflect the person's values. In these moments, the goal is not to recreate the past but to affirm the present. Trauma-informed occupational therapy in older adulthood is not only a clinical approach, but also a form of respect, recognizing that healing and meaning remain possible at every stage of life.

Widowhood, Grief, and the Loss of Relational Anchors

The death of a spouse or long-term partner is one of the most disorienting events in older adulthood. For many women, this loss disrupts more than emotional connection. It dismantles routines, isolates social engagement, and alters the flow of daily occupations that once gave life structure and meaning. Shared meals become solitary, familiar conversations fall silent and long-held roles such as managing a home or caring for a partner suddenly dissolve. In some cases, the loss reveals previously hidden dependencies in areas like financial planning, transportation, or home maintenance. For others, it reactivates early trauma, as the absence of a relational anchor reopens wounds of fear, abandonment, or vulnerability.

Grief is not only emotional. It is deeply occupational. Occupational therapists can support older women through this transition by helping them reconstruct meaning and autonomy through small, personalized interventions. This may begin with morning practices that encourage grounding and orientation, such as opening windows for natural light, preparing a comforting beverage, or engaging in a short movement sequence. Mealtime interventions may include adapting a favorite shared recipe for solo preparation or creating new social opportunities around food, such as attending a community lunch program or hosting a weekly meal with a neighbor.

When former partner roles included managing finances or home systems, therapists can offer task-specific training with compensatory tools such as visual checklists, memory aids, or simplified budgeting templates. For women who retreat from community or leisure activities, graded reentry may include structured scheduling, social coaching, or participating in events with therapist support to reduce anxiety and promote safe engagement. Therapists can also facilitate narrative occupations such as journaling, storytelling, or creating legacy projects that honor the lost relationship while supporting identity reconstruction.

Rather than prescribing coping strategies, occupational therapy allows grief to unfold through meaningful doing. It helps women reclaim agency, discover new forms of participation, and reconnect with parts of themselves that may have been set aside during caregiving or partnership. In this way, therapy becomes not just a space for healing but a process of rediscovering life after loss.

Abuse, Neglect, and Medical Trauma in Late Life

Older women are particularly vulnerable to forms of abuse that go unrecognized, including emotional manipulation, financial exploitation, medical neglect, and physical or sexual violence. These forms of harm often occur in settings where older adults are expected to feel safe, such as within families, residential facilities, and healthcare systems. For women with a history of relational trauma, the experience of being spoken over, ignored, or handled without consent may echo earlier violations in ways that are deeply distressing yet difficult to articulate.

In addition to interpersonal abuse, many older women experience trauma within the medical system itself (Ghneim & Stein, 2024). Invasive procedures, institutional routines that prioritize efficiency over dignity, and environmental factors such as lack of privacy or noise overload can erode a sense of safety and control. Occupational therapists can intervene by advocating for trauma-aware care practices, creating environments that emphasize respect and consent, and helping clients reestablish a sense of control over their bodies and choices. Supporting self-efficacy, even in small decisions, is often a critical step in healing.

Displacement, Dependency, and Occupational Erasure

Transitions in later life are often marked by forced displacement, whether due to the death of a spouse, financial instability, medical crises, or caregiving needs. Moving into a daughter's home, entering assisted living, or leaving a long-held residence after a fall may be necessary, but it often comes with the loss of familiar spaces, roles, and routines. For many older women, these transitions are experienced as more than logistical. They are experienced as identity dislocations. The spaces that once affirmed autonomy now feel unfamiliar or controlled by others.

Dependency in this context is both a physical and emotional reality. It can be accompanied by shame, frustration, or passive withdrawal, especially when decisions are made without a woman's input. Occupational therapy can play a vital role in mitigating the trauma of these transitions by ensuring that older women are not only physically supported but also empowered to participate in decisions about their care, daily routines, and social life. Therapists can help rebuild a sense of authorship over the day. Decisions like what time to wake, what to wear, and what to eat are not trivial details. They are essential markers of self-determination. Understanding the layered trauma and occupational disruption that can emerge across both midlife and older adulthood sets the foundation for trauma-informed occupational therapy that is responsive, relational, and grounded in everyday function.

Applying Trauma-Informed Care Across the Second Half of the Lifespan

Occupational therapy in the second half of life must extend beyond restoring lost function to address the layered impacts of trauma on identity, regulation, and occupational engagement. Trauma-informed care during these years requires attunement to the survival strategies that often emerge after decades of relational rupture, systemic inequity, caregiving fatigue, and cumulative health challenges (Santoro et al., 2022). Rather than focusing solely on performance deficits, interventions must scaffold nervous system regulation, support role renegotiation, and create opportunities for occupational reinvention that align with each woman's values, needs, and capacities.

Effective assessment strategies are essential to this approach. Screening for trauma history should be done respectfully and indirectly, avoiding methods that risk retraumatization or pathologizing. Tools that examine occupational disruption—such as inventories of lost roles, disengaged patterns, or restricted environments—can surface critical insights without requiring explicit disclosure. Meaning-centered assessments that explore shifts in purpose, connection, or future goals are particularly useful when identity is in flux, whether due to menopause, widowhood, retirement, or institutional relocation.

Regulation must be prioritized before reengagement in cognitively or emotionally demanding roles. Many women navigating trauma in midlife or older adulthood present with elevated autonomic arousal, chronic fatigue, or persistent somatic distress. Stabilizing the nervous system through sensory-based grounding, paced breathing, environmental adjustments, and consistent co-regulatory relationships creates a foundation for sustainable occupational participation. When role reentry is rushed without addressing regulation, the result is often overwhelm, disengagement, or perceived treatment failure.

Narrative and future-oriented approaches play a central role in trauma-informed care during this stage of life. Supporting women in reconstructing personal narratives that frame midlife and older adulthood not as periods of loss, but as developmental phases rich with possibility, helps foster occupational hope and self-determination (Khan, 2025). Future-directed goal setting, life review with meaning making, and narrative reconstruction allow women to imagine new occupational identities—even when prior roles have been altered or erased by trauma. See Table 5.3 for examples of goals and corresponding trauma-informed occupational therapy strategies that support recovery and reengagement across midlife and older adulthood.

Integrating these strategies into occupational therapy practice requires more than the application of techniques. It calls for sustained attunement to the lived

Table 5.3 Trauma-Informed Occupational Therapy Goals and Strategies for Midlife and Older Adulthood

Client Goal	Underlying Challenge	Trauma-Informed Occupational Therapy Strategy
Rebuild daily structure after role loss	Loss of occupational rhythm due to job change, retirement, or widowhood	Co-create time-based routines anchored in sensory regulation and meaningful activities; use visual schedules and gentle behavioral activation
Regain confidence in social engagement	Withdrawal after chronic relational trauma or systemic exclusion	Scaffold graded exposure to affirming social spaces; integrate identity-affirming groups or community programs aligned with client values
Manage emotional dysregulation interfering with function	Autonomic reactivity from unresolved trauma; disrupted sleep, eating, or attention	Implement environmental modifications, paced breathing, sensory-based grounding; build awareness of nervous system cues through psychoeducation
Restore purpose after major life transition	Disconnection from previous roles (e.g., caregiver, professional, partner)	Use narrative reconstruction to explore identity shifts; engage in future-oriented goal setting and strengths-based life review
Participate meaningfully in home and community	Avoidance due to fear, chronic fatigue, or institutional disempowerment	Start with context-based participation goals (e.g., mail, meals, outdoor walks); integrate trauma-aware pacing and control over task timing and location
Reclaim voice and decision making in daily life	Feelings of helplessness or loss of autonomy from abuse or displacement	Prioritize shared decision making; embed micro-choices in sessions; validate preferences as functional outcomes in themselves

experiences, survival strategies, and evolving identities of women navigating trauma across midlife and older adulthood. Trauma-informed care during these stages is not solely about restoring lost function, but about rebuilding occupational coherence, relational trust, and a sense of future possibility. Through individualized assessment, regulation support, narrative reconstruction, and scaffolded reengagement, occupational therapy can create conditions where healing is not defined by returning to prior roles, but by forging new pathways that honor resilience, accommodate changing capacities, and support meaningful participation in everyday life.

Culturally Responsive Care and Advocacy in Midlife Health and Older Adulthood

At 63, Khadijah Fadel had been living with ALS for four years. Before her diagnosis, she worked as a high school counselor and was a well-known advocate in her Muslim community. But her professional life had not been without hardship. After 9/11, she endured years of subtle and overt discrimination at work—comments about her headscarf, coworkers questioning her loyalty, students mimicking Arabic words in mocking tones. She had filed complaints at times, but nothing changed. "You learn to keep your head down," she told her occupational therapist, "and you learn not to expect anyone to protect you." Since her illness progressed, the loss of independence reopened old wounds. Hospital staff often addressed her son instead of her. Her hijab was once removed during a procedure without permission. Male aides entered her room without knocking. "The hardest part isn't the weakness," she explained. "It's feeling like I don't get to have boundaries anymore."

By the time women reach the second half of life, many are navigating not only physical changes such as menopause or fatigue, but also the accumulated weight of being overlooked. For women of color, LGBTQIA+ women, and those living with disabilities, these years often bring a compounded burden. Past traumas were never addressed, systems were never built for them, and care models continue to overlook the whole person.

What too often gets missed is that these women are still showing up every day—in their families, at work, and in their communities—while managing symptoms that are not just biological, but structural. In a 2022 study published in *Women's Midlife Health*, researchers analyzing the 25-year Study of Women's Health Across the Nation cohort found that Black women reported more severe menopause symptoms, poorer sleep, worse mental health, and greater declines in physical function than White women. The authors connected these disparities to cumulative stress and structural racism (Harlow et al., 2022). A 2023 study in *The Journals of Gerontology: Series B* found that LGBTQIA+ individuals were significantly more likely to report discrimination in medical settings, directly impacting care access and follow-through (Bayram et al., 2023). Women with disabilities remain almost entirely excluded from menopause and aging research, despite clear evidence that chronic illness, neurodivergence, and physical impairments shape health experiences in distinct and profound ways. These are not secondary concerns; they are central to achieving equity in care.

Addressing Compounded Trauma in Marginalized Women

Culturally responsive care requires more than surface-level inclusion. It calls for acknowledgment of the structural harm embedded in many women's life histories. Midlife and older adulthood often mark a convergence of stressors, including caregiving for aging parents, job instability, menopause, retirement, medical complexity, and the loss of long-held roles. For marginalized women, these transitions are often shaped by a lifetime of bias, systemic exclusion, and intergenerational trauma.

Occupational therapists must bring an intersectional lens to care, one that sees beyond diagnosis and recognizes the social, historical, and structural forces shaping identity, access, and function. This includes validating a woman's understanding of her own body, co-creating meaningful routines, and advocating for care delivery that honors autonomy and lived experience. Culturally responsive practice recognizes that fatigue may stem from chronic emotional labor, that attention difficulties may reflect prolonged stress exposure, and that routines must be built around what is sustainable, not just what is ideal. See Table 5.4 for an overview of common barriers encountered by marginalized women in the second half of life and strategies occupational therapists can use to support advocacy and equitable care.

These disparities are not incidental. They are the result of long-standing systemic patterns that require intentional disruption. While individualized interventions can support symptom management, true occupational justice demands that therapists engage the broader forces shaping access, participation, and well-being. This means not only helping women navigate care systems, but amplifying their voices in policy, advocating for workplace protections, and ensuring that services are informed by lived experience. Culturally responsive occupational therapy is not only about treating the woman in front of you, but also about transforming the conditions around her.

Table 5.4 Common Barriers and Occupational Therapy Advocacy Strategies for Marginalized Women in Midlife and Older Adulthood

Group	Key Barriers in Midlife Health	Occupational Therapy Response
Black Women	Earlier menopause onset, more severe symptoms, and lower likelihood of receiving hormone therapy	Use culturally affirming assessments, validate symptom reports, support inclusion in decision making, and advocate for equitable treatment access
LGBTQIA+ Women	Discrimination and care avoidance due to stigma and exclusion	Provide gender-affirming care, support chosen family involvement, and create safety for disclosure and advocacy
Women with Disabilities	Exclusion from menopause research and limited support for emotional or sensory needs	Prioritize access and autonomy, modify environments, and co-create health routines that reflect evolving needs
Immigrant Women	Language barriers, cultural mistrust, and lower rates of preventive screening	Use interpreters, integrate cultural health beliefs, and build care plans connected to trusted community supports
Multi-marginalized Women	Intersecting trauma, chronic stress exposure, and systemic barriers	Address trauma history within evaluation, scaffold role redefinition, and apply an equity lens to treatment planning

The Role of Occupational Therapy in System-Level Advocacy

Individual care is necessary, but without broader advocacy, its reach is limited. Women in the second half of life do not just need support managing symptoms— they need systems that affirm their identities, adapt to their changing needs, and remove the barriers that have historically excluded them. Occupational therapy is uniquely positioned to drive this change, not only by supporting function, but by challenging the institutional and policy-level forces that shape it.

At the system level, this includes advocating for inclusive clinical guidelines, calling for research that reflects the diversity of aging women, and helping to shape workplace policies that consider cognitive shifts, caregiving burdens, and chronic health concerns. It means intervening when a woman's concerns are minimized or misinterpreted and providing documentation and support for accommodations that promote occupational participation with dignity.

Cultural responsiveness in the second half of life is not passive. It is a proactive, justice-aligned stance. It asks clinicians to move beyond awareness and toward action—designing, documenting, and demanding systems that reflect the realities of those they serve. In doing so, occupational therapy becomes not only a space for recovery, but a force for reform. When advocacy becomes standard rather than supplementary, we move closer to true equity in care for aging women.

Case Vignettes and Clinical Reflections

The following vignettes illustrate how trauma, identity, and structural barriers converge in midlife—and how occupational therapy can offer more than symptom management. These are not stories of transformation through discipline or mindset shifts. They are stories of women navigating invisible labor, role loss, and systemic exclusion. The role of the therapist in each case is not to restore a past version of function, but to co-create space for coherence, stability, and redefinition of what participation can look like.

Case Example 1: Diane, Age 52—Corporate Executive Managing Cognitive Shifts and Racialized Workplace Stress

Diane was a senior marketing executive known for her strategic leadership and high performance. Over the past year, she began experiencing intermittent difficulty with focus, word retrieval, and sustained attention during high-stakes meetings. She also reported increased irritability, sleep disruption, and physical fatigue. While her physician attributed these changes to menopause, Diane sensed there was more at play. She was balancing an intense workload, caring for her mother with early-stage dementia, and navigating daily racial microaggressions in her predominantly White corporate environment. Although she originally sought occupational therapy for time management support, her initial evaluation revealed chronic role strain, emotional depletion, and cognitive inefficiency under stress.

The occupational therapist utilized performance-based assessments, including executive-function screeners and contextual activity logs, to identify specific breakdowns in her attention regulation and task sequencing. Together, they restructured Diane's daily routines to include restorative occupations tailored to her sensory preferences and energy patterns. These included early morning walks without devices, a structured ten-minute breathing protocol before meetings, and a protected lunch hour involving time in a botanical park near her office. These activities were intentionally embedded to support autonomic regulation and cognitive reset throughout the day.

In parallel, the therapist collaborated with Diane to identify workplace modifications that could improve sustainability without compromising professional identity. This included scripting language for accommodation requests, such as moving high-demand planning meetings to late morning when her cognitive stamina was stronger and implementing visual planning tools for project oversight that reduced dependence on memory recall. The therapist documented these needs using function-centered terminology to support a formal request to human resources.

Recognizing the impact of racialized stress on Diane's overall occupational performance, the therapist also integrated mindfulness strategies that were grounded in culturally affirming environments. Instead of traditional mindfulness apps, Diane engaged with guided meditations and storytelling through a Black women's wellness collective that emphasized ancestral strength and collective rest. These approaches honored her cultural identity while supporting nervous system regulation in a way that felt authentic and empowering. Over time, Diane reported increased clarity, emotional steadiness, and a sense of authorship over her routines. Occupational therapy did not resolve all external pressures, but it equipped her with strategies to function effectively within them—on her terms.

Case Example 2: Elena, Age 48—LGBTQIA+ Advocate Recovering From Surgical Trauma and Occupational Disconnection

Elena was a former nonprofit director and long-time advocate for LGBTQIA+ health equity. After years of enduring chronic pelvic pain that had been repeatedly misattributed to stress and anxiety, she underwent a total hysterectomy. Although the procedure brought physical relief, it also initiated a period of deep emotional disruption. Elena described feeling estranged from her body, disconnected from her identity as a leader, and uncertain about how to return to the advocacy work that had once given her purpose. Her primary care provider referred her to occupational therapy after noting significant withdrawal from daily routines, irregular sleep, limited food intake, and diminished participation in social life.

The occupational therapist conducted a structured occupational history and used the Canadian Occupational Performance Measure to identify areas of disruption that mattered most to Elena. Through this process, it became clear that her occupational disengagement was not rooted in apathy, but in unresolved trauma related to previous medical invalidation and a loss of connection to her roles and identity. The therapist prioritized regulation first, integrating a sensory-based plan that included evening use of deep pressure through foam roller techniques, warm water immersion for muscle relaxation, and rhythmic movement practices that supported vestibular input and grounding. These tools helped reestablish a baseline of safety and connection between Elena's body and her daily environment.

Therapeutic goals focused on restoring self-directed routines. Elena began with small, time-structured tasks such as preparing a single meal each afternoon and completing a reflective writing prompt in the evening. As her engagement improved, the therapist helped her scaffold a return to values-based activities by volunteering ten hours per week at a local LGBTQIA+ community center. This was framed not as a return to productivity, but as a reentry into relational and purpose-driven spaces that affirmed her identity and allowed for gradual occupational rebuilding.

Importantly, the therapist also addressed the emotional terrain of surgical recovery within the context of queer identity. Elena was encouraged to explore narrative reconstruction work through journaling and audio storytelling formats that allowed her to make meaning from her experience without retraumatization. She chose to work through a curated workbook developed by LGBTQIA+ clinicians that offered reflective prompts aligned with themes of embodiment, grief, and resilience. By the end of her therapy process, Elena described feeling more anchored, both in her daily structure and in her evolving identity. Occupational therapy gave her more than coping tools, it offered a way to rebuild a life that honored her body, her voice, and the work she was still capable of doing.

Case Example 3: Maria, Age 76—Retired Caregiver Navigating Widowhood and Institutional Displacement

Maria had spent most of her adult life caring for others, raising five children, supporting her husband through chronic illness, and helping to raise her grandchildren. After her husband passed away unexpectedly, her children encouraged her to move into an assisted living facility, hoping to ease her caregiving load. But Maria struggled with the transition. She reported persistent exhaustion, poor appetite, and a reluctance to participate in group activities. Once deeply engaged in church and family life, she now spent most of her time alone in her room, unsure how to occupy her days.

Her intake with occupational therapy revealed multiple layers of disruption. Maria was grieving not only the loss of her husband, but the loss of her home, her routines, and her role as the person others depended on. She described feeling invisible in the facility, where schedules were rigid and personal preferences often ignored. Although her physical health was stable, her sense of purpose had eroded.

The therapist began by helping Maria reestablish a sense of structure and continuity in her day—small, chosen routines that reconnected her to her values. Maria began preparing her own morning coffee with music she enjoyed, taking brief walks at her preferred times, and participating in a life review group where she could share stories from her past. These routines were not just activities; they were symbolic acts of reclaiming time, voice, and control.

Recognizing the trauma of institutional displacement, the therapist worked with facility staff to advocate for more autonomy in Maria's care plan. This included greater flexibility in mealtimes, access to a private journaling space, and consistent staff assignments to reduce the emotional toll of unfamiliarity. The therapist also introduced narrative prompts that helped Maria integrate her identity as a caregiver into her current life stage. It was not something lost, but something that could evolve into mentorship, storytelling, and quiet leadership within the community. By the end of their work together, Maria reported fewer episodes of anxiety and more days that "felt like her." Occupational therapy had not only supported her adjustment to a new environment, but it had also helped her rediscover her role within it.

Therapist Reflections on Clinical Decision Making

The experiences of Diane, Elena, and Maria reflect the diverse ways trauma can shape a woman's occupational life in the second half of adulthood. Their stories did not begin with trauma, but with subtle expressions of disconnection such as fatigue, loss of motivation, and difficulty with roles that once came easily. These were not simply signs of aging, stress, or recovery. They were evidence of deeper disruptions in regulation, safety, and meaning that demanded clinical curiosity and structural sensitivity.

In Diane's case, the therapist addressed how racialized stress and role overload affected her cognitive performance and occupational identity. With Elena, the focus was on reestablishing a sense of embodiment and agency after medical trauma, while honoring her queer identity and relationship to advocacy. In Maria's story, trauma emerged through displacement and institutional invisibility. Her care required a reassertion of personal rhythm, relational continuity, and culturally rooted self-determination.

Across these cases, occupational therapy offered more than tools or strategies, it provided a framework for reentering life on new terms. This work is not about restoring a prior version of function. It is about helping women inhabit who they are now, with clarity, dignity, and control. Each case illustrates the need for therapists to attend not only to performance and regulation, but to power, place, and possibility.

Trauma-informed care in midlife and older adulthood requires deep listening, cultural humility, and clinical precision. It means holding space for grief and identity change, while scaffolding the routines and environments that make reengagement feel possible. It also means challenging the systems that continue to marginalize the very women we are here to serve, including those that are medical, institutional, and societal in nature. When occupational therapy is practiced through this lens, it becomes not just a site of recovery, but a practice of repair.

Summary and Implications

The second half of a woman's life is often marked by transitions that are invisible to the systems designed to support her. These transitions such as menopause, caregiving shifts, widowhood, retirement, and relocation carry with them not only physiological change, but layers of accumulated trauma, role loss, and systemic exclusion (Harlow et al., 2023). For women who live at the margins of gender, race, disability, or socioeconomic status, these disruptions are further compounded by medical gaslighting, cultural invisibility, and reduced access to responsive care. These are not isolated experiences. They are patterned, predictable, and preventable.

Occupational therapy offers a lens uniquely suited to this complexity. It allows us to move beyond symptom tracking and toward narrative reconstruction, nervous system stabilization, and the rebuilding of daily life on a woman's own terms. It also requires us to challenge the structural barriers that limit what aging, healing, or participation are allowed to look like. Whether supporting a midlife professional navigating cognitive shift, a queer woman recovering from surgical trauma, or an elder redefining her role after displacement, the work remains the same: to hold space for occupational reinvention that is grounded in safety, shaped by identity, and defined by the woman herself.

References

Bayram, E., Weigand, A. J., & Flatt, J. D. (2023). Perceived discrimination in health care for LGBTQIA+ people living with Parkinson's disease. *The Journals of Gerontology: Series B, Psychological Sciences and Social Sciences, 78*(9), 1459–1465. https://doi.org/10.1093/geronb/gbad046

Cook, J. M., & Simiola, V. (2018). Trauma and aging. *Current Psychiatry Reports, 20*(10), 93. https://doi.org/10.1007/s11920-018-0943-6

Fakhry, S. M., Morse, J. L., Garland, J. M., Wilson, N. Y., Shen, Y., Wyse, R. J., & Watts, D. D. (2021). Redefining geriatric trauma: 55 is the new 65. *The Journal of Trauma and Acute Care Surgery, 90*(4), 738–743. https://doi.org/10.1097/TA.0000000000003062

Ghneim, M. H., & Stein, D. M. (2024). Age-related disparities in older adults in trauma. *Surgery, 176*(6), 1771–1773. https://doi.org/10.1016/j.surg.2024.08.038

Håkansson, C., Eklund, M., Lidfeldt, J., Nerbrand, C., Samsioe, G., & Nilsson, P. M. (2005). Well-being and occupational roles among middle-aged women. *Work (Reading, Mass.), 24*(4), 341–351.

Harlow, S. D., Burnett-Bowie, S. M., Greendale, G. A., Avis, N. E., Reeves, A. N., Richards, T. R., & Lewis, T. T. (2022). Disparities in reproductive aging and midlife health between Black and White women: The Study of Women's Health Across the Nation (SWAN). *Women's Midlife Health, 8*(1), 3. https://doi.org/10.1186/s40695-022-00073-y

Harlow, S. D., Sievert, L. L., LaCroix, A. Z., Mishra, G. D., & Woods, N. F. (2023). Women's midlife health: The unfinished research agenda. *Women's Midlife Health, 9*(1), 7. https://doi.org/10.1186/s40695-023-00090-5

Infurna, F. J., Gerstorf, D., & Lachman, M. E. (2020). Midlife in the 2020s: Opportunities and challenges. *The American Psychologist, 75*(4), 470–485. https://doi.org/10.1037/amp0000591

Khan, S. (2025). *Occupational therapy and women's health: A practitioner guide* (1st ed.). Routledge.

Lee, J., & Lee, J. E. (2022). Psychological well-being of midlife women: A structural equation modeling approach. *Menopause (New York, N.Y.)*, *29*(4), 440–449. https://doi.org/10.1097/GME.0000000000001933

Saadedine, M., Faubion, S. S., Kling, J. M., & Kapoor, E. (2024 [2002]). Cognitive health update in midlife women. *Journal of Women's Health*, *33*(1), 5–9. https://doi.org/10.1089/jwh.2023.0642

Santoro, N. F., Coons, H. L., El Khoudary, S. R., Epperson, C. N., Holt-Lunstad, J., Joffe, H., Lindsey, S. H., Marlatt, K. L., Montella, P., Richard-Davis, G., Rockette-Wagner, B., Salive, M. E., Stuenkel, C., Thurston, R. C., Woods, N., & Wyatt, H. (2022). NAMS 2021 utian translational science symposium September 2021, Washington, DC charting the path to health in midlife and beyond: The biology and practice of wellness. *Menopause (New York, N.Y.)*, *29*(5), 504–513. https://doi.org/10.1097/GME.0000000000001995

Thurston, R. C., Chang, Y., Buysse, D. J., Hall, M. H., & Matthews, K. A. (2019). Hot flashes and awakenings among midlife women. *Sleep*, *42*(9), zsz131. https://doi.org/10.1093/sleep/zsz131

Verburgh, M., Verdonk, P., Muntinga, M., van Valkengoed, I., Hulshof, C., & Nieuwenhuijsen, K. (2024). "But at a certain point, the lights literally went out": A qualitative study exploring midlife women's experiences of health, wellbeing, and functioning in relation to paid work. *Work (Reading, Mass.)*, *77*(3), 799–809. https://doi.org/10.3233/WOR-220567

Chapter 6

The Spectrum of Violence Against Women

Chapter Objectives

Upon completing this chapter, readers will be able to:

1. Describe the diverse forms of violence women may experience across the lifespan, including intimate, sexual, psychological, institutional, and digital violence.
2. Analyze how violence affects nervous system regulation, emotional expression, and occupational participation across daily life domains.
3. Identify trauma-related signs that may emerge during occupational therapy sessions, including avoidance, hyperarousal, altered routines, and difficulty with trust or body-based tasks.
4. Apply trauma-informed strategies that promote safety, autonomy, and reengagement in meaningful roles and environments.
5. Evaluate the role of occupational therapy in both direct care and system-level advocacy to support survivors and reduce barriers within healthcare and community systems.

Francesca Moreau, a 36-year-old graphic designer, was admitted to the hospital with a traumatic brain injury following an assault by her former partner. Traumatic brain injury is a known consequence of intimate partner violence, often overlooked in clinical care (Colantonio & Valera, 2022). It was not the first time she had experienced violence, but it was the first time she sought medical attention. In the acute care unit, she presented with headaches, dizziness, memory lapses, and difficulty organizing her thoughts. During occupational

DOI: 10.4324/9781003658559-6

therapy sessions, she appeared alert but anxious. When asked to complete grooming tasks at the sink, she stood rigidly and avoided looking in the mirror. She startled easily at noises in the hallway and pulled her arm away when the therapist offered a washcloth. She hesitated before sitting on the edge of the bed, repeatedly asked for permission to begin, and avoided discussing preferences related to clothing or hygiene products. Although she complied with the session, she frequently apologized and asked if she was doing things correctly. The medical chart emphasized fall risk and cognitive rehabilitation, but the therapist recognized indicators of trauma. Francesca showed signs of discomfort with body-based care, difficulty making choices, and emotional withdrawal during basic routines. These patterns are common among survivors of intimate partner violence and may reflect occupational deprivation resulting from trauma-related disruption (Ballan & Freyer, 2020). These responses reflected more than brain injury alone. They pointed to a nervous system shaped by fear and a daily life interrupted by violence.

Francesca's experience highlights the way violence can reshape a woman's routines, sense of control, and capacity to engage in care. These patterns often emerge in clinical settings as anxiety, avoidance, or difficulty with daily tasks. Occupational therapy must recognize how different forms of violence affect participation across home, work, healthcare, and community life.

Across every country, income level, and life stage, women experience violence at disproportionately high rates. Gender-based violence is not an outlier. It is one of the most pervasive and under-addressed public health emergencies of our time (Campbell, 2002). Nearly one in three women worldwide has experienced physical or sexual violence, most often at the hands of an intimate partner. In the United States, more than one in four women report severe intimate partner violence, and over 81 percent have experienced sexual harassment or assault. These numbers do not reflect isolated incidents. They reveal structural patterns of harm shaped by power, gender, and societal silence.

The impact of violence does not end when the event is over. It embeds itself in the nervous system, in patterns of avoidance and hypervigilance, in the disruption of routines and roles that once brought meaning. Many survivors never disclose their histories, but the effects often show up in clinical care as:

- Disrupted sleep, emotional volatility, or difficulty focusing
- Withdrawal from work, caregiving, or social participation

- Chronic pain or fatigue that cannot be fully explained by pathology
- Reluctance to engage with healthcare, touch, or group environments

Violence alters a woman's relationship to her body, her sense of safety, and her capacity to engage in daily life with autonomy and ease. These are not only psychological or physical consequences. They are occupational disruptions that require trauma-awareness, justice-centered, and functionally grounded responses across disciplines.

Forms of Violence and Their Occupational Impact

When Mariela Leroy stopped attending her weekly dance class, her instructor assumed she had lost interest. In reality, she had not left her apartment in three days. A 42-year-old mother of two, Mariela had come to the United States five years earlier as a refugee after fleeing violence in her home country. During that time, she witnessed armed troops raid her village, burn homes, and detain neighbors. Although she and her children escaped, the memories remained vivid. Now living in low-income housing and working unpredictable shifts at a bakery, Mariela described her days as blurry and disjointed. At her occupational therapy intake related to fibromyalgia, she reported chronic back pain, frequent nightmares, and a racing heart whenever she heard loud noises or sirens. She no longer cooked traditional meals, avoided mirrors, and found it difficult to complete basic daily tasks. "I do not feel like a person right now," she said. "I feel like I am holding my breath all the time."

Mariela had not disclosed the full scope of her trauma to her doctor or employer, but her body and daily routines communicated what she could not say aloud. Her sleep was shallow and interrupted. Her caregiving routines felt mechanical. She withdrew from activities that once brought her comfort. Her nervous system remained on high alert, constantly preparing for danger that never fully ended. Her case illustrates how the effects of violence persist long after the immediate threat is gone, often showing up in the ways a woman moves through her day, engages with her surroundings, and carries out roles that once defined her sense of self. These patterns are particularly complex among immigrant and Caribbean women, where migration-related stressors compound trauma (Lacey et al., 2021).

Violence against women is not confined to a single relationship, setting, or moment in time. It unfolds across intimate partnerships, workplaces, digital spaces, and institutions, often beginning early in life and persisting into older adulthood. For many women, especially refugees and those displaced by conflict, violence is not only interpersonal but also structural and state-inflicted. It may involve exposure to armed conflict, forced displacement, detention, sexual exploitation, or the loss of community and protective networks. Each form of violence carries distinct harm, but all interfere with a woman's ability to engage in daily life with safety, autonomy, and purpose. A 2023 global report by UN Women estimated that 736 million women, or nearly one in three, have experienced physical or sexual violence by an intimate partner, non-partner, or both (UN Women, 2024). In the same year, approximately 51,100 women and girls were killed by intimate partners or family members, highlighting the lethal consequences of gender-based violence.

In the United Kingdom, over one million cases of violence against women and girls were recorded in 2022–2023, equating to nearly 3,000 crimes each day. This violence represents nearly 20 percent of all recorded crime, excluding fraud. In the United States, more than one in four women report severe intimate partner violence, and over 81 percent have experienced sexual harassment or assault in their lifetime. In Australia, 23 women were killed by male violence in the early months of 2025, with seven fatalities occurring in just one week. Despite the severity, political leaders have remained virtually silent during election campaigns, focusing instead on other issues. In Spain's film and audiovisual industry, a 2025 report revealed that 60.3 percent of women have experienced sexual violence in work-related settings. Of those affected, 49.5 percent reported physical assaults, 81.4 percent verbal abuse, and 22.3 percent faced digital or virtual abuse. These statistics highlight the pervasive nature of violence against women and its profound impact on their daily lives and occupational engagement.

Sexual Violence and Coercion

Sexual violence includes rape, harassment, unwanted sexual contact, and reproductive control. More than one in five women in the United States reports completed or attempted rape during their lifetime, and these numbers are even higher among marginalized populations. Survivors often disengage from activities that require body awareness, physical exposure, or interpersonal trust. It is common to see avoidance of intimacy, discomfort with grooming or dressing, and heightened distress in clinical or touch-based environments (Leblanc et al., 2020).

Occupational therapists may encounter these patterns long before a history of violence is disclosed. Recognizing that disconnection, hypervigilance, or silence around certain tasks may reflect trauma rather than noncompliance is essential. Therapists can adjust their approach by offering clear choices, narrating steps before physical contact, and reducing exposure during dressing or hygiene routines. Evidence suggests that multicomponent interventions improve both physical and psychological recovery for survivors of violence (Calle-Guisado et al., 2023). Body-based interventions like yoga, breath practices, or sensory-calming strategies should be introduced slowly and always with consent. For some clients, reclaiming control through simple acts such as choosing their clothing, setting the pace of a grooming task, or creating a personalized dressing sequence can begin to restore safety and autonomy. Trauma-informed care does not require disclosure. It requires attunement, flexibility, and a deep respect for the ways the body holds memory. Meta-analyses have shown that trauma-informed approaches enhance psychological outcomes among survivors (Chu et al., 2024).

Intimate Partner Violence

Nearly one in four women in the United States has experienced severe physical violence by an intimate partner. Intimate partner violence includes physical harm, emotional manipulation, sexual coercion, and financial control. Survivors often navigate daily life under chronic surveillance or fear, which impacts their ability to maintain employment, access healthcare, or engage in community life. Some become socially isolated, while others remain in survival mode—overextending themselves in caregiving roles or suppressing emotional expression to preserve safety.

Occupational therapy can support reestablishment of routines, gradual community reentry, and adaptation of the home and work environments to enhance autonomy and reduce risk (Ballan et al., 2022). Unlike other trauma exposures that may stem from a single event or external circumstance, intimate partner violence unfolds within the fabric of daily life—embedded in routines, relationships, and environments that may outwardly appear stable. This proximity creates unique occupational challenges. The same kitchen where meals were prepared may also be where threats occurred. The same schedule used to care for children may have been shaped around anticipating a partner's mood or movements. Therapists must understand that even routine-based interventions can feel threatening if they mirror past control dynamics. In this context, restoring choice is therapeutic. Offering clients opportunities to decide what task to begin with, how a session is paced, or which space feels most comfortable to work in can begin to rebuild internal safety. Occupational therapy does not simply help survivors resume activity. It also creates opportunities for women to reclaim ownership over their time, space, and roles after those domains have been repeatedly violated. This reclamation is a core outcome described in women's experiences of trauma-informed care (Liu et al., 2024).

Digital, Institutional, and Psychological Abuse

Technological and psychological abuse are increasingly common and deeply destabilizing. An estimated 10 percent of women have experienced digital abuse from a partner, including cyberstalking, online harassment, or nonconsensual sharing of images (Earl et al., 2022). Psychological abuse, including gaslighting, intimidation, or humiliation, can be just as damaging. In healthcare systems, institutional trauma may occur when women are dismissed, over-pathologized, or forced to navigate services that invalidate their identities. Survivors may withdraw from online platforms, delay healthcare, or avoid advocacy settings entirely.

Occupational therapy can play a key role in rebuilding digital confidence, supporting emotional safety in healthcare participation, and restoring a sense of personal agency in decision making. For survivors of digital abuse, therapists can support safe technology use by helping clients establish boundaries with devices, create structured online routines, or relearn digital tasks in ways that reduce anxiety and promote control. In cases of institutional harm, occupational therapists can help clients prepare for appointments by developing scripts, co-writing questions, or role-playing advocacy interactions. Therapists may also serve as collaborative partners during healthcare navigation—helping clients decode forms, access accommodations, or choose environments that align with their sensory and emotional needs. Such roles are increasingly recognized in rehabilitation literature as essential to trauma-informed care (Toccalino et al., 2024). Psychological abuse often leaves behind confusion and self-doubt, which can undermine even basic decision making. Research shows that access to resources significantly influences recovery trajectories (Weaver et al., 2021). In these cases, occupational therapy offers structured opportunities for clients to practice autonomy through low-pressure choices, self-reflection tools, and identity-based occupations that reinforce self-trust. The goal is not only functional restoration, but the rebuilding of internal authority in the face of systems and relationships that have tried to erase it.

Violence in Later Life

Approximately one in ten adults over the age of 60 experience elder abuse each year, and older women are particularly at risk due to longer life expectancy, social isolation, and increased reliance on caregivers. Violence in later life may involve neglect, physical harm, emotional abuse, or financial exploitation. Older women may experience a loss of control over their environment, changes in sleep or eating patterns, or decreased interest in activities that once held meaning. Prior trauma may also be reactivated during medical procedures or institutional transitions.

Occupational therapy can support older women by promoting environmental safety, sustaining meaningful daily structure, and preserving autonomy within care settings. Therapists may use personalized routines, visual schedules, and sensory-based strategies to support orientation and emotional regulation, especially for clients with cognitive change. They can also facilitate life review activities, digital storytelling, or legacy projects that affirm personal identity and restore dignity after experiences of silencing or control. In care planning, occupational therapists can advocate for communication access, choice in daily tasks, and respectful touch to prevent retraumatization. These strategies do not just enhance function. They create relational and sensory conditions that help older women feel safe, seen, and respected.

The Long-Term Ripple Effects of Violence on Occupation

The aftermath of violence is often more enduring than the incident itself. For women who have experienced interpersonal violence, either directly as primary survivors or indirectly as witnesses or caregivers to survivors, the consequences extend far beyond physical injury or acute stress. These forms of trauma often reshape a woman's relationship to her body, her roles, and her environment in ways that are persistent but not always recognized.

Unlike other forms of trauma, such as medical events, environmental disasters, or grief, violence often carries with it a violation of trust, autonomy, and relational safety. The perpetrator is frequently known, the setting is familiar, and the memory is embodied. As a result, women who have experienced violence may present with patterns of occupational disruption that differ in tone, complexity, and persistence. These may include:

- Hypervigilance during caregiving or parenting, often expressed as over-monitoring, emotional rigidity, or difficulty delegating responsibility
- Avoidance of routine medical care or physical touch, not due to generalized anxiety, but due to body-based reminders of coercion or boundary violation
- Grooming and self-care habits that fluctuate sharply, such as excessive control over appearance or complete disengagement from hygiene practices
- Difficulty establishing consistent routines, particularly in environments with unclear boundaries or perceived power imbalances
- Persistent distrust in professional relationships, which may appear as nonadherence, deflection, or difficulty with therapeutic alliance

In secondary trauma, such as witnessing domestic violence or supporting a survivor, the signs may appear more covert: chronic fatigue, guilt linked to perceived inaction, or emotional shutdown in situations that resemble the original context. These women may struggle to name what they experienced, especially if their role was peripheral, but their nervous systems have adapted around the need to monitor and protect.

The occupational implications are often misinterpreted. Sleep disturbances may be attributed to stress. Interpersonal withdrawal may be labeled as depression. Delayed responses to follow-up care may be seen as noncompliance. Without a trauma-informed lens, the patterns linked to violence are pathologized rather than contextualized.

Occupational therapy plays a critical role in long-term recovery after violence by addressing the tangible, daily consequences that persist even after the threat has passed. For many women, reengagement does not begin with goals or graded exposure—it begins with safety. This includes working collaboratively on personalized safety planning, whether the client is actively in a harmful environment or managing the residual effects of past violence. Safety planning may involve identifying triggers in the home or workplace, creating discreet exit strategies, structuring routines around predictable environments, and ensuring access to emergency contacts or confidential transportation when needed.

Evidence supports the use of occupation-based strategies to rebuild a sense of agency, including scheduling decision-making tasks during times of day when the client feels most grounded, integrating relational repair through safe and chosen connections, and developing rituals that mark control over personal time, space, and body. In cases of long-term coercion or identity erosion, therapists may support clients in reclaiming interrupted roles—not by returning to them exactly as they were, but by redefining them in ways that prioritize autonomy, values, and dignity. These interventions are not one-size-fits-all. They must be responsive to the specific dynamics of the violence experienced, whether interpersonal, institutional, or community-based, and grounded in practices that center safety, trust, and control as therapeutic outcomes in their own right.

Interdisciplinary and Occupational Therapy Responses

Recovery after violence does not begin with performance. It begins with protection. For many survivors, especially those navigating chronic coercion or betrayal within caregiving systems, occupational therapy may be one of the few clinical environments where safety and control are prioritized. While trauma-informed care often emphasizes emotional processing or mental health stabilization, occupational therapy addresses the daily structures that reinforce or undermine a survivor's sense of agency. Recovery is not simply about what a woman can do—it is about what she feels safe doing, and under what conditions.

Occupational therapy practitioners must consider three parallel objectives in this work:

- Restoring daily rhythm through predictable, choice-based routines
- Supporting nervous system regulation through task design and pacing
- Embedding control and autonomy into environments, schedules, and interpersonal interactions

These objectives are not static. They evolve based on the survivor's environment, access to resources, and history of violence. In interdisciplinary teams, OTs are uniquely positioned to notice when a client withdraws from therapy, avoids tasks with sensory triggers, or uses hyper-productivity as a survival strategy. Therapists must not only treat the visible disruption but also understand the history it is rooted in and the systems that may continue to reproduce harm.

Collaboration with Advocacy Organizations and Health Providers

Occupational therapists rarely work in isolation when supporting survivors of violence. Effective intervention requires seamless collaboration with shelters, social workers, mental health providers, primary care physicians, and sometimes legal advocates. OTs can contribute valuable insight into a survivor's real-world function, which can inform housing decisions, court reports, and care transitions.

In hospital discharge planning, therapists can advocate for trauma-aware referrals, sensory accommodations, or community reintegration supports. In outpatient settings, collaboration with case managers or domestic violence counselors may allow for more realistic expectations about role demands or schedule flexibility. OTs can also ensure that survivors are not retraumatized during care planning by clearly defining consent, ensuring transparency, and upholding the survivor's right to decline or defer tasks. These collaborations work best when clinicians maintain open communication and avoid assumptions about capacity, safety, or goals.

Occupational Therapy Specific Tools and Approaches

Occupational therapists bring a unique set of tools to post-violence care. Unlike traditional crisis interventions, OT practice focuses on daily routines, environmental structure, and meaningful occupation. Therapists can offer practical tools that are embedded into real-life decisions—how to plan a day, navigate space, or choose what matters most when everything feels disoriented. One foundational tool is the personalized safety planning template, which can be adapted to any context: clinical, residential, or community-based. A well-designed safety plan is more than a list of emergency contacts—it includes occupational patterns, sensory preferences, support roles, and backup plans that are specific to the survivor's daily life. See Table 6.1 for an example of a safety planning template that can be adapted to support occupational engagement and emotional regulation following experiences of violence.

Safety planning is not a one-time conversation. It is a dynamic process that evolves alongside the survivor's daily life and changing context. For many women, knowing when and where they feel most stable is the foundation for rebuilding participation. When these plans are grounded in occupation—through

Table 6.1 Safety Planning Template for Occupational Therapy Practice

Component	Example or Prompt
Predictable Safe Timeframes	When do you feel most grounded during the day? What hours feel most difficult?
Environmental Anchors	What spaces feel calming or safe? How can you access them regularly?
Exit and Communication Strategy	Do you need a nonverbal signal, backup phone, or silent alert app?
Regulation and Grounding Toolkit	Which sensory inputs help you feel steady (e.g., warm water, pacing, music)?
Trusted Roles and Support	Who can support you without requiring explanation? When and how do you want to reach them?
Identity Reminders	What rituals, objects, or routines help you feel most like yourself?

structured routines, regulation strategies, and clearly identified support roles—they allow for more than emergency readiness. They create space for restored authorship. With safety scaffolds in place, the therapeutic focus can gradually shift from crisis navigation to deeper work around occupational identity, values, and role reintegration.

Life Redesign Maps and Values-Based Scheduling

Another approach involves co-constructing a life redesign map, a visual tool that helps survivors externalize their disrupted roles, redefine priorities, and identify areas for reengagement. This map is not chronological or linear. It is layered, relational, and based on lived experience. It might include roles that feel dormant, identities the client wants to explore, and goals that are anchored in healing rather than productivity. Clients often benefit from this process because it allows them to see their lives as adaptable rather than broken.

Values-based scheduling builds on this map by embedding priorities into the day. Rather than pushing for full routines, therapists work with clients to anchor one or two meaningful actions around core values such as safety, connection, learning, or rest. This process makes use of time-blocking, energy mapping, and negotiated pacing to restore occupational rhythm without overwhelm. Over time, these micro-decisions support both autonomy and resilience.

Survivor-Centered Adaptations for Daily Tasks

Women recovering from violence may need task adaptations that reflect not only physical or cognitive needs but also emotional, sensory, and relational boundaries. Occupational therapy can offer alternative pathways to engage in daily tasks without triggering distress. This might include:

- Dressing in layers to minimize sensory vulnerability and reduce discomfort during transitions
- Preparing food without knives or using pre-chopped ingredients to limit exposure to triggering tools
- Using noise-control tools, such as headphones, white noise, or door draft blockers, to reduce startling stimuli in shared spaces
- Installing soft lighting or indirect light sources in kitchens and bathrooms to avoid overstimulation or disorientation during morning or nighttime routines
- Rearranging home environments to allow for escape routes, sightlines to doors, or the removal of objects associated with trauma
- Replacing mirrors in grooming spaces with calming imagery or covering them temporarily during body-care tasks to reduce dissociation or distress
- Offering alternatives to direct physical touch in therapeutic sessions or group work (e.g., using weighted objects or visual cues to support presence without physical contact)
- Using scheduling apps or visual planners with gentle reminders instead of alarms or loud notifications to reduce startle responses
- Encouraging the use of familiar music or guided audio during tasks like cooking, folding laundry, or bathing to anchor time and support grounding
- Creating buffer zones in routines, such as transition rituals between work and home, can help reorient the nervous system after high-demand tasks
- Allowing for asynchronous participation in group programs, journaling, or communication activities, giving clients control over how and when they share their voice

These adaptations help reframe occupation as a space of empowerment rather than performance. By reducing demands on the nervous system and supporting personal choice, therapists can create safer ways for women to reengage in the everyday tasks that hold meaning, connection, and identity. These occupational strategies are most effective when embedded within an interdisciplinary care framework. Collaboration with social workers, advocates, housing coordinators, mental health providers, and trauma-informed medical teams ensures that adaptations are supported across settings. For example, an OT may work with a domestic violence advocate to align home modifications with safety planning, or with a primary care provider to schedule appointments during calmer parts of the day. When teams communicate and center the survivor's lived experience, they reinforce consistent safety signals, reduce reactivation risk, and create continuity of care that allows occupational recovery to unfold with dignity and control.

System-Level Advocacy and Occupational Justice

Eleni Samar arrived in the United States after fleeing conflict in Sudan, carrying with her the trauma of forced displacement, gender-based violence, and the loss of nearly everything familiar. Although granted asylum, her new reality was shaped by institutional barriers—long delays in accessing health services, clinics without interpreters, and intake forms that left no room for her story. When she sought occupational therapy for chronic joint pain and disrupted sleep, she was given a handout on posture and told to return if it got worse. No one asked about trauma. No one connected her symptoms to the violence she had endured or the grief she still carried. "I survived war," she later told a caseworker. "But here, it feels like I have to keep surviving silence." Eleni's experience reveals how structural neglect and cultural invisibility can compound trauma, even in settings meant to provide care.

Violence against women is not only perpetuated by individuals. It is maintained through systems that normalize harm, overlook survivors, and restrict access to meaningful recovery. While trauma-informed care often focuses on the therapeutic relationship, true healing also depends on the environment around the survivor—how institutions respond to disclosure, how policies shape participation, and how services either restore or deny a sense of justice. For occupational therapists, this means stepping beyond individualized treatment plans and confronting the conditions that constrain occupational choice.

Occupational justice calls on practitioners to recognize the ways structural violence limits a woman's ability to engage fully in society. A survivor who avoids clinics because her pain was repeatedly dismissed is not noncompliant. She is responding to institutional betrayal. A woman who cannot attend work without risking retaliation from a violent partner is not unmotivated. She is navigating systems that offer no viable protection. In these contexts, therapy must extend beyond task modification. It must include systems-level intervention.

Therapists can engage in system-level advocacy by identifying patterns of exclusion and pushing for upstream solutions. This might involve revising intake forms to better capture trauma histories, ensuring that documentation includes functional impacts of violence for use in court or benefits applications, or advocating for the inclusion of trauma survivors in program design and evaluation. It also includes educating colleagues about how trauma shows up in occupation—not just as fear or distress, but as flattened affect, inconsistent attendance, or subtle resistance to touch, sound, or authority.

System-level work also requires political and policy fluency. Therapists who understand the laws and structural barriers surrounding housing, employment, education, and healthcare access for survivors are better positioned to advocate for systemic change. Occupational therapy is not neutral—it exists within systems that can either reinforce or challenge injustice. When therapists name and respond to the institutional factors that silence, retraumatize, or exclude survivors, they shift from service providers to social change agents. This shift is essential if the field is to live up to its ethical commitment to health, equity, and full participation for all.

Challenging Institutional Violence

Institutional violence occurs when systems designed to provide care instead become sites of harm. This includes patterns of dismissal in healthcare, punitive policies in schools or shelters, and bureaucratic barriers in social services that retraumatize or silence survivors. For many women, institutional violence does not feel like a dramatic event. It feels like being talked over, not believed, or asked to prove pain. It feels like receiving fewer options, less time, or no follow-up. These experiences can accumulate over time and lead to functional disengagement from essential services.

Occupational therapists are often on the front lines of institutional care, whether in hospitals, home health, correctional facilities, or educational settings. As a result, they are uniquely positioned to challenge practices that perpetuate trauma. This might include calling out how a discharge policy places survivors at risk, questioning why trauma is excluded from standard evaluation protocols, or advocating for procedural changes that allow for more choice, privacy, and pacing in clinical encounters.

Documentation is also a powerful tool for resisting institutional harm. Therapists can ensure that their notes reflect not just task performance, but contextual factors like safety concerns, emotional regulation, and environmental control. By clearly articulating the occupational impact of institutional practices, therapists can build evidence that supports systemic redesign. See Table 6.2 for examples of institutional barriers and how occupational therapists can support systemic change through targeted actions.

These examples reflect just a fraction of the institutional patterns that contribute to ongoing occupational disruption for women impacted by violence. While many of these barriers fall outside traditional definitions of clinical care, they shape whether and how survivors access services, disclose trauma, or sustain participation over time. Occupational therapists are often the first to notice when policies fail to match lived realities. By documenting patterns, challenging default procedures, and proposing practical alternatives rooted in function and safety, therapists can directly influence how institutions operate. This is not supplemental work. It is foundational to restoring occupational justice in systems that too often overlook the survivors they serve.

Table 6.2 Institutional Barriers and OT Strategies for System-Level Redesign

Institutional Barrier	OT Opportunity for System-Level Advocacy or Redesign
Standardized intake forms that ignore trauma history or do not ask about safety	Collaborate with administration to revise forms to include trauma-sensitive questions about environment and daily function
Lack of private spaces for evaluation or goal setting	Advocate for designated low-stimulation, private rooms in clinical and educational settings
Mandatory reporting practices that discourage disclosure due to fear of retaliation	Educate teams on alternate phrasing, voluntary check-ins, and timing of disclosure to protect client autonomy
Inflexible attendance or productivity metrics in rehab or day programs	Propose flexible attendance policies and functional outcome tracking that reflect regulation and readiness
Gaps in service coordination between healthcare and domestic violence agencies	Develop shared care plans and secure release protocols to connect survivors to housing, legal, and safety services
Discharge planning based solely on medical stability	Integrate occupational participation criteria into discharge decisions (e.g., ability to navigate daily routine safely)
Staff training limited to physical safety or compliance	Co-develop continuing education focused on trauma-informed practice, institutional betrayal, and occupational justice

Advocacy in Practice Settings

Amina Begum was referred to school-based occupational therapy for sensory processing difficulties and focus issues related to her ADHD. Teachers described her as fidgety, inattentive, and sometimes defiant. In OT sessions, Amina rarely made eye contact. She flinched at sudden noises, avoided seated tasks, and often asked to go to the bathroom when asked to write about herself. Her therapist noticed she carried her backpack everywhere, even to short sessions, and became visibly tense when it was moved. Over time, it became clear that what had been labeled as executive dysfunction and behavioral resistance were also signs of trauma. Amina had witnessed domestic violence and was currently living in transitional housing with her mother and siblings. The OT adjusted goals to prioritize regulation, added a trauma-informed sensory plan to her IEP, and advocated for flexible scheduling that allowed Amina to access quiet space before high-demand classes. Her needs weren't just neurological, they were environmental, relational, and shaped by survival.

Occupational justice is not just a theory. It is a practice that must show up in daily decisions—in how therapists write goals, structure interventions, and speak in team meetings. Advocacy within practice settings begins with disrupting every-day assumptions: that all clients have access to quiet recovery environments, that "noncompliance" means lack of motivation, or that routines should be restored exactly as they were before the trauma occurred.

Therapists can advocate for trauma-informed policy changes such as flexible scheduling, sensory-friendly clinic design, and routine screening for violence and trauma exposure. They can help establish referral pathways to community organizations that support survivors or co-develop care plans that reflect legal, cultural, and emotional safety, not just clinical improvement. More broadly, therapists can use their voice to influence program design, staff training, and leadership decisions. Joining or forming trauma-informed care committees, pushing for data collection on survivor outcomes, or collaborating with community advocates are all ways to ensure that the voices and needs of women impacted by violence shape the systems intended to serve them. See Table 6.3 for setting-specific examples of how occupational therapists can advocate for systemic change in practice.

Table 6.3 Systemic Advocacy Opportunities for Occupational Therapists Across Practice Settings

Practice Setting	Type of Advocacy	Examples of Systemic Occupational Therapy Advocacy Opportunities
Pediatrics	Trauma-sensitive intake and environmental design	Integrate trauma-informed questions into caregiver intake forms; recommend staggered scheduling and quiet spaces for children with violence exposure.
School-Based OT	Policy and program reform	Advocate for restorative justice practices over punitive discipline; co-create trauma-responsive IEP goals with mental health teams; propose sensory-safe calming rooms in lieu of seclusion.
Inpatient Hospital	Discharge planning and staff training	Recommend consistency in provider assignments for survivors; add trauma-informed notes to discharge summaries; train teams on signs of medical retraumatization.
Inpatient Rehab	Institutional policy adaptation	Promote trauma training for all disciplines; adjust therapy intensity to match regulation capacity; recommend flexible room-sharing or gender-sensitive spaces.

(Continued)

Table 6.3 (Continued)

Practice Setting	Type of Advocacy	Examples of Systemic Occupational Therapy Advocacy Opportunities
Outpatient Clinics	Referral systems and procedural change	Establish partnerships with advocacy groups for warm handoffs; propose narrative or values-based intake assessments; modify attendance policies to account for safety disruptions.
Home Health	Risk identification and interdisciplinary coordination	Collaborate with social work or case managers on home safety exits or emergency contacts; document trauma-related occupational barriers such as disordered pacing, start-initiation delays, or shutdowns.
Community-Based OT	Cross-sector collaboration and systems navigation	Facilitate joint sessions with legal or housing advocates; co-develop education sessions with survivors for service providers; support organizing around occupational justice issues (e.g., access to care, transit, safe housing).

These examples reflect how advocacy is not reserved for policy meetings or leadership roles. It happens during documentation, during goal writing, during hallway conversations with nurses or teachers, and in the ways therapists respond to patterns that others may overlook. When a therapist notices that a parent flinches in a noisy clinic, or that a client avoids appointments after interacting with a particular provider, those observations are not just therapeutic—they are diagnostic of the system. And when addressed with intention, they can become the starting point for structural change.

Occupational therapists are not only agents of adaptation but also agents of accountability. Within every practice setting, there are policies, routines, and cultural norms that either support or suppress a survivor's ability to engage. Naming these dynamics, advocating for changes that reflect lived experience, and designing interventions that prioritize autonomy and safety are all part of trauma-informed occupational justice. Advocacy does not distract from clinical work, it deepens it. When systems are redesigned with survivors in mind, occupation becomes more than recovery. It becomes a pathway back to power.

Case Vignettes and Clinical Reflections

Survivors of violence often enter occupational therapy not with a clear diagnosis, but with a pattern of disconnection—missed appointments, disrupted routines, diminished participation, or somatic complaints that do not align neatly with clinical categories. What lies beneath is often a history of harm that has gone unspoken or unrecognized. For women impacted by violence, occupational disruption is rarely about motivation or skill. It is about survival. The following cases illustrate how interpersonal violence, institutional dismissal, and systemic barriers converge to shape function—and how occupational therapy can respond with safety, structure, and advocacy woven into every step of care.

Case Example: Talia, Age 36—Survivor of Intimate Partner Violence and Systemic Dismissal

Talia was referred to outpatient occupational therapy after multiple work absences and a recent emergency department visit for what was documented as "nonspecific abdominal pain" and decline in daily function. A single mother and certified nursing assistant, Talia had been in an on-and-off relationship with her partner for nearly a decade. Over the past year, she reported frequent gastrointestinal distress, poor sleep, and difficulty concentrating at work, especially during high-pressure caregiving tasks. Though she had been to multiple providers, her symptoms were repeatedly minimized or reframed as stress-related, without further screening for violence or trauma history.

During her OT intake, the therapist asked about daily routines and noticed significant pauses when Talia described her mornings. With permission, the therapist gently explored her sense of safety at home. Talia eventually disclosed that her partner's behavior had escalated, including limiting her access to transportation, interfering with her work schedule, and frequently monitoring her phone. She described feeling like she had to "shrink" herself at home and "stay ahead of what could go wrong."

Rather than beginning with traditional work endurance goals, the occupational therapist focused on helping Talia reestablish basic occupational safety and regulation. Together, they developed a personalized safety plan, which included a silent text alert for her sister, a visual planner with commute alternatives, and grounding strategies she could use during moments of high emotional arousal at home or work. Talia was also supported in identifying sensory-calming routines she could implement discreetly, such as handwashing with scented soap at work or wearing a textured bracelet she could use for self-soothing.

Recognizing the need for coordinated care, the therapist collaborated with Talia's primary care provider to include language in her documentation that clearly articulated the functional impact of trauma on her ability to manage shift work and childcare responsibilities. This interdisciplinary effort helped support a modified schedule and reduce attendance-related disciplinary action. The occupational therapist also connected Talia with a local advocacy group for legal and housing resources, extending trauma-informed care beyond the clinic and into the community.

Over time, Talia began to regain a sense of authorship over her day. She resumed baking with her daughter on weekends, returned to journaling, and expressed interest in rejoining a church group she had once loved. She described the therapy process as "a way to make my days make sense again," and emphasized that the strategies were not about getting back to normal. Instead, they were about building a life where she no longer had to live in reaction to fear.

Case Example: Marisol, Age 60—Survivor of Medical Neglect and Institutional Retraumatization

Marisol was referred to home-based occupational therapy following a hospitalization for complications related to diabetes and chronic pain. She had a long history of inconsistent medical care due to insurance limitations, provider turnover, and repeated experiences of racial and gender bias in clinical settings. During her hospital stay, she reported that staff often spoke over her, failed to explain procedures, and dismissed her requests for pain management. She described feeling "invisible and handled" rather than included in her care. This was not new—Marisol had stopped attending preventive appointments years earlier, after a clinician questioned her credibility and implied her symptoms were exaggerated.

During the initial OT visit, the therapist noticed that Marisol hesitated before answering most questions and repeatedly apologized for taking up time. When asked about her daily routine, she disclosed that she often avoided bathing or dressing until late afternoon and ate only once a day, saying it "felt safer not to need anything." The therapist recognized signs of institutional retraumatization—patterns of occupational withdrawal shaped not by physical limitations alone, but by longstanding relational harm in healthcare systems.

Intervention began with validating Marisol's experiences and reframing her occupational needs through a lens of dignity and control. Together, they co-created a flexible daily structure that preserved energy while anchoring essential tasks in moments of calm. Bathing was reframed as a midday reset rather than a morning requirement. Meal prep involved pre-portioned options and preferred sensory cues, including culturally familiar ingredients and music. Marisol was also invited to create a "consent checklist" for future healthcare visits, which she could share with providers to outline communication preferences, touch boundaries, and support needs.

The occupational therapist collaborated with Marisol's case manager to document her trauma-related occupational barriers in a way that would support service extensions and avoid future discharge due to "noncompliance." They also submitted a referral to a community-based health navigator program that pairs medically underserved patients with culturally responsive providers. Marisol's goals eventually expanded to include short outdoor walks with her granddaughter and contributing to a community recipe project through her senior center. As she described it, "Therapy didn't just help me move. It helped me feel like I could say no, and that no one would punish me for it."

Therapist Reflections on Clinical Decision Making

Talia and Marisol's experiences reflect two distinct but interconnected pathways of violence. Talia navigated coercion and surveillance within an intimate relationship, while Marisol lived with the long-term effects of institutional dismissal and medical neglect. Both stories illustrate how violence can reshape not only what a woman does, but how she relates to her body, her environment, and the systems she depends on.

In both cases, occupational therapy did not begin with productivity or role performance. It began with listening. In Talia's case, therapy offered a space where disclosure could occur without pressure, and where safety planning became part of functional treatment. In Marisol's case, it offered an opportunity to name patterns of harm that had never been recognized as trauma, and to rebuild daily life around agency and choice. The therapists in both examples worked across disciplines, documenting functional impact, coordinating with advocates and medical teams, and adjusting expectations to center the survivor's sense of readiness.

These cases serve as reminders that trauma-informed care must be more than accommodating. It must be actively anti-oppressive. Occupational therapists must ask not only what tasks are disrupted, but *why*—and whether the conditions surrounding a woman's life are safe enough to support participation in the first place. Recovery from violence is not a return to baseline. It is a process of reentering life with tools, boundaries, and systems that finally make daily occupation possible.

Summary and Implications

Violence against women affects far more than physical health. It reshapes daily function, decision making, and engagement in routines that once felt safe. Whether the violence is intimate, digital, institutional, or psychological, its impact often surfaces in therapy as avoidance, difficulty with trust, or distress during everyday tasks. Occupational therapists are well positioned to notice these patterns and respond with care that centers safety, consent, and emotional presence.

Rather than focusing solely on performance or compliance, trauma-informed occupational therapy restores autonomy in spaces where control was taken. This may involve adjusting session pacing, offering choice during care tasks, or supporting clients in navigating systems that have previously silenced or harmed them. These interventions are not just supportive. They are reparative. They create conditions where recovery becomes possible and where women can reconnect with their roles, values, and capacity for participation.

References

Ballan, M. S., & Freyer, M. (2020). Occupational deprivation among female survivors of intimate partner violence who have physical disabilities. *The American Journal of Occupational Therapy: Official Publication of the American Occupational*

Therapy Association, *74*(4), 7404345010p1–7404345010p7. https://doi.org/10.5014/ajot.2020.038398

Ballan, M. S., Freyer, M., & Romanelli, M. (2022). Occupational functioning among intimate partner violence survivors with disabilities: A retrospective analysis. *Occupational Therapy in Health Care*, *36*(4), 368–390. https://doi.org/10.1080/07380577.2021.1994684

Calle-Guisado, V., Adsuar, J. C., Barrios-Fernandez, S., Mendoza-Muñoz, M., Muñoz-Bermejo, L., Domínguez-Muñoz, F. J., Ortiz-González, L., & Rojo-Ramos, J. (2023). Effects of a multicomponent programme for improving physical and psychological health in victims of intimate partner violence: Study protocol for a randomised control trial. *International Journal of Environmental Research and Public Health*, *20*(4), 2815. https://doi.org/10.3390/ijerph20042815

Campbell, J. C. (2002). Health consequences of intimate partner violence. *Lancet (London, England)*, *359*(9314), 1331–1336. https://doi.org/10.1016/S0140-6736(02)08336-8

Chu, Y. C., Wang, H. H., Chou, F. H., Hsu, Y. F., & Liao, K. L. (2024). Outcomes of trauma-informed care on the psychological health of women experiencing intimate partner violence: A systematic review and meta-analysis. *Journal of Psychiatric and Mental Health Nursing*, *31*(2), 203–214. https://doi.org/10.1111/jpm.12976

Colantonio, A., & Valera, E. M. (2022). Brain injury and intimate partner violence. *The Journal of Head Trauma Rehabilitation*, *37*(1), 2–4. https://doi.org/10.1097/HTR.0000000000000763

Earl, J., Maher, T. V., & Pan, J. (2022). The digital repression of social movements, protest, and activism: A synthetic review. *Science Advances*, *8*(10), eabl8198. https://doi.org/10.1126/sciadv.abl8198

Lacey, K. K., Parnell, R., Drummond-Lewis, S. R., Wood, M., & Powell Sears, K. (2021). Physical intimate partner violence, childhood physical abuse and mental health of U.S. Caribbean women: The interrelationship of social, contextual, and migratory influences. *International Journal of Environmental Research and Public Health*, *19*(1), 150. https://doi.org/10.3390/ijerph19010150

Leblanc, N. M., Alexander, K., Carter, S., Crean, H., Ingram, L., Kobie, J., & McMahon, J. (2020). The effects of trauma, violence, and stress on sexual health outcomes among female clinic clients in a small northeastern U.S. urban center. *Women's Health Reports (New Rochelle, N.Y.)*, *1*(1), 132–142. https://doi.org/10.1089/whr.2019.0027

Liu, V. C., Nelson, L. E., & Shorey, S. (2024). Experiences of women receiving trauma-informed care: A qualitative systematic review. *Trauma, Violence, & Abuse*, *25*(4). https://doi.org/10.1177/15248380241234346

Toccalino, D., Asare, G., Fleming, J., Yin, J., Kieftenburg, A., Moore, A., Haag, H. L., Chan, V., Babineau, J., MacGregor, N., & Colantonio, A. (2024). Exploring the relationships between rehabilitation and survivors of intimate partner violence: A scoping review. *Trauma, Violence & Abuse*, *25*(2), 1638–1660. https://doi.org/10.1177/15248380231196807

UN Women. (2024, November 25). *Facts and figures: Ending violence against women.* www.unwomen.org/en/what-we-do/ending-violence-against-women/facts-and-figures

Weaver, T. L., Kelton, K., & Riebel, J. (2021). The relationship between women's resources and health-related quality of life in a sample of female victims of intimate partner violence. *Journal of Social Service Research*, *47*(4), 565–578. https://doi.org/10.1080/01488376.2020.1859433

Chapter 7

Health Implications of Violence Against Women

Chapter Objectives

By the end of this chapter, readers will be able to:

1. Identify the multisystem health consequences associated with chronic exposure to interpersonal and structural violence in women.
2. Analyze how trauma-related disruptions to the nervous, immune, and endocrine systems impact occupational performance.
3. Apply trauma-informed clinical reasoning to differentiate between functional deficits related to chronic disease versus trauma adaptations.
4. Develop occupational therapy intervention strategies that address cognitive, physiological, and emotional manifestations of violence in daily life.
5. Advocate for system-level approaches that integrate trauma history into healthcare planning, access, and recovery for women impacted by violence.

Jane Rogers was 42 when she was referred to occupational therapy for chronic fatigue, difficulty following through on daily tasks, and low stamina. Over the past five years, she had been diagnosed with fibromyalgia, irritable bowel syndrome, migraines, and, more recently, insulin resistance and hypertension. Her lab results showed elevated inflammatory markers and a concerning cholesterol profile, yet no one could explain why her symptoms kept progressing. She moved with hesitation, startled at loud sounds, and described feeling foggy and detached during even simple activities like cooking or answering email. In the third session, Jane revealed that she had survived

DOI: 10.4324/9781003658559-7

over a decade of intimate partner violence, something that had never been asked about in any previous medical visit. Her therapist shifted focus from performance goals to physiological stabilization, using autonomic tracking, interoceptive awareness, and functional pacing to reduce symptom flares and reestablish body trust within daily routines. Sessions prioritized energy conservation, choice-based activity engagement, and clinical education that reframed her symptoms as adaptations rather than failures.

Violence against women is not only a personal violation. It is a health event with measurable biological consequences that extend across the lifespan. It has been formally recognized as a global public health issue with multisystem consequences (Stöckl & Sorenson, 2024). Repeated exposure to physical, sexual, or psychological harm has been shown to accelerate disease onset, disrupt hormonal and immune regulation, and significantly elevate the risk of both chronic and acute medical conditions. Yet these effects are often misattributed, poorly documented, or entirely missed in routine care. What begins as interpersonal trauma frequently becomes an undetected variable in complex diagnoses.

A 2023 study in the *American Journal of Preventive Medicine* found that women who experienced both childhood and adult interpersonal violence had a 35 percent higher risk of developing adult-onset diabetes, even after controlling for other factors (Sanderson et al., 2023). These findings held across race and sex, reinforcing the biological burden that long-term trauma places on endocrine and metabolic systems.

Research has consistently shown that women who experience violence face higher rates of heart disease, stroke, autoimmune illness, gastrointestinal disorders, and reproductive health complications. Many live with untreated traumatic brain injuries, sexually transmitted infections, and chronic pain syndromes that are never directly linked back to the original harm. These health consequences are not only severe. They are compounded by fragmented systems, provider bias, and medical environments that often fail to ask about or address the root cause.

Occupational therapists have a critical role in bridging the gap between symptom presentation and lived experience (Barreca & Wagner, 2024). Survivors of violence may present with chronic fatigue, cognitive inefficiency, or occupational withdrawal, yet beneath these patterns lies a health history shaped by long-term physiological stress, disrupted care access, and unacknowledged trauma. A trauma-informed approach requires therapists to interpret these symptoms through both biomedical and psychosocial lenses. For example, in women with autoimmune or cardiometabolic conditions, therapists can support task pacing and graded engagement while monitoring physiological thresholds like fatigue onset, orthostatic changes, or post-exertional symptoms (Corso et al., 2023). In the context of chronic pain, occupational therapists may introduce body awareness through postural alignment, joint protection strategies, or adaptations that reduce overactivation without reinforcing avoidance. When addressing nutrition, medication management, or health routines, therapists can explore the relational and emotional meaning behind each task—especially when adherence is inconsistent—not assuming noncompliance but investigating overwhelm, mistrust, or executive disruption.

Cognitive symptoms often emerge as reduced initiation, slowed processing, or difficulty shifting attention. Therapists can integrate functional cognitive strategies, including visual sequencing tools, external cueing systems, and contextual memory supports into daily routines. Rather than overemphasizing productivity, interventions should be rooted in capacity building—supporting self-regulation, flexible engagement, and restoration of agency. Clinical goals should center on reestablishing a sense of control within everyday environments, not just restoring task completion. Most importantly, therapists must be willing to ask about meaning, safety, and preference—and not just about performance. By holding space for the full story behind the diagnosis, occupational therapy becomes a site of recovery where physiology, lived experience, and occupation are addressed in equal measure.

Violence as a Catalyst for Disease and Multisystem Dysregulation

Violence does not end with physical harm. It initiates a prolonged physiological cascade marked by chronic activation of the stress response system, which over time disrupts hormonal balance, weakens immune regulation, and contributes to the development of autoimmune and inflammatory diseases that occur more frequently in women with histories of intimate partner violence and other forms of trauma. Research across disciplines has confirmed that women exposed to interpersonal violence are more likely to develop disease involving multiple body systems earlier in life, with more severe symptoms and reduced access to care (Köhler-Forsberg et al., 2025). These are not just consequences of stress. They reflect the long-term effects of sustained biological disruption and persistent threat perception.

The body responds to violence with precision. When a woman is in danger, her nervous system activates protective responses designed to keep her alive. These include elevated heart rate, reduced digestive function, increased cortisol, and heightened vigilance. When the threat is ongoing or unresolved, these responses become the default setting. Over time, they deplete the body, disrupt metabolic balance, and increase the likelihood of chronic illness. This is not theoretical. It is observable in blood pressure patterns, glucose control, hormone fluctuations, and levels of systemic inflammation.

Women who have experienced violence often live with invisible illnesses that are slow to develop and difficult to treat. These include autoimmune disorders, fibromyalgia, chronic fatigue syndrome, irritable bowel disease, migraines, and a range of cardiometabolic conditions. Many of these diagnoses are approached through siloed treatments—pain management, endocrinology, rehabilitation—without recognition of the original trauma that shaped their onset or exacerbated their progression.

Occupational therapists are uniquely positioned to support women who live at the intersection of trauma and complex illness. While traditional healthcare often emphasizes diagnosis and symptom reduction, occupational therapy focuses on restoring function, safety, and engagement in everyday life. This requires a shift in approach when working with women whose symptoms reflect not only biological dysfunction but years of living in survival mode. For example, in cases of chronic fatigue or autoimmune flare, energy conservation is not just about physical endurance, it becomes a way to titrate nervous system demand. Therapists may structure activity logs that track energy dips alongside emotional triggers, helping clients identify patterns that reflect both physiological depletion and trauma-related reactivity. For women with cardiometabolic conditions, interventions might include planning meals and physical activity around emotional safety and physiological thresholds, rather than rigid health protocols.

Cognitive strategies should reflect the realities of trauma-related executive disruption. Instead of generic memory exercises, therapists can integrate task sequencing into real routines—like breaking down medication management into tactile steps using visual cues, checklists, and verbal scripting to reduce overwhelm and build mastery. When self-care tasks like bathing or dressing provoke avoidance due to pain or body distrust, therapists can offer adaptations in timing, positioning, or sensory input while preserving client choice. They can also use narrative methods, like timeline mapping or symbolic journaling, to process how chronic illness has shaped identity and routines over time.

Participation goals should be calibrated for safety, not just independence. A return to caregiving or employment may require practicing boundary-setting or scripting responses to invasive questions. Social reentry may involve rehearsal of relational skills or scheduling participation in smaller, emotionally regulated spaces. Therapists should conduct contextual interviews to determine which aspects of a woman's environment feel unsafe and develop realistic strategies to reduce exposure or build protective structures. This approach is not about doing less. It is about doing what is necessary to support nervous system recovery and restore occupational agency. In the lives of women managing both trauma and disease, therapy is not just about regaining function. It is about rebuilding trust—in the body, in care relationships, and in the possibility of living without fear.

Neuroendocrine and Immune System Impact

At 27, Shandora Cooper was referred to occupational therapy after a recent autoimmune flare made it difficult for her to manage daily responsibilities. Diagnosed with lupus five years earlier, she had lived with waves of fatigue and joint pain, but the past several months brought new symptoms—sensory sensitivity, memory lapses, and sudden emotional shutdowns during routine occupational tasks. During the intake, Shandora shared that she had recently started trauma counseling related to a history of intimate partner violence in her early twenties. Her occupational therapist used a trauma-informed approach that emphasized predictability and choice, inviting Shandora to co-create an energy contour map that tracked her physical and emotional capacity throughout the day. By rating her energy and stress levels in two-hour increments for one week, patterns emerged: her fatigue peaked between noon and 3 p.m., and she felt most alert shortly after waking and again in the early evening. This helped identify when she was most regulated and capable of engagement, allowing therapy sessions and priority tasks to be scheduled during those windows.

Her occupational therapist then used micro-routine scaffolding, breaking down key daily occupations into gentle, manageable steps. For example, instead of expecting full morning routines, Shandora began her days with a short breathing sequence while holding a warm compress, followed by one low-demand task such as preparing breakfast or opening mail. These early successes supported confidence and reduced shutdowns. Sensory supports like weighted lap pads and scented hand cream were introduced slowly and always with consent, reinforcing body awareness and grounding. Weekly check-ins allowed the therapist to adjust the structure based on flare patterns and emotional stressors. Within a month, Shandora reported fewer afternoon crashes, improved task follow-through, and greater confidence in pacing herself without shame. Rather than focusing on productivity, therapy centered on restoring safety, predictability, and a sense of choice within her body and her daily life.

Violence significantly disrupts the body's stress regulation systems, particularly the HPA axis and the sympathetic nervous system (Katrinli et al., 2022). Chronic activation of these systems leads to elevated cortisol, impaired immune function, and systemic inflammation. This biological profile is associated with higher rates of autoimmune disorders including lupus, rheumatoid arthritis, multiple sclerosis, and Hashimoto's thyroiditis. Women with trauma histories often report flares in these conditions that correlate with psychological stress, relational conflict, or anniversary reactions.

Occupational therapists working with these clients must be aware that fatigue, sensory sensitivity, and unpredictable pain may reflect physiological dysregulation rather than lack of motivation. Interventions should begin with stabilization—not productivity. This includes developing personalized **"energy contour maps"** to identify times of day when fatigue or pain are least disruptive and using those windows for priority tasks. Therapists can also implement **micro-routine scaffolding**, helping clients build flexible daily rhythms that reduce demand on the HPA axis. For example, alternating cognitively or emotionally taxing tasks with restorative occupations—such as patterned drawing, warm water immersion, or guided nature exposure—can buffer sympathetic overdrive and promote parasympathetic recovery.

Sensory modulation kits, co-designed with clients, can support immune-regulatory alignment by calming the vagus nerve. These may include textured objects, temperature tools, or movement-based regulation like slow vestibular input. For clients reporting autoimmune flares, therapists can trial **rhythm-based occupational dosing**, pacing activities across the week in sync with flare patterns and immune medication cycles (Olmos-Ochoa et al., 2023).

Additionally, therapists can coordinate with medical providers to ensure that occupational plans integrate clinical realities—such as medication-induced fatigue or post-infusion crashes. Health journals that combine **daily functional logs with flare tracking** offer therapists and physicians data that can inform both pacing strategies and clinical decision-making. Ultimately, the goal is not just participation but regulation. Interventions grounded in body trust, sensory attunement, and context-responsive pacing enable women to reclaim function not by overriding their bodies, but by working with them. Healing in this context is less about restoration of pre-trauma capacity and more about re-patterning daily life around what is biologically sustainable and emotionally safe.

Cardiometabolic and Chronic Pain Disorders

At 45, Lenora Bennett had been diagnosed with hypertension, Type 2 diabetes, and high cholesterol by the time she was referred to occupational therapy for fatigue, disorganization, and difficulty managing her daily routine. These diagnoses had accumulated slowly, beginning six years after she left an emotionally and financially abusive marriage.

During those years, Lenora had no regular healthcare provider and few supports, and she coped by working long hours, suppressing emotion, and ignoring her own physical discomfort. What appeared to be lifestyle-related conditions were, in fact, the long-term outcomes of prolonged stress activation, disrupted eating and sleep patterns, and chronic nervous system dysregulation.

When she finally entered therapy, Lenora was exhausted, overwhelmed, and unsure how to regain control over her daily life. Sessions focused not just on disease management, but on helping her rebuild safe and sustainable routines from the inside out. The therapist introduced visual planning tools, flexible scheduling, and strategies to scaffold health behaviors without triggering shame. Regulation supports included paced breathing, guided movement before complex tasks, and tools for managing emotional activation during family conflict. Over time, therapy also helped Lenora explore the link between her health symptoms and her trauma history, using narrative reflection, cognitive reframing, and values-based decision making. Unlike standard care models that treat chronic illness as isolated pathology, occupational therapy recognized that Lenora's functional challenges were rooted in her body's long-standing adaptations to stress and survival. Early intervention could have mitigated the progression of disease, but even now, a trauma-responsive approach helped restore engagement, choice, and hope.

Violence has been linked to significantly higher rates of cardiovascular disease, obesity, metabolic syndrome, and Type 2 diabetes in women. These outcomes are driven by a combination of chronic stress, cortisol disruption, poor sleep, limited access to care, and, often, health avoidance due to fear or medical mistrust. Some survivors may also develop disordered eating or compulsive exercise patterns in response to trauma, further complicating metabolic regulation. Pain is another common thread. Fibromyalgia, migraines, and complex regional pain syndrome often emerge in women with unresolved trauma histories, particularly those who experienced early or prolonged abuse. These conditions can create cyclical occupational withdrawal, where the absence of structure or activity further intensifies pain and reduces participation.

Occupational therapy can intervene by helping women reestablish safe, graded routines that do not rely on pain elimination. For Teresa, this meant anchoring her day with what she called "low-demand wins"—predictable, meaningful tasks that didn't activate performance pressure or sensory overload. She and her therapist co-designed a "capacity map" instead of a standard daily planner. This visual aid used color-coded windows based on Teresa's energy patterns (rather than time slots), allowing her to choose tasks when her body was most available for engagement. Laundry became a two-step activity split between days. Phone calls were reserved for "green energy" hours. When flares occurred, the map helped her reframe modification as adaptability, not failure.

Sleep disruption, a frequent complaint among trauma survivors with metabolic or inflammatory conditions, was addressed through environmental scripting. Instead of starting with standard sleep hygiene advice, the OT conducted a sensory scan of Teresa's bedtime space, identifying overbright lighting and unpredictable noise from a neighbor's unit as key arousal triggers. Together, they developed a tactile-based downregulation routine using a warm compress, dim amber lighting, and a grounding playlist with low-frequency tones. These cues were layered with a transitional activity—putting away folded towels—which signaled safety and closure without emotional intensity.

For nutritional re-engagement, OT addressed not meal prep alone, but Teresa's emotional and sensory relationship with food. She had developed rigid rules about when and what she could eat, shaped by years of control-oriented coping. Her therapist did not immediately challenge the rules. Instead, they explored the function behind them—safety, predictability, and agency—and reframed nutrition not around macros, but around nervous system needs. Meals became "stability anchors," and the focus shifted to choosing foods that felt warming, easy to digest, and emotionally neutral. The kitchen space was also adapted: instead of long cooking sessions, OT introduced a three-bowl system (prep, eat, clean) to break tasks into manageable phases that supported follow-through without overwhelm.

In movement planning, traditional exercise goals were replaced by "mobility moments" tied to function. Rather than prescribing 30 minutes of walking, the therapist helped Teresa link movement to roles she still valued such as watering plants on the balcony, stretching while heating tea, or using a step stool to rearrange books for a reading nook. These low-load, role-based movements supported circulation, joint mobility, and body awareness without triggering pain escalation. Each was monitored not only for physical response but for affective feedback, felt easeful, tolerable, or emotionally charged—and the plan adjusted accordingly.

Ultimately, occupational therapy in this context is not just about pain or fatigue management. It is about re-establishing rhythm, safety, and meaning within the nervous system's bandwidth. For survivors like Teresa, effective care hinges on precision: aligning interventions with sensory thresholds, emotional history, and daily life constraints, while avoiding the common trap of "fixing" what is, in fact, a well-adapted survival system. With clinical creativity and relational depth, therapists can offer not only relief but repair—supporting women to live in bodies that no longer feel like battlegrounds, but like homes.

Physical Injury and Long-Term Structural Damage

Not all violence leaves visible marks. Many of the most debilitating injuries experienced by survivors are internal, cumulative, or entirely missed at the time they occur. In women, physical trauma resulting from intimate partner violence, sexual assault, and other forms of gendered harm frequently leads to orthopedic injuries, pelvic damage, neurological impairment, and traumatic brain injuries—yet these are often underdiagnosed, undertreated, or excluded from the survivor's medical record altogether.

Estimates suggest that up to 92 percent of injuries from intimate partner violence occur to the head, neck, and face, and recent studies indicate that one in four women who experience ongoing partner violence has sustained at least one brain injury. These injuries are particularly underrecognized in women, who are less likely than men to be screened for concussion or TBI when presenting with cognitive or emotional symptoms.

Gender disparities also exist in post-injury care, with women more frequently misdiagnosed with anxiety or depression when functional deficits stem from unacknowledged physical trauma. For occupational therapists, recognizing and responding to these injuries requires a lens that is both clinical and trauma-responsive—one that considers not only what happened to the body, but how that injury was received, reported, and documented. Therapists should be alert to subtle indicators such as delayed response time, difficulty with visual tracking, light sensitivity, unexplained dizziness, or inconsistent motor planning that may point to undiagnosed brain injury. Reports of pelvic discomfort during transfers or hesitancy with toileting and grooming tasks may also indicate trauma to the pelvic floor. If a client struggles to sequence basic routines, avoids head movement, or frequently loses track of conversation flow, these may signal neurological disruption rather than cognitive fatigue alone. Trauma-responsive occupational therapy does not assume a complete history—it listens to the body, observes patterns in occupational engagement, and integrates clinical reasoning with sensitivity to what may never have been disclosed.

Traumatic Brain Injury and Neurological Sequelae

When Elizabeth Foster, a 48-year-old high school art teacher, began occupational therapy after a reported fall down the stairs, her referral focused on safety during dressing and bathing following a mild traumatic brain injury. But during ADL retraining, the therapist noticed behaviors that went beyond physical precaution. Elizabeth hesitated before entering the bathroom, startled at sudden sounds, and repeatedly apologized for taking too long, even when tasks were completed safely. When asked to select clothing, she froze mid-decision and later disclosed feeling anxious in enclosed spaces. Her medical history included past urgent care visits for migraines and dizziness, yet no imaging had ever been completed. The therapist paused retraining goals and shifted toward a trauma-informed approach—introducing step-by-step visual cues, minimizing verbal corrections, and creating a consistent routine that began each session with three minutes of guided breathing paired with light hand movement exercises. These brief regulation practices helped orient Elizabeth to time and space, reduce anticipatory anxiety, and prepare her nervous system for task engagement. With Elizabeth's consent, the therapist also advocated for a neurological consultation, recognizing that untreated symptoms of brain injury were likely layered with unresolved trauma.

Traumatic brain injury is one of the most overlooked physical consequences of violence against women. Although TBI is frequently associated with sports or military contexts, recent research has revealed that intimate partner violence is one of the leading causes of brain injury among women worldwide. A 2022 study published in *The Lancet Public Health* estimated that over 24 million women in the United States alone have experienced at least one TBI resulting from partner violence, often through direct blows to the head, strangulation, falls, or violent shaking. Despite these numbers, most survivors never receive imaging, formal diagnosis, or rehabilitative care.

The underdiagnosis of TBI in women is shaped by gendered clinical assumptions. Symptoms such as memory lapses, executive dysfunction, irritability, dizziness, and fatigue are frequently dismissed or misattributed to stress, menopause, or mood disorders. Strangulation in particular—a common tactic of control in abusive relationships—can lead to hypoxic brain injury even in the absence of visible trauma, yet it is rarely screened for during emergency or follow-up care. Women may also minimize or normalize their symptoms, either out of fear of retaliation or because cognitive disruption has become part of their daily life.

The long-term occupational consequences of TBI in this context are significant. Survivors may struggle with attention to task, organizing daily routines, regulating emotional responses, or tolerating sensory input—all of which can interfere with work, caregiving, and independent living. These challenges may arise gradually or fluctuate over time, making it difficult for survivors to explain or anticipate their own limitations. For occupational therapists, the role is not only to support functional recovery, but to recognize TBI symptoms that have been previously ignored and create treatment plans that honor the survivor's pace, context, and safety.

Effective interventions may include memory aids, energy pacing, visual cueing, and simplified task environments. Therapists should use observational tools and trauma-sensitive communication to identify cognitive barriers and avoid assumptions based on medical documentation alone. In cases where formal TBI diagnosis is absent, therapists can still address the lived impact of cognitive disruption through contextual performance-based assessments. By reframing TBI as both a physical and relational injury, OT can provide both functional strategies and validation for survivors who have been living with invisible damage for years.

Pelvic, Visceral, and Orthopedic Trauma

Michelle Brooks, a 32-year-old elementary school principal, was referred to pelvic floor occupational therapy after years of unresolved dyspareunia—pain during or after sexual intercourse—that had not improved despite multiple consultations with gynecologists and urologists. During the initial evaluation, she maintained a professional demeanor but sat stiffly in her chair, her voice overly controlled. As the therapist introduced the pelvic floor assessment process, Michelle became increasingly withdrawn, avoiding direct questions about symptoms and tensing during guided breathing exercises. Although the referral described chronic pelvic pain, the therapist noticed signs of distress, such as rigid posture, flat affect, and a tendency to deflect whenever care touched on internal awareness. Recognizing the possibility of trauma, the therapist paused the session, provided clear choices about next steps, and introduced a gentle grounding strategy using rhythmic tapping and verbal pacing. As trust developed, Michelle disclosed a history of sexual coercion in her early twenties, a detail absent from her medical record. Her therapy plan shifted to emphasize safety, emotional regulation, and choice-centered body awareness, focusing less on pelvic correction and more on restoring autonomy and comfort within her own body.

Violence against women often involves targeted injury to the abdomen, pelvis, and musculoskeletal system—yet these injuries are frequently overlooked, underreported, or explained away as unrelated conditions. Survivors of sexual violence may live with chronic pelvic pain, dyspareunia, incontinence, or pelvic organ prolapse without ever disclosing the origin of their symptoms. In some cases, women have been repeatedly referred to gastrointestinal or gynecological specialists with no resolution, because the root of their dysfunction—violence—is never identified.

Physical trauma to the visceral organs may present later as gastrointestinal dysregulation, interstitial cystitis, or constipation that impacts daily function. These conditions can significantly disrupt a woman's occupational life, particularly in roles involving caregiving, work, or community participation. Functional limitations may include difficulty with toileting, fatigue related to chronic discomfort, or avoidance of environments where access to restrooms or privacy is limited.

Orthopedic injuries are also common. Rib fractures, wrist sprains, dislocated shoulders, or cervical strain may result from being grabbed, pushed, or thrown. For many women, these injuries do not lead to emergency care due to fear, coercion, or lack of access. When care is eventually sought, it may occur long after the injury, leading to persistent pain, joint instability, or altered range of motion that affects mobility and self-care. Therapists must be alert to the history behind "old" orthopedic injuries and recognize that a delayed presentation may reflect more than just time—it may reflect a trauma history.

In occupational therapy, addressing these injuries requires a trauma-informed approach that centers consent, predictability, and dignity. Therapists may support clients in modifying toileting and hygiene routines, implementing pelvic floor-safe movement plans, or using assistive devices that reduce strain while preserving autonomy. For some survivors, even seemingly benign physical tasks can be triggering, especially if they replicate the postures or environments associated with violence. Intervention must always be client-paced, with adaptations that are both functionally appropriate and emotionally safe. See Table 7.1 for key differences in how brain injury, pelvic, visceral, and orthopedic conditions may present in survivors of violence compared to non-trauma-related cases, along with examples of trauma-sensitive questions occupational therapists can use during evaluation.

For women who have survived violence, the body often becomes both a site of injury and a site of silence. Traumatic brain injuries may be minimized or reframed as emotional instability, while pelvic pain and visceral dysfunction are quietly absorbed into daily routines without explanation. Orthopedic injuries may heal physically but continue to shape movement patterns, pain tolerance, and emotional responses to certain postures or tasks. These conditions do not always present as linear or logical. Instead, they are filtered through years of threat, self-protection, and medical dismissal. For occupational therapists, the ability to differentiate between injury rooted in violence and that which stems from other causes is not just a diagnostic skill—it is a form of advocacy. Recognizing these patterns allows clinicians to ask the right questions, pace interventions with sensitivity, and restore function in ways that do not retraumatize. When physical symptoms are shaped by coercion, assault, or systemic harm,

Table 7.1 Differentiating Health Conditions Related to Trauma and Violence from Non-Trauma Presentations

Condition Type	Typical Presentation Without Trauma History	Common Presentation in Survivors of Violence	Trauma-Sensitive Questions for OT Evaluation
Traumatic Brain Injury	Reports of recent impact, visible trauma, formal diagnosis via imaging, straightforward symptom awareness	Delayed or no diagnosis, vague or minimized symptoms, memory gaps, emotional dysregulation, fear of "getting it wrong"	"Have you noticed changes in focus, memory, or mood that others have dismissed or misunderstood?"
Pelvic Pain/ Dysfunction	Linked to childbirth, aging, or known musculoskeletal cause; relatively open discussion of symptoms	Discomfort discussing symptoms, unexplained avoidance of toileting or intimacy, body detachment	"Are there parts of your daily routine— like dressing or using the bathroom—that feel more difficult or uncomfortable than they used to?"
Visceral or GI Distress	Related to diet, infection, or anatomical issue; typically disclosed and medically followed	Functional GI symptoms with unclear medical findings; linked to emotional stress, fear of meals or food prep	"When symptoms like pain or cramping show up, are there patterns in your routine or stress that seem connected?"
Orthopedic Injury	Clear mechanism of injury (e.g., sports, fall), consistent timeline, focus on joint or muscle function	History of "old injury," unclear mechanism, hypervigilance during movement, inconsistent performance under pressure	"Are there movements or tasks that feel safe in some settings but overwhelming or painful in others?"

rehabilitation must go beyond biomechanics—it must rebuild trust, autonomy, and control through every therapeutic encounter.

Reproductive and Sexual Health Consequences

Violence against women has profound and often unacknowledged consequences on reproductive and sexual health. While injuries and trauma to these systems may be acute, their effects are frequently chronic, showing up not only in gynecological and obstetric complications, but also in the routines and relationships that make up a woman's daily life. Women who have experienced sexual assault, coercion, or long-term control often disengage from healthcare systems entirely, avoiding reproductive screenings, birth control management, or sexual activity due to fear, shame, or unresolved trauma (Güler et al., 2024). These disruptions are compounded by provider bias and clinical environments that fail to create emotional safety or recognize the signs of sexual trauma.

Occupational therapy, apart from pelvic floor rehabilitation, is not typically at the forefront of care for women experiencing reproductive or sexual health challenges, yet the consequences of violence in this area are profoundly occupational. Survivors may experience disruptions in dressing, hygiene, intimacy, toileting, and in fulfilling romantic or caregiving roles. For women whose reproductive trauma intersects with childbirth, infertility, or chronic pelvic conditions, the ripple effects often reach into identity, regulation, and routine. Therapists working in any setting must be equipped to recognize these challenges and respond with interventions that are both clinically grounded and trauma responsive.

Sexually Transmitted Infections and Reproductive Trauma

Women who have experienced violence are at significantly higher risk of acquiring sexually transmitted infections, including Human Immunodeficiency Virus, Human Papillomavirus, gonorrhea, and chlamydia. This risk is not only due to forced sexual contact, but also to the ways coercive control disrupts access to protection, consent, and medical care. In abusive relationships, contraception may be withheld or sabotaged. Appointments may be canceled, tracked, or used as a point of threat. Even after the violence ends, survivors often avoid sexual health screenings due to discomfort with invasive procedures, fear of judgment, or shame tied to prior trauma.

Sexually transmitted infections that go untreated can have long-term occupational consequences. Chronic pelvic pain, fatigue, urinary complications, and discomfort during movement or intimacy are common. These symptoms affect routines related to hygiene, toileting, dressing, and rest, and may also impact relationships and self-perception. Women may begin to withdraw from valued activities—not because of pain alone, but because of how trauma has altered their relationship to their body.

Occupational therapists can offer critical support in navigating these consequences. This includes adapting hygiene and toileting routines to reduce discomfort, introducing noninvasive sensory strategies to restore a sense of safety, and supporting access to care by helping clients plan, prepare for, and recover from appointments. Therapists may also use visual supports, scripting, or graded exposure to help clients resume routines related to sexual health. For some, this work will include reconnection to intimacy in ways that feel physically and emotionally safe. For others, it may involve supporting abstinence or disengagement from sexual roles while maintaining autonomy and dignity.

Obstetric and Postpartum Complications in the Context of Violence

Interpersonal violence during the perinatal period is a major but underrecognized contributor to poor maternal and neonatal outcomes. Women exposed to chronic stress and caregiving strain are more likely to develop autoimmune rheumatic diseases and adverse obstetric outcomes (Parks et al., 2023). Survivors are at significantly higher risk of complications such as placental abruption, preterm labor, low birth weight, and perinatal loss. Physical assaults to the abdomen, forced sex during pregnancy, and prolonged exposure to threat-related stress can lead to life-threatening conditions (Bookwalter et al., 2020), yet women are rarely screened for violence in obstetric care. In many cases, survivors navigate pregnancy in silence, fearing retaliation, dismissal, or involvement from child protective services if they disclose.

The risk does not end at birth. Survivors of violence are more likely to experience postpartum hemorrhage, surgical complications, infections, and delayed wound healing—often while caring for a newborn in environments that feel emotionally or physically unsafe. For some, the postpartum period is marked by repeated hospital visits, unrecognized infections, or unmanaged pain that interferes with daily function. For others, the trauma is institutional: being ignored during labor, not believed about pain, or subject to coercive interventions without informed consent. These forms of violence may not leave visible injuries, but they leave enduring occupational disruption.

Maternal Health Disparities and Medical Trauma

Pregnant and postpartum women who experience violence also face heightened medical risk due to systemic failures in maternal healthcare. Black, Indigenous, and other women of color are disproportionately affected by maternal mortality and morbidity, often due to a combination of delayed care, provider bias, and lack of culturally responsive services. When survivors present with fatigue, dizziness, wound pain, or functional decline, these symptoms are too often dismissed as exaggeration or labeled as anxiety, rather than explored through the lens of medical trauma or delayed healing.

Occupational therapists can play a critical role in addressing the functional and psychosocial impact of obstetric and postpartum complications, particularly for survivors of violence. Therapy may involve task-specific modifications to reduce strain on healing tissues, such as teaching adaptive strategies for infant lifting, breastfeeding positions that minimize abdominal pressure, or toileting routines that account for pelvic floor pain. Therapists can support clients in pacing household and caregiving tasks to manage anemia-related fatigue or infection-related discomfort, while promoting postural alignment and joint protection in cases of pelvic girdle dysfunction. For clients recovering from coercive or traumatic birth experiences, occupational therapy can also facilitate narrative processing through structured storytelling, values-based activity planning, and safe reengagement in daily occupations that restore a sense of agency. By integrating trauma-informed strategies with evidence-based rehabilitation, occupational therapy helps bridge the gap between medical recovery and meaningful life participation during a period of profound vulnerability.

Institutional Harm and Postpartum Occupational Disruption

For many survivors, the postpartum experience is shaped not only by physical recovery but by the lingering impact of institutional harm. Some women report being denied adequate pain relief, pressured into procedures without full consent, or treated with suspicion when expressing distress. These experiences reflect systemic violence that can influence how a woman engages with healthcare, parenting, and her own body long after hospital discharge. Reactions such as avoiding medical appointments, withdrawing from caregiving routines, or showing discomfort during physical touch may stem from unresolved trauma rather than disinterest or noncompliance.

Occupational therapists are uniquely positioned to support healing in these complex contexts by creating therapeutic environments that rebuild trust, foster predictability, and emphasize personal control (Jackson & Jewell, 2021). Support may include scripting and rehearsal for follow-up visits, positioning adaptations that reduce exposure and increase comfort during infant care, and daily routines that align with emotional readiness as well as physical recovery. Expressive interventions—such as guided journaling, story mapping, or symbolic object creation—can support narrative processing and help women reclaim their postpartum identity. For incarcerated or formerly incarcerated women, who often face elevated risks of trauma, isolation, and healthcare neglect, occupational therapy can support role continuity, individualized care planning, and the safe integration of maternal tasks within restricted environments. In all cases, recovery should be defined not by institutional timelines or productivity, but by a woman's own sense of safety, dignity, and agency.

Reproductive and postpartum complications linked to violence are often framed as isolated health events, when in reality they are embedded in longer histories of control, harm, and medical dismissal. For many survivors, the postpartum period is not simply one of recovery, but of reckoning—with the body, with systems, and with roles that now feel unstable or unsafe. Occupational therapy offers a pathway toward function that centers not only physical healing, but the restoration of autonomy, dignity, and daily coherence. As we turn to the psychiatric and cognitive consequences of violence, it becomes even more clear

Table 7.2 Occupational Therapy Strategies for Reproductive and Postpartum Complications Linked to Violence

Violence-Linked Health Issue	Functional Consequences	Trauma-Informed OT Strategies
Postpartum wound complications in context of assault or unsafe home	Hesitancy to move freely at home, toileting difficulties, delay in healing due to environmental stress	ADL modification for hygiene and toileting, movement plans that minimize pain and exposure, coordination with nursing or wound care in home settings
History of sexual violence triggering birth trauma response	Avoidance of infant care, distress with pelvic exams, difficulty with breastfeeding or body positioning	Choice-based caregiving routines, adaptive positioning for feeding, scripting for clinical visits, graded exposure to body-based tasks
Intimate partner violence during pregnancy	Unpredictable schedule disruptions, poor prenatal care access, lack of safe rest or nutrition	Routine building for sleep and nourishment, mobile-based appointment prompts, safety-integrated ADL planning
Forced or coerced birth interventions (e.g., withheld consent, dismissal)	Emotional withdrawal, mistrust of medical providers, fear of future pregnancy	Medical system navigation coaching, narrative reconstruction work, referral to advocacy groups or trauma doulas
Violence-linked miscarriage or perinatal loss	Profound grief, disengagement from social and occupational roles, disrupted sleep and eating routines	Grief-informed scheduling, expressive occupations, reintegration into meaningful routines with attention to pacing
Coercive control impacting postpartum follow-up	Missed appointments, underreporting of symptoms, passive healthcare compliance	Visual health tracking tools, collaborative planning with social work or legal supports, scripting to reclaim agency
Chronic pelvic pain from prior assault or obstetric trauma	Sexual avoidance, disrupted toileting, reluctance to seek help	Sensory-based body work, pelvic-safe mobility plans, integration of trauma-informed pelvic health referrals

that the body and mind are not separate domains—they are co-regulated systems that require care rooted in safety, precision, and trust. Table 7.2 outlines trauma-informed occupational therapy strategies used to address reproductive and post-partum complications in the context of violence.

Psychiatric and Cognitive Health Consequences

Violence is not only a bodily threat—it is a sustained neurological assault that reshapes how a woman experiences memory, mood, attention, and identity. Long after physical wounds have healed, survivors of violence often live with invisible symptoms that affect every domain of daily life. The psychiatric effects of violence can include major depressive disorder, generalized anxiety, posttraumatic stress disorder, dissociation, and suicidal ideation. In many cases, these conditions co-occur and evolve over time, altering the survivor's ability to function across roles and environments. Yet mental health consequences of violence are frequently mischaracterized as personality flaws or treatment resistance, rather than recognized as rational responses to prolonged threat and disruption.

In parallel, many survivors experience cognitive disruption that does not meet diagnostic criteria for brain injury but significantly interferes with daily functioning. These impairments in attention, working memory, task initiation, or emotional modulation are often dismissed—especially in women—as disorganization, burnout, or noncompliance. When viewed through a trauma-informed lens, however, these disruptions are recognized as downstream effects of dysregulated nervous systems, chronic cortisol exposure, and unresolved hypervigilance. Occupational therapists are uniquely equipped to address these psychiatric and cognitive consequences not as pathology to be fixed, but as adaptive responses that require reorganization of routine, rhythm, and environment.

Post-Traumatic Stress Disorder, Complex Trauma, and Mood Disorders

PTSD is one of the most common psychiatric outcomes among women who have experienced violence. While PTSD can follow a single traumatic incident, many survivors, especially those subjected to intimate partner violence, sexual abuse, or coercive control—develop more diffuse and persistent symptoms over time. Complex trauma does not always look like flashbacks or panic attacks. It can surface as difficulty managing emotions, disconnection from self or others, chronic hyperarousal, or a sense of emptiness that undercuts daily life. These patterns often interfere with a woman's ability to carry out routines, maintain roles, or feel capable in the spaces she once moved through with confidence.

Depression and anxiety frequently accompany trauma, especially when compounded by exhaustion, grief, or a long history of invalidation. These conditions don't just affect how someone feels, they change what they can manage. Even simple tasks like preparing meals or making appointments can feel overwhelming when the brain is still wired for survival. Survivors often describe a fog that is hard to name and harder to work through. What looks like disinterest or low motivation may in fact be the aftershock of trying to function while carrying invisible weight.

Occupational therapy offers a distinct contribution to trauma recovery by translating emotional healing into functional, concrete action. For women with PTSD or complex trauma, therapists can use task grading to reintroduce daily activities that feel manageable and affirming. For example, instead of assigning a full morning routine, a therapist might begin with helping the client identify one task such as brushing teeth or preparing a preferred breakfast that feels safe and achievable. Activity analysis allows the therapist to identify and modify specific sensory, cognitive, or emotional triggers embedded in those tasks. For a woman who becomes overwhelmed with appointments, therapy might involve scripting phone calls, rehearsing communication scenarios, or integrating visual scheduling systems that reduce decision fatigue.

For clients with mood disorders and executive dysfunction, therapists can use backward chaining to support task initiation or embed mindfulness-based strategies into occupations such as cooking, walking, or creative projects. In each case, the focus is not just on completing a task but restoring a sense of agency in how, when, and why it is done. Occupational therapy can also facilitate identity reconstruction through values clarification, narrative journaling, or symbolic object creation that helps women reclaim roles lost during prolonged survival. These interventions help transform abstract therapeutic goals into lived, embodied routines that connect emotional insight with meaningful daily participation.

Functional Manifestations of Trauma and Occupational Therapy Response

In survivors of violence, trauma often reveals itself through subtle patterns in occupational performance that are easily overlooked in conventional assessment. These may include excessive time spent organizing a simple task, reluctance to begin activities that require self-direction, or heightened agitation when routines are interrupted. A woman may complete a cooking task but insist on repeating steps in a fixed order with visible tension, reflecting a need for control in response to past unpredictability. Others may reject offers of help or defer entirely to the therapist during sessions, indicating disruptions in autonomy or conditioned compliance from past coercion. Difficulty tolerating silence, persistent scanning of the room, or emotional detachment during meaningful occupations can reflect underlying hypervigilance or dissociation. Therapists must observe not only whether tasks are completed but how the individual modulates affect, tolerates uncertainty, and relates to the activity itself. By analyzing these nuanced behaviors, occupational therapists can differentiate performance difficulties rooted in trauma from those stemming from cognitive or physical limitations, and design interventions that prioritize safety, relational repair, and voluntary engagement.

Cognitive Impacts and Executive Dysfunction

Survivors of violence frequently experience disruptions in executive functioning, even in the absence of a diagnosed brain injury. Difficulties with focus, memory, decision making, and organization are common and yet often misunderstood. These challenges may not present as dramatic impairments, but as subtle, chronic barriers to everyday tasks: forgetting appointments, losing track of steps in a routine, or feeling unable to initiate even simple actions. When the nervous system has spent years in survival mode, cognitive efficiency is often sacrificed for vigilance and self-protection.

Research suggests that repeated exposure to trauma alters the function of brain regions responsible for planning, working memory, and emotional regulation. The prefrontal cortex may become less accessible during moments of stress, while the amygdala remains overactive. In practice, this means that under pressure—or even in unfamiliar environments—survivors may freeze, shut down, or struggle to follow through. These are not signs of resistance. They are signs that the brain is prioritizing threat detection over task completion.

For occupational therapists, this cognitive profile requires a shift in how executive function is assessed and supported. Survivors may do well in a structured clinic but falter at home, where triggers are present and unpredictability is high. Therapists can provide functional assessments in context, identify breakdowns in real-world performance, and design interventions that compensate without pathologizing. This may include external cueing systems, simplified task flows, or sensory-regulated workspaces. Just as importantly, therapists can help clients build cognitive resilience—not by pushing harder, but by aligning tasks with capacity, pacing demands, and teaching strategies for navigating overload before it becomes shutdown.

Executive dysfunction in survivors of violence is not a personal failure. It is a physiological adaptation to chronic threat, and it deserves the same nuance, creativity, and clinical rigor we apply to any other form of cognitive disruption. With the right scaffolding, survivors can rebuild confidence in their ability to manage, plan, and participate—not as they once did, but in ways that reflect the person they are becoming. See Table 7.3 for examples of psychiatric and cognitive health consequences commonly experienced by survivors of violence, and corresponding occupational therapy strategies to support function, regulation, and daily engagement.

Even in the absence of a formal psychiatric diagnosis or confirmed brain injury, survivors of violence often carry enduring patterns of emotional and cognitive disruption that affect how they live, work, and connect with others. A woman may avoid cooking not because she lacks interest, but because the smell of oil on the stove triggers memories of past harm. She may miss appointments or deadlines because initiating tasks in the morning requires a level of emotional regulation her nervous system cannot yet sustain. Some survivors

Table 7.3 Occupational Therapy Strategies for Psychiatric and Cognitive Health Impacts of Violence

Presentation	Functional Impact	Occupational Therapy Strategies
Complex trauma (emotional dysregulation, hypervigilance, or detachment)	Difficulty maintaining routines, emotional overwhelm in daily tasks, disrupted relational engagement	Establish regulatory anchors in daily schedule, use co-regulation and grounding, integrate values-based activity planning
Depression and grief related to violence	Fatigue, withdrawal from roles, lack of interest in meaningful occupations	Behavioral activation rooted in choice and pacing, modified routine building, reintroduction of restorative activities
Anxiety or fear-based avoidance	Avoidance of tasks or environments, reduced participation in self-care or community roles	Graded exposure plans, safety mapping, collaborative problem-solving to reduce perceived threat and restore agency
Executive dysfunction (task initiation, planning, working memory)	Missed steps in multi-tasking, disorganized routines, reduced task follow-through	External cueing systems, visual task sequencing, scripting and pacing supports adapted to fluctuating capacity
Medical mistrust and emotional reactivity in care settings	Missed appointments, difficulty following through on treatment plans, shutdown in clinical interactions	Appointment scripting, healthcare system navigation supports, co-authored documentation language for medical teams

describe feeling numb in caregiving roles, not due to apathy, but because their bodies are still conditioned to suppress emotion for self-protection. These symptoms are shaped not just by what happened, but by what was required to survive—and what was denied in the aftermath, whether that was safety, support, or space to heal without being judged.

When occupational therapists respond with attunement, structure, and flexibility, they create more than a care plan; they build a framework for rebuilding agency. That might mean replacing rigid schedules with flexible scaffolding, introducing task cues that reduce decision fatigue, or offering language for describing internal states that have long been unnamed. It may also mean honoring a survivor's pause, rather than pushing for performance, and adapting environments so that the nervous system can begin to feel what safety actually is. These clinical acts are not small. They are invitations to re-enter life with a renewed sense of ownership and on the survivor's own terms.

System Navigation and Medical Mistrust

A 2024 systematic review published in *Child Abuse & Neglect* identified multiple socioecological barriers that prevent survivors of childhood sexual abuse from disclosing their experiences, including fear of not being believed, emotional avoidance, and mistrust of authority figures. These same patterns persist in adulthood, especially when survivors of violence interact with healthcare systems (Latiff et al., 2024). For many women, accessing medical care is not a neutral act. It is a process that often requires survivors to assess risk, anticipate invalidation, and weigh whether disclosure will lead to support or further harm. Studies have shown that women with histories of intimate partner violence, sexual assault, or systemic abuse are significantly more likely to delay care, avoid routine screenings, or disengage from follow-up services, particularly when they have previously felt dismissed or blamed by providers. These patterns are not evidence of poor compliance. They are rational adaptations to systems that have failed to recognize the long-term consequences of violence on health and behavior.

Medical mistrust among survivors is especially pronounced in women from historically marginalized communities. Black, Indigenous, immigrant, and LGBTQIA+ women are more likely to experience implicit bias, language exclusion, and provider skepticism—barriers that often compound existing trauma and reduce the likelihood of returning for care. When a woman is told that her pain is exaggerated or that her history is irrelevant to her current symptoms, she may begin to edit what she says in medical settings, not out of avoidance, but as a form of self-protection. Over time, these experiences accumulate and result in reduced access to care, poorer health outcomes, and a pervasive sense of vulnerability within healthcare systems.

Occupational therapists can play a critical role in helping survivors re-engage with healthcare in ways that feel structured, supported, and empowering. This may involve preparing clients for upcoming appointments using scripting or visual mapping, developing tools that track symptoms in nonclinical language, or identifying moments in care that have previously felt unsafe. Therapists may also serve as intermediaries, facilitating communication between survivors and their healthcare teams to ensure that histories of violence are acknowledged in functionally meaningful ways. In practice, this could mean recommending flexible scheduling for medical visits to accommodate trauma-related fatigue, helping survivors request consistent providers, or addressing sensory sensitivities that make clinical environments feel overwhelming.

Supporting medical system navigation is not limited to task management. It requires occupational therapists to understand medical mistrust as a consequence of trauma exposure and to frame advocacy as a core part of treatment. By providing structure around health-related routines, clarifying decision-making processes, and naming the emotional toll of clinical encounters, therapists can increase both access to and engagement with essential services. When care is approached through a relational and trauma-informed lens, occupational therapy becomes more than a support—it becomes a corrective experience that allows survivors to participate in health-related decision making without fear of dismissal or retraumatization.

Occupational Therapy Approaches to Stability and Autonomy

Violence against women leaves an imprint that extends far beyond the moment of harm. It reconfigures physiological systems—disrupting circadian rhythms, overactivating the stress response, and impairing immune, endocrine, and cardiovascular regulation. These biological shifts do not remain confined to the body. They reverberate into how a woman eats, sleeps, works, and moves through the routines that once sustained her. For many survivors, the experience of illness—chronic pain, fatigue, digestive instability, cognitive fog—is inseparable from the experience of trauma. Yet clinical interventions too often isolate one domain from the other, overlooking the essential question: how does a woman live, and what does her body now require to feel stable?

Occupational therapy is uniquely positioned to answer that question, not by focusing on productivity, but by addressing the functional implications of dysregulation across systems (Goldstein et al., 2024). Research has demonstrated that exposure to interpersonal violence is linked to disruptions in autonomic balance, inflammatory load, and hormonal rhythms (Baldwin-White, 2019; Berke et al., 2023). These physiological stress cascades impact occupational performance in subtle but persistent ways: reduced stamina, diminished stress tolerance, sleep fragmentation, and delayed recovery from exertion. A trauma-informed occupational therapist begins by assessing not only what tasks are difficult, but when, why, and under what conditions. Instead of starting with performance goals, therapy may begin with recalibrating daily energy distribution or identifying physiological thresholds beyond which function begins to unravel.

Stability emerges when the body can anticipate its demands without tipping into survival mode. Therapists can co-create routines that prioritize regulatory anchors—periods of rest, sensory integration, structured nutrition, or guided movement—to reduce allostatic load. These routines are not generalized wellness advice. They are precision-based strategies tailored to the survivor's clinical presentation and occupational context. For example, a woman managing trauma-related irritable bowel symptoms may benefit from environmental control during meals and flexible work schedules that reduce social exposure during flare-ups. Another navigating post-traumatic insomnia might build in a layered evening sequence: visual dimming, thermal regulation, and nonverbal tasks designed to signal neurological downshifting. These are not lifestyle enhancements. They are recovery tools.

Autonomy—true autonomy—requires more than informed decision-making. It requires a body that can metabolize information, regulate arousal, and support sustained engagement without collapse. As women re-enter roles that once defined them—caregiver, professional, partner—occupational therapy helps renegotiate those roles with clearer boundaries, new pacing, and structures that reflect current capacities rather than prior demands. Tools such as values-based scheduling, body budgeting, and interoceptive mapping allow survivors to scaffold their days with intention and agency, even in the presence of chronic health conditions or residual trauma symptoms. Healing after violence is often framed in psychological or relational terms. But for many women, healing begins when their body becomes a predictable partner again. See Table 7.4 for examples of

Table 7.4 Occupational Therapy Strategies for System-Level Dysregulation Following Violence

Physiological System Affected	Trauma-Linked Dysregulation	Occupational Therapy Strategy
Autonomic Nervous System	Heightened arousal, poor vagal tone, sympathetic dominance (fight, flight, or freeze patterns)	Establish daily regulatory anchors (e.g., breath pacing, sensory modulation, structured transitions)
Endocrine System	Cortisol imbalance, hormonal dysregulation, fatigue, sleep-wake disruption	Map energy fluctuations and co-develop activity pacing; introduce pre-sleep routines to support melatonin regulation
Immune System	Chronic inflammation, autoimmune flare-ups, pain syndromes	Support energy conservation, symptom journaling, and adaptation of routines during flare periods
Gastrointestinal System	Irritable bowel symptoms, appetite loss or dysregulation, somatic stress responses	Modify food prep routines for safety and pacing, recommend private meal settings, support consistent nourishment
Musculoskeletal System	Pain sensitization, tension, disuse patterns, activity avoidance	Integrate graded movement, ergonomic supports, body mechanics training, and relaxation-based mobility interventions
Cognitive-Executive Function	Working memory disruption, task initiation difficulty, disorganized thinking	Use visual task plans, external cueing systems, decision-mapping, and context-sensitive structuring
Sleep-Wake Regulation	Delayed sleep onset, fragmented sleep, nonrestorative rest	Design sleep routines tied to sensory input, temperature, and pre-bed wind-down tasks tailored to nervous system needs

how occupational therapy strategies can be aligned with specific physiological systems affected by violence-related trauma, supporting both stabilization and functional reengagement (Khan, 2025).

These strategies translate directly into clinical care. For example, a woman navigating post-traumatic fatigue, chronic inflammation, and dysregulated cortisol patterns after years of intimate partner violence may struggle with morning disorientation, delayed task initiation, and poor follow-through on health routines. Rather than framing this as low motivation, the occupational therapist might implement targeted executive supports such as tiered task sequencing, voice-activated reminders linked to prescribed medications, and pre-assembled care kits that minimize decision burden. Sessions could also include training in compensatory energy conservation techniques—such as completing tasks from seated positions, task clustering during periods of increased alertness, and the use of environmental light cues to support consistent waking routines without overreliance on alarms. These adjustments are small in appearance but clinically significant in building reliability and engagement in daily roles.

In another case, a woman recovering from pelvic and orthopedic trauma after sexual assault may experience functional pain, muscle guarding, or aversion to routine physical movement, particularly when activities involve body exposure or internal awareness. The occupational therapist might introduce mirror-free dressing strategies, structured pelvic mobility exercises with external cueing instead of introspective instruction, or introduce bathing equipment that allows complete physical control over water temperature and flow. For women who avoid community spaces due to past surveillance or control, therapists can co-develop exposure plans that scaffold reentry, such as starting with brief, time-defined walks in predictable routes followed by low-stimulation environments like libraries or botanical gardens. These are not simply accommodations. They are precision-based interventions grounded in the understanding that occupational recovery after violence must account for the physiology of trauma, not just the narrative.

System-Level Advocacy and Health Equity

While individual recovery is critical, the broader landscape that shapes women's health after violence cannot be ignored. Interpersonal harm is compounded by institutional responses that often fail to recognize, document, or accommodate its occupational consequences. Women who have survived violence frequently navigate fragmented systems—silos between physical health, mental health, and social care—that not only overlook their trauma history but actively disrupt healing through procedural rigidity, racial or gender bias, and lack of continuity. Occupational therapists have a responsibility to not only treat the survivor in front of them, but to examine and challenge the structures that limit her access to meaningful care.

System-level advocacy in this context means interrogating how violence is—or is not—accounted for in the pathways that shape healthcare delivery, reimbursement, and policy. This includes advocating for trauma-informed screening practices during hospital intake, ensuring that histories of violence are considered during rehabilitation goal setting, and pushing for the inclusion of trauma-related diagnoses in medical documentation that affects access to services. For instance, a therapist working with a client recovering from repeated head injuries due to intimate partner violence may advocate for the coding of traumatic brain injury, rather than attributing symptoms solely to anxiety or non-specific fatigue—securing eligibility for cognitive rehabilitation services that would otherwise be denied.

Equity-focused occupational therapy also means elevating the lived realities of women who fall through the cracks of standard protocols. Therapists can participate in quality improvement teams, contribute to research on violence and occupational health outcomes, and collaborate with institutional partners to revise workflows that disadvantage survivors. In school-based settings, this might involve advocating for trauma-responsive behavior support plans rather than punitive interventions for students living with domestic instability. In home health, it could mean documenting not just a woman's ability to perform hygiene tasks, but the structural barriers—such as shared bathrooms with unsafe cohabitants—that inhibit participation. By naming and recording the occupational effects of violence in clinical language, therapists create documentation that has power beyond the therapy session.

Ultimately, health equity cannot be achieved without confronting the systemic forces that perpetuate violence-related harm. Occupational therapists, as experts in function, environment, and participation, are uniquely positioned to bridge the gap between individual recovery and structural reform. The work extends beyond one-on-one care—it includes reshaping how systems recognize trauma, allocate resources, and define recovery itself.

Case Vignette and Clinical Reflections

The long-term health impacts of violence are often diffuse, episodic, and easily overlooked in systems that prioritize acute illness or isolated diagnoses. Yet for many women, these consequences shape the pace and pattern of daily life, affecting everything from digestive regulation to executive functioning, immune response, and mobility. Pain may not follow anatomical logic. Fatigue may appear disconnected from activity. Symptoms often fluctuate with no clear biomedical cause, leading providers to label them as psychological or exaggerated. In this clinical gray area, occupational therapy becomes essential, not as a substitute for medical care, but as a lens through which complex, body-based trauma can be observed, named, and addressed in the context of function. The following cases illustrate how violence shapes disease progression and occupational performance, and how trauma-informed practice can translate that understanding into meaningful interventions.

Case Example 1: Nyla, Age 41—Chronic Health Decline and Fragmented Recovery After Intimate Partner Violence

Nyla, a 41-year-old mother of two, was referred to occupational therapy by her rheumatologist due to worsening fatigue, declining functional participation, and reported nonadherence to treatment plans. Her diagnoses included systemic lupus erythematosus, fibromyalgia, and irritable bowel syndrome—each accompanied by a long history of flare cycles, ER visits, and fragmented care. What her chart did not capture was the decade she spent in a violent relationship, during which she experienced repeated physical assaults, reproductive trauma, and prolonged emotional coercion. She had never disclosed the full scope of her history to any provider. "I just got good at saying 'fine', even when everything was falling apart," she said during her second therapy session.

Nyla described mornings as unpredictable and laborious, often requiring two hours to complete basic hygiene, dress, and prepare her children for school. Cooking had become intolerable due to pain and lightheadedness, and she avoided social or community activities due to fear of collapse or public embarrassment. The therapist initiated a multi-day occupational routine audit that helped identify key points of physiological dysregulation, including early morning temperature intolerance, postprandial fatigue, and hypersensitivity during ADLs that required bending or lifting. Intervention focused on preserving functional energy through targeted adaptations: sit-to-stand transfer supports in the kitchen and bathroom, thermoregulation layers to manage dysautonomia, and pain-responsive pacing cues linked to hygiene and meal preparation.

Recognizing that Nyla's health history had been repeatedly reframed as psychosomatic or noncompliant, the therapist supported her in preparing language she could use during provider visits—integrating functional observations into a structured symptom-impact matrix. Together, they drafted documentation that connected her occupational performance patterns (e.g., meal skipping due to anticipatory nausea, collapse in executive function after pain spikes) to underlying autonomic instability and trauma-related triggers. These notes were co-signed and submitted with her OT progress report, which emphasized occupation-based evidence of functional decline tied to trauma-related mechanisms, including probable central sensitization and post-exertional symptom exacerbation.

The therapist also directly contacted her rheumatologist and primary care provider, advocating for re-evaluation of diagnostic categories that had excluded Nyla from receiving cognitive rehabilitation and pelvic floor therapy. The communication highlighted how her occupational disengagement was not due to lack of interest or effort, but to untreated trauma sequelae that were interfering with activities essential to recovery. This reframing led to updated referrals and, for the first time in her care trajectory, formal recognition of trauma exposure as a clinically significant variable in her medical record.

Case Example 2: Ana, Age 37—Missed Diagnosis of Traumatic Brain Injury After Workplace Assault

Ana, a 37-year-old public transit employee, was referred to occupational therapy for support with "work stress and return-to-duty adjustment" following a workplace sexual assault that had occurred eight months prior. Although she had been medically cleared to return after an initial emergency room visit, she reported ongoing headaches, dizziness, irritability, and difficulty concentrating. Her supervisors had observed frequent errors in safety protocols and noted that Ana was increasingly withdrawn, often appearing confused or fatigued mid-shift. She had begun skipping meals, forgetting tasks, and experiencing what she described as "a complete shutdown" when too many instructions were given at once.

In her first two OT sessions, Ana minimized her symptoms, attributing them to anxiety and "not being the same person" since the assault. But through structured activity observation, the therapist noted indicators of post-concussive impairment, including reduced auditory tolerance, poor dual-task sequencing, and visual tracking delays. When asked about prior history, Ana revealed a past head injury from a physically abusive partner in her early twenties that was never formally treated. No provider had explored the possibility of cumulative brain injury, and Ana had been referred exclusively for mental health support.

Using the Rivermead Post-Concussion Symptoms Questionnaire and functional observation of job-simulated tasks, the therapist identified red flags for traumatic brain injury layered onto trauma-induced nervous system dysregulation. An interdisciplinary referral to a neuropsychologist was initiated, and OT documentation clearly articulated how Ana's current impairments were affecting her ability to meet essential job functions and maintain safe participation in her role. This documentation was key in securing accommodations, including modified shift lengths, protected sensory recovery breaks, and a gradual increase in task complexity.

The therapist also introduced occupational strategies to help Ana reestablish confidence and autonomy in daily life. These included structured checklists for morning routines, noise-reducing earwear for public transit environments, and external cueing tools to manage cognitive fatigue during transit inspections. With ongoing support, Ana began to reengage with her work identity in a way that felt safe and sustainable. Perhaps more importantly, she no longer saw her symptoms as weakness—but as signals her body had been trying to communicate all along.

Therapist Reflections on Clinical Decision Making

Nyla and Ana's stories reflect a reality that many women live but few healthcare systems fully recognize: the long-term health impacts of violence are complex, cumulative, and often mislabeled. What appeared on the surface as nonadherence, cognitive disorganization, or vague somatic complaints were, in fact, adaptive responses to chronic trauma and underacknowledged physiological disruption. In both cases, occupational therapy was not simply a supportive service—it was the clinical entry point where function, health, and trauma finally intersected.

For Nyla, the therapeutic focus was not on increasing productivity but on identifying how her body was communicating overload. The use of routine mapping, co-authored documentation, and provider advocacy allowed trauma to be understood as a driver of systemic inflammation and performance variability—not a background detail, but a central feature of her health trajectory. For Ana, early use of occupation-based cognitive screening revealed a missed diagnosis that had dramatically shaped her sense of capacity, confidence, and safety. What began as support for "stress management" became a mechanism for medical reclassification, workplace protection, and cognitive healing.

These cases reaffirm that occupational therapists are not just facilitators of daily activity, they are translators of lived experience into clinical language that can reshape diagnoses, unlock services, and challenge institutional blind spots. When therapists move beyond surface-level task support and approach performance as an expression of underlying neurophysiological and psychosocial patterns, they become powerful advocates for equity and repair.

Summary and Implications

The physiological consequences of violence against women are not limited to acute injuries or psychological trauma—they ripple across systems, disrupting immune function, hormonal balance, neurological processing, and everyday occupational engagement. These health impacts are frequently misunderstood, misdiagnosed, or attributed to character flaws or noncompliance, especially in women who are managing invisible or chronic symptoms without formal trauma documentation. Yet when viewed through a trauma-informed, body-aware lens, these patterns begin to make clinical sense.

Occupational therapists are uniquely positioned to uncover and interpret the functional manifestations of trauma—whether it shows up as missed meals, disrupted routines, fatigue masking executive dysfunction, or silent disengagement from care. By grounding intervention in daily life and collaborating across disciplines, therapists can ensure that violence is no longer seen as an isolated event, but as a health determinant that requires precise, long-term, and occupation-based responses. In doing so, occupational therapy becomes a conduit for system correction—connecting the dots between lived experience, clinical outcomes, and pathways to sustainable recovery.

References

Baldwin-White, A. (2019). "When a girl says no, you should be persistent until she says yes": College students and their beliefs about consent. *Journal of Interpersonal Violence, 36*(19–20), NP10629–NP10652. https://doi.org/10.1177/0886260519875552

Barreca, J., & Wagner, A. (2024). A pilot survey of pediatric occupational and physical therapy providers' confidence, attitudes, barriers, and education regarding trauma-informed care. *Physical & Occupational Therapy in Pediatrics, 44*(6), 765–782. https://doi.org/10.1080/01942638.2024.2360457

Berke, D. S., Tuten, M. D., Smith, A. M., & Hotchkiss, M. (2023). A qualitative analysis of the context and characteristics of trauma exposure among sexual minority survivors: Implications for posttraumatic stress disorder assessment and clinical practice. *Psychological Trauma: Theory, Research, Practice, and Policy, 15*(4), 648–655. https://doi.org/10.1037/tra0001464

Bookwalter, D. B., Roenfeldt, K. A., LeardMann, C. A., Kong, S. Y., Riddle, M. S., & Rull, R. P. (2020). Posttraumatic stress disorder and risk of selected autoimmune diseases among US military personnel. *BMC Psychiatry, 20*(1), 23. https://doi.org/10.1186/s12888-020-2432-9

Corso, A., Engel, H., Müller, F., Fiacco, S., Mernone, L., Gardini, E., Ehlert, U., & Fischer, S. (2023). Early life stress in women with autoimmune thyroid disorders. *Scientific Reports, 13*(1), 22341. https://doi.org/10.1038/s41598-023-49993-3

Goldstein, E., Chokshi, B., Melendez-Torres, G. J., Rios, A., Jelley, M., & Lewis-O'Connor, A. (2024). Effectiveness of trauma-informed care implementation in health care settings: Systematic review of reviews and realist synthesis. *The Permanente Journal, 28*(1), 135–150. https://doi.org/10.7812/TPP/23.127

Güler, A., Maas, M. K., Mark, K. P., Kussainov, N., Schill, K., & Coker, A. L. (2024). The impacts of lifetime violence on women's current sexual health. *Women's Health Reports (New Rochelle, N.Y.), 5*(1), 56–64. https://doi.org/10.1089/whr.2023.0089

Jackson, M. L., & Jewell, V. D. (2021). Educational practices for providers of trauma-informed care: A scoping review. *Journal of Pediatric Nursing, 60*, 130–138. https://doi.org/10.1016/j.pedn.2021.04.029

Katrinli, S., Oliveira, N. C. S., Felger, J. C., Michopoulos, V., & Smith, A. K. (2022). The role of the immune system in posttraumatic stress disorder. *Translational Psychiatry, 12*(1), 313. https://doi.org/10.1038/s41398-022-02094-7

Khan, S. (2025). *Occupational therapy and women's health: A practitioner guide.* Routledge.

Köhler-Forsberg, O., Ge, F., Aspelund, T., Wang, Y., Fang, F., Tomasson, G., Thordadottir, E., Hauksdóttir, A., Song, H., & Valdimarsdottir, U. A. (2025). Adverse childhood experiences, mental distress, and autoimmune disease in adult women: Findings from two large cohort studies. *Psychological Medicine, 55*, e36. https://doi.org/10.1017/S0033291724003544

Latiff, M. A., Fang, L., Goh, D. A., & Tan, L. J. (2024). A systematic review of factors associated with disclosure of child sexual abuse. *Child Abuse & Neglect, 147*, 106564. https://doi.org/10.1016/j.chiabu.2023.106564

Olmos-Ochoa, T. T., Speicher, S., Ong, L. E., Kim, J., Hamilton, A. B., & Cloitre, M. (2023). Supporting equitable engagement and retention of women patients in a trauma-informed virtual mental health intervention: Acceptability and needed adaptations. *Psychiatric Rehabilitation Journal, 46*(1), 26–35. https://doi.org/10.1037/prj0000531

Parks, C. G., Pettinger, M., de Roos, A. J., Tindle, H. A., Walitt, B. T., & Howard, B. V. (2023). Life events, caregiving, and risk of autoimmune rheumatic diseases in the women's health initiative observational study. *Arthritis Care & Research, 75*(12), 2519–2528. https://doi.org/10.1002/acr.25164

Sanderson, M., Cook, M., Brown, L. L., Mallett, V., & Coker, A. L. (2023). Lifetime interpersonal violence or abuse and diabetes rates by sex and race. *American Journal of Preventive Medicine, 65*(5), 783–791. https://doi.org/10.1016/j.amepre.2023.06.007

Stöckl, H., & Sorenson, S. B. (2024). Violence against women as a global public health issue. *Annual Review of Public Health, 45*(1), 277–294. https://doi.org/10.1146/annurev-publhealth-060722-025138

Chapter 8

Trauma in the Lives of Women of Color

Chapter Objectives

Upon completion of this chapter, the reader will be able to:

1. Describe the multifaceted ways trauma manifests in the occupational lives of women of color, including relational, cultural, and systemic contributors that are often overlooked in traditional models of care.
2. Analyze the role of intergenerational trauma and culturally inherited roles in shaping occupational identity, role performance, and help-seeking behavior among racially and ethnically marginalized women.
3. Differentiate between occupation as coping and occupation as healing by identifying signs of reenactment, over-functioning, and protective withdrawal within daily routines.
4. Apply trauma-informed, culturally responsive strategies in occupational therapy that support role renegotiation, values-based participation, and liberation-centered intervention.
5. Advocate for equity in clinical assessment and documentation by integrating culturally attuned evaluation tools, addressing implicit bias, and contextualizing occupational performance through systemic and historical frameworks.

At 29, Ayanna Owens was the person everyone relied on—at work, at home, and in her community. As a program coordinator at a busy social services agency, she managed multiple caseloads, deescalated tense situations, and always stepped in when someone else dropped the ball. But beneath the competence was exhaustion. Ayanna, a Black woman raised by a mother who survived domestic violence, had

DOI: 10.4324/9781003658559-8

learned early that staying ahead of harm meant staying quiet, composed, and overprepared. She came to occupational therapy for help with chronic pain, migraines, and what her doctor called burnout, but the therapist noticed deeper patterns. During ADL retraining, Ayanna struggled to prioritize her own needs, avoided eye contact when discussing rest, and became visibly tense when offered choices. Her schedule was packed, but none of it reflected care for herself. Instead of focusing on productivity, her therapist co-created a daily energy map to track where emotional effort was being spent, introduced rhythmic movement for regulation, and used culturally meaningful occupations for Ayanna-like Afro-Caribbean dance to support agency and embodiment. Together, they worked to reframe Ayanna's narrative not as a failure of self-care, but as the cost of carrying generations of survival in silence.

In a 2024 qualitative study published in *Birth*, researchers explored the intersection of traumatic childbirth and obstetric racism among Black, Latina, and Asian mothers in the United States. Women in the study described feeling dismissed, stereotyped, and disempowered during labor, often reporting lasting impacts such as postpartum anxiety, depression, and medical mistrust. Their stories revealed that trauma was not only tied to the intensity of pain or medical complications, but to the way they were treated or ignored during one of the most vulnerable moments of their lives.

Across the United States, Black women face disproportionately high rates of trauma exposure, yet their suffering is often minimized, misdiagnosed, or pathologized rather than understood. According to the National Center for PTSD, women of color are significantly more likely to experience both interpersonal violence and institutional betrayal, with Black women in particular facing a dual burden of racial and gender-based stressors. This chronic exposure does not only shape emotional well-being but affects how women participate in daily life, access care, and engage in occupational roles. And yet, the frameworks used to understand trauma often leave their stories on the margins.

Trauma in the lives of women of color is often overlooked because it does not always conform to the dominant narratives clinicians are trained to recognize. It is not always loud or immediate. It may not arrive as a single event, but as a steady, accumulating pressure—a lifetime of being interrupted, corrected, or erased. Trauma can be embedded in institutions that are supposed to help, in communities shaped by generational inequity, and in the quiet decisions women make every day about where to go, what to say, and how much of themselves it is safe to reveal.

A 2024 study by Crouch and colleagues, which examined women of color enrolled in urban adult basic education programs, found that those with higher exposure to trauma (particularly sexual assault and sudden death) also reported significantly greater symptoms of anxiety and depression. These women were not receiving specialized care. They were simply trying to access education. This research highlights a critical truth: trauma does not only show up in mental health clinics or emergency rooms. It shows up in classrooms, waiting rooms, job interviews, and daily routines that become harder to manage when the body is carrying unacknowledged harm.

For women of color who have experienced trauma, survival has been earned through constant vigilance. But that vigilance comes at a cost. The ability to endure is often mistaken for resilience, while the physical, emotional, and cognitive toll is dismissed. Without a lens that accounts for racialized stress, cultural invisibility, and the occupational consequences of long-term threat, providers risk mislabeling survival strategies as dysfunction.

This invisibility extends into professional settings where the consequences of trauma are compounded rather than addressed. In a 2024 narrative review published in *Teaching and Learning in Medicine*, Johnson and colleagues examined the first-person accounts of Black women faculty across higher education. These narratives revealed a recurring pattern of racial trauma that included being the only Black woman in a department, navigating unspoken expectations, and experiencing repeated invalidation or neglect. Many described the psychological toll of having to remain composed while enduring what one author called "the cloak of invisibility." The weight of this labor is not merely emotional. It is physical, cognitive, and occupational. It interferes with rest, with clarity, and with one's ability to engage meaningfully in work or community life.

Such stories are critical not only because they validate the lived experiences of women of color, but because they expose how systems normalize their suffering. What may look like disengagement in a faculty meeting, missed assignments in an adult classroom, or emotional shutdown in a clinic is often a signal of cumulative trauma that has gone unacknowledged for too long. These are not signs of poor coping. They are adaptations to surviving in environments where being overlooked is routine and being believed is rare.

Understanding trauma through the voices of those most impacted offers a necessary corrective to standard models of care. It shifts the clinical gaze from what is missing in a client to what has been endured. It reframes silence, perfectionism, or exhaustion not as deficits, but as evidence of systems that have required too much for too long. When occupational therapists can recognize these patterns as functional, protective, and deeply contextual, they are better positioned to offer care that affirms the whole person—not just what she does, but what she has carried to get here.

Identity and Trauma in Women of Color

Trauma in women of color is shaped not only by what happens to them, but by how those experiences are filtered through the lens of race, gender, and culture—often simultaneously. The emotional toll of surviving a traumatic event is compounded when systems fail to believe the survivor or pathologize her response through a racially biased lens. A Latina woman navigating a predominantly White workplace may endure both sexual harassment and cultural stereotyping, but fear that reporting either will result in retaliation or being labeled "too sensitive" or "difficult." A Black woman who discloses partner violence in a healthcare setting may be met with suspicion or apathy, especially if the provider holds implicit biases about Black families or assumes strength means resilience without support.

For women of color, trauma is often followed by a second wound: erasure. After experiencing violence, many face culturally coded silencing, being told not to shame the family, not to draw negative attention to the community, or not to confirm dominant stereotypes about their race or culture. This is particularly common among Asian and Middle Eastern women, who may be discouraged from speaking openly about trauma due to community pressures around honor, reputation, or family loyalty. The result is a form of occupational withdrawal that is often misread: these women may disengage not because they lack motivation, but because their trauma has been met with invisibility, minimization, or cultural betrayal.

Cultural Roles and Compounded Burden

In many communities of color, women are expected to carry cultural continuity. They are traditional bearers, caregivers, and translators of institutional systems for their families—roles that become especially heavy after trauma. A first-generation Caribbean woman navigating a chronic illness may avoid disclosing pain because she feels responsible for appearing strong, especially in front of elders who have survived migration or racial discrimination. In some Indigenous communities, historical trauma is transmitted alongside cultural knowledge, and women may feel responsible for both preserving heritage and healing wounds they did not cause. Occupational therapy in these contexts must do more than support function—it must respect the meaning behind the roles women are holding and help redistribute that labor without cultural invalidation.

For example, a Haitian grandmother recovering from joint replacement may be skipping pain management routines because she feels obligated to maintain morning prayer rituals, cook ceremonial meals, and supervise grandchildren's care before school. Instead of framing this as nonadherence, the occupational therapist can offer a culturally attuned occupational profile that explores how spiritual and familial obligations are prioritized in her daily structure. Together, they might develop energy-conserving adaptations for meal prep, co-create inter-generational routines where grandchildren assist with morning rituals, or use visual timetables that pace her prayer and medication schedules in alignment.

Similarly, a South Asian woman living in a multigenerational household may refuse outside help despite clear signs of burnout. Her refusal may not be rooted in pride but in fear of community judgment or disrupting family hierarchy. Here, the therapist might explore culturally respectful language for boundary-setting, use values clarification to distinguish obligation from desire, and offer narrative tools such as letter writing or guided journaling to externalize the emotional toll of her caregiving role.

These interventions are not intended to erase culturally meaningful roles but to reestablish the client's sense of agency within them. When a woman is given the space to define how she continues a role, rather than feeling bound by inher-ited expectations, the therapeutic process becomes less about compliance and more about conscious participation. Healing is more likely to endure when the client sees herself as the author of her routines, rather than a character locked into someone else's script. Occupational therapists can facilitate this shift by using tools such as occupational storytelling, legacy mapping, or structured decision-making grids that help clients examine how their current roles align or conflict with their core values and health needs. The deeper goal is not just functional independence but functional alignment, where daily actions reflect both cultural identity and self-preservation. In this way, therapy becomes a place not just for recovery, but for reclamation.

Surveillance and Silencing in Public Systems

Unlike White women, women of color who seek help after trauma are often entering systems that already view them with suspicion. For example, a Black mother reporting abuse may be more likely to have child protective services involved—not as support, but as surveillance. Latina immigrants may avoid hos-pitals altogether due to fear of documentation inquiries, regardless of their legal status. Indigenous women may hesitate to disclose violence out of fear that their children will be removed or their parental capacity questioned. These realities are not secondary to trauma but central to how trauma is processed, healed, or further deepened.

Occupational therapists working in these contexts must move carefully, building trust through transparency, checking assumptions, and recognizing how institutional harm informs every aspect of participation. This includes how goals are framed, how questions are asked, and how much a client feels safe to reveal. Therapists must be attuned to the subtle signs of institutional trauma, such as avoidance of services, hypervigilance during assessments, or hesitancy around documentation, and interpret these not as resistance, but as adaptive strategies shaped by systemic exposure to harm.

In practice, this means clarifying what will and will not be shared with other agencies, offering choices around how and when to engage in sensitive topics, and creating space for clients to co-author their narratives without fear of consequence. For example, an OT supporting a mother in a home health setting might prioritize routines that enhance family safety and emotional regulation while advocating behind the scenes for less intrusive service delivery. Trust-building is not a soft skill, it is a therapeutic intervention in itself, especially for clients who have experienced care as a threat rather than a refuge.

Harm in the Health System

Whitney James, a thirty-eight-year-old Black woman, arrived at the emergency room one morning in February 2024 with sharp abdominal pain, bloating, and nausea that had persisted for several days. She was told by the attending physician that it was "probably just gas" and advised to adjust her diet. No imaging was ordered. Feeling dismissed but unsure how to advocate for herself without being labeled "difficult," Whitney returned home, only to collapse days later and be rushed back to the hospital. This time, a CT scan revealed a large tumor pressing against her intestines. The delay in diagnosis led not only to physical complications but to a deep erosion of trust in the medical system. In therapy sessions weeks later, she described the ER visit as a turning point—when she stopped believing she would be taken seriously. That dismissal stayed with her, shaping how she approached every health-related task afterward, from scheduling appointments to disclosing symptoms. Her experience highlights a common reality for many Black women—the risk lies not only in the condition itself, but in how often serious symptoms are dismissed or ignored until it is too late.

For many women of color, healthcare is not experienced as a site of safety or healing. Instead, it is often a place of dismissal, misdiagnosis, and retraumatization. While all trauma survivors are vulnerable to poor clinical encounters, women of color face an added burden: they are more likely to have their symptoms questioned, their pain minimized, and their bodies viewed through racialized assumptions. Hispanic women frequently encounter language barriers, cultural misunderstandings, and assumptions about pain tolerance that delay diagnosis or compromise care. Asian American women often face a damaging presumption of emotional silence or stoicism, which can lead providers to underestimate distress or overlook signs of trauma entirely. Studies have shown that Black women are less likely to receive adequate pain treatment, more likely to be misdiagnosed with psychiatric conditions when reporting somatic symptoms and often face provider disbelief when disclosing trauma histories.

In a 2022 study published in *The Journal of Racial and Ethnic Health Disparities*, researchers explored perceived discrimination in medical settings among Black women using both the Discrimination in Medical Settings scale and qualitative interviews. The findings were striking: most participants reported experiencing discrimination during healthcare encounters, leading to medical mistrust and damaged patient-provider relationships. Despite the majority having been recently screened for cervical cancer, the women described care interactions as dismissive, invalidating, and sometimes overtly discriminatory. These patterns did not merely impact satisfaction; they shaped health behaviors, screening uptake, and overall willingness to seek preventive services.

Medical mistrust among women of color is not irrational. It is a learned and lived response to decades of harm—forced sterilizations, biased diagnostic practices, language barriers, and exclusion from research. This mistrust influences occupational engagement in subtle but profound ways. A woman who stops going to follow-up visits may not be "noncompliant"; she may be protecting herself from repeated invalidation. A woman who avoids mental health care may be navigating cultural stigma and fear of being pathologized by a clinician who does not understand her context.

Occupational therapists must be attuned to these dynamics, especially when working with clients from communities historically marginalized by the healthcare system. This means going beyond rapport-building to actively incorporate structural awareness into care. Therapists can screen for medical trauma using validated tools, adapt treatment pacing to address mistrust or reactivity, and co-create plans that honor a client's healthcare boundaries. Advocacy may include preparing clients for appointments with scripts or role-play, writing support letters to mitigate bias in provider interactions, and documenting prior medical harm in ways that legitimize—not pathologize—their experiences. Trauma-informed occupational therapy in this context must recognize that recovery is not just about function; it is about restoring safety, power, and dignity in systems that have too often eroded all three.

Culturally Discordant Care and Misdiagnosis

Clinicians often interpret trauma symptoms through frameworks that do not account for racial or cultural expression. For instance, somatic symptoms such as headaches, fatigue, body tension are common trauma responses among Latina and Asian women but may be dismissed as "stress" or cultural exaggeration. Black women expressing anger or protectiveness may be misread as aggressive or paranoid, especially when clinical teams lack racial literacy. These misinterpretations are not just diagnostic errors, they shape treatment access, disrupt therapeutic rapport, and reinforce internalized shame.

In a 2023 study published in *Journal of Racial and Ethnic Health Disparities*, Washington and Randall found that Black women frequently experience perceived discrimination in medical settings, contributing to delayed care, damaged provider trust, and increased emotional burden. Many participants described feeling unheard or dismissed when communicating symptoms or concerns, particularly in preventive care contexts like cervical cancer screening. These findings underscore how cultural misrecognition and racial bias in clinical encounters can have direct and lasting impacts on women's health decisions and outcomes.

Occupational therapy practitioners must also remain committed to ongoing education in racial equity, cultural humility, and the historical context of medical mistrust. This includes staying informed about current research on disparities in diagnosis and treatment, engaging in continuing education related to racialized trauma, and building clinical reflexivity to examine their own biases. Beyond learning, occupational therapists should actively educate clients of color about their rights within healthcare systems, including the right to be heard, to request a different provider, to bring an advocate to appointments, and to access culturally responsive services. Therapists can help clients script difficult conversations with providers, rehearse advocacy language in safe spaces, or use visual tools to support communication when verbal exchanges are overwhelming. They can also support clients in identifying and connecting with community-based health resources that reflect their cultural background, values, and needs. By combining relational care with system navigation, occupational therapy becomes not only a space of healing, but a platform for justice and empowerment.

Invisible Labor and Health Avoidance

Mei Lin is a thirty-seven-year-old Chinese Canadian woman referred to occupational therapy after experiencing postpartum complications and chronic shoulder pain. Although she expressed a desire to improve her health, she missed multiple follow-up sessions. When the therapist reached out, Mei Lin explained that she is caring for her newborn child while also managing the health needs of her aging parents who live with her. As the only English-speaking adult in her household, she often translates medical information and handles all health appointments for her family. "My pain can wait," she said. "I need to make sure everyone else is taken care of first." Though soft-spoken, her exhaustion was palpable.

Women of color often carry invisible labor within healthcare settings. They translate for family members, navigate complex health systems, and coordinate intergenerational care needs during their own appointments. This additional responsibility is not accounted for in most clinical models. It leads many to delay or disengage from their own care. A Southeast Asian mother raising a child with medical complexity may skip physical therapy because it conflicts with hospital visits for her child. An Afro-Caribbean elder may avoid rehabilitation settings that remind her of past experiences of institutional control or medical disregard.

This avoidance is not simply a matter of access or awareness. It is rooted in a long history of structural racism, institutional betrayal, and medical neglect. In a 2022 article published in *Health in Color*, researchers Elizabeth Dayo, Kayonne Christy, and Ruth Habte traced the maternal health disparities among Black women to both historical and contemporary sources of harm. They document how present-day inequities in obstetric care are shaped by the legacy of experimental surgeries on enslaved Black women, as well as current patterns of delayed diagnosis, inadequate pain treatment, and provider disbelief. The authors emphasized that even Black women with higher education are significantly more likely to experience severe maternal complications than White women with less formal education.

These patterns are compounded by what Geronimus has described as the weathering effect, the physiological impact of prolonged exposure to discrimination and racial stress. Studies show that Black women in midlife may present with biological profiles of someone several years older, reflecting the cumulative toll of living under racialized pressure. In Canada, a lack of race-based health data further masks these disparities. The ideology of race-evasive care, often framed as colorblindness, assumes equity without ever measuring it. As a result, the health interests of Black women and other racially marginalized groups remain underrepresented in research, policy, and clinical response.

Health avoidance among women of color is not disengagement. It is often an act of preservation. Many choose self-management over exposure to disrespect or disbelief. They opt out not from apathy but from an understanding that care is not always caring. Occupational therapists must recognize that this invisible labor and historical injury influence how and when a client engages.

In practice, occupational therapy can respond by building routines around cultural and familial roles instead of asking clients to choose between wellness and responsibility. This includes offering flexible scheduling, co-designing plans that honor caregiving dynamics, and using care mapping tools to visualize and redistribute labor where possible. Therapists must also be willing to advocate beyond the session. This might mean partnering with culturally aligned providers, writing letters that contextualize a missed appointment, or supporting systemic change within the institution itself. Above all, practitioners should enter each interaction with the humility to understand that being present in care may require tremendous personal and cultural negotiation for the client.

Relational Wounds and Cultural Pressures

For many women of color, trauma is not confined to individual incidents. It is embedded within relational dynamics shaped by culture, migration, colonial histories, and survival expectations. Emotional abuse, boundary violations, and intergenerational conflict often go unnamed because they are normalized within cultural or family systems. A daughter may be expected to sacrifice education for caretaking. A woman may remain silent about intimate partner violence to protect family reputation. These forms of harm are not less real because they are relationally complex—they are often more enduring, especially when the trauma is minimized by both cultural norms and clinical frameworks.

Within these contexts, trauma is frequently maintained by silence and shaped by loyalty. The expectation to protect family members, even those who caused harm, can result in profound emotional compartmentalization. For example, a young Afro Latina woman may feel guilt for disclosing abuse that her family insists is a private matter. A Filipina caregiver may tolerate emotional neglect from siblings because her cultural role demands obedience and self-sacrifice. These experiences often result in chronic stress, self-blame, and difficulty establishing personal boundaries—core areas where occupational therapy can provide intervention.

In a 2023 study published in the *Journal of Substance Use and Addiction Treatment*, researchers examined how intergenerational trauma and substance use shaped outcomes for Black women involved in the criminal justice system. Using longitudinal data, they found that women who reported parental or grandparental substance use had significantly higher odds of both personal substance use and open child protective services cases. Although only a subset of participants reported intergenerational trauma directly, the effects of those experiences were amplified when compounded by socioeconomic and relational pressures, including caregiving demands and histories of incarceration. These findings illustrate how trauma transmitted across generations, particularly when shaped by systemic inequities, can disrupt family roles, increase surveillance, and entrench cycles of harm.

Occupational therapists must be prepared to address the occupational consequences of these inherited dynamics. Trauma-informed care in this context means recognizing how relational wounds are encoded into daily routines, role expectations, and help-seeking behavior. For many clients, therapy must include validating the invisible costs of caregiving, supporting boundary formation, and gently exploring internalized guilt that comes from placing personal needs above family obligation. Therapists can use tools like role mapping, values clarification, and trauma narratives to help clients deconstruct relational identities shaped by both cultural pressure and survival.

The Cost of Expected Strength

Women of color are often socialized to be strong, resilient, and self-sacrificing. These traits, while protective in oppressive systems, can also prevent emotional processing and delay healing. The "strong Black woman" trope, for example, may lead to the internalization of unrealistic expectations where expressing vulnerability is framed as weakness. This cultural schema encourages women to endure silently, suppress emotion, and prioritize the needs of others over their own. Similarly, immigrant daughters may adopt perfectionism and over-functioning in response to the sacrifices their families made to survive.

In a 2018 study published in *Sex Roles*, researchers Abrams, Hill, and Maxwell examined how the perceived obligation to manifest strength contributes to depression among Black women in the United States. They found that self-silencing, defined as the suppression of one's emotional needs, opinions, or discomfort to preserve relationships or meet cultural expectations, played a mediating role in this relationship. Women who identified with the Strong Black Woman schema reported higher levels of depressive symptoms, particularly when they felt pressure to appear composed and capable at all times. Rather than a source of empowerment, the chronic need to conceal vulnerability often created a cycle of internalized distress, emotional isolation, and reduced help-seeking behavior.

These findings have important implications for occupational therapy practice. Therapists may encounter clients who consistently downplay pain, refuse to rest, or resist mental health referrals not because they lack insight, but because their sense of identity is tightly bound to the performance of strength. In this context, therapeutic progress requires more than behavioral change and it calls for a reconstruction of belief systems around worth, wellness, and visibility.

Occupational therapists can intervene by validating the toll of performing strength and gently exploring how societal, familial, and cultural pressures have shaped the client's relationship with self-care. This may include narrative work focused on shifting survival scripts, establishing permission for rest, and co-creating routines that center joy rather than performance. Interventions might also include reclaiming leisure as a site of agency, using expressive occupations to externalize guilt or grief, and developing daily structures that integrate self-prioritization—often for the first time. Practitioners should approach this work with deep cultural humility and an understanding that strength, while admirable, is not always sustainable when it comes at the cost of wellness.

Attachment Disruption and Role Diffusion

In multigenerational households or transnational families, attachment patterns are often shaped by separation, migration, or role reversal. A child raised by extended family may experience insecure attachment despite receiving physical care. A young woman who becomes the translator, financial planner, and emotional anchor for her household may lose access to developmentally appropriate roles. This role diffusion, where boundaries between child, sibling, and adult become blurred, can lead to burnout, identity confusion, and difficulty with self-definition in adulthood.

Recent research also shows how these disrupted attachments can carry forward in complex and damaging ways. In a 2022 study published in *Child Abuse & Neglect*, Miljkovitch and colleagues investigated the intergenerational transmission of child sexual abuse among male survivors and found that disorganized attachment, particularly to fathers, was associated with a higher risk of perpetration in adulthood. Importantly, the study emphasized the potential protective role of secure adult romantic relationships, suggesting that attachment disruptions in early life may be mitigated through later experiences of emotional security. While this research focused on male survivors, its implications for occupational therapy extend across gender. It reinforces the idea that insecure and disorganized attachments formed in childhood can influence relational functioning, emotional regulation, and role engagement well into adulthood.

For women of color, these attachment disruptions are often compounded by cultural expectations of caretaking and emotional labor. The fusion of identity with family responsibility, especially in contexts shaped by immigration, poverty, or trauma, can result in clients who appear highly competent yet internally depleted. Therapists may find that clients express difficulty identifying personal goals, trusting peers, or expressing unmet needs, not due to pathology but because their roles were shaped by necessity rather than choice.

Occupational therapy can support the reorganization of relational roles through targeted, trauma-informed interventions. This may include helping clients distinguish between culturally valued caretaking and enmeshed obligation, restoring emotional clarity without disregarding cultural norms. Therapists might guide role-mapping exercises that clarify responsibilities, support boundary-setting through scripting and advocacy tools, and co-develop routines that reallocate energy toward self-defined goals. Above all, practitioners must validate the survival logic behind these roles while creating safe therapeutic space to imagine new patterns of connection, identity, and rest.

Barriers to Healing and Accessing Support

For many women of color, healing is not only about recovering from trauma; it is about navigating the systems that have contributed to it. Medical bias, cultural stigma, and economic barriers all shape the degree to which women can access meaningful care. Even when services are available, they are often rooted in frameworks that do not account for racialized stress, intergenerational trauma, or culturally specific expressions of pain. Healing, in this context, becomes a labor of translation: explaining, justifying, and often defending one's experience to providers who may not fully understand it.

In a 2023 study examining barriers to trauma recovery among Black and Latina women, participants described feeling "talked over," "disbelieved," or "made to feel dramatic" in medical and mental health settings. Others noted that family expectations and cultural taboos around mental illness made it difficult to name or seek help for trauma. These obstacles do not reflect personal resistance; they are structural exclusions that have shaped entire lifetimes of silence.

What many occupational therapists may not realize is that therapeutic non-engagement is often an act of protection, not avoidance. When a woman of color resists talking about trauma or misses appointments, she may be safeguarding herself from re-experiencing harm in a clinical setting that lacks cultural safety. This self-protective stance can emerge from prior interactions where her voice was minimized, her pain was discredited, or her survival strategies were pathologized. Understanding this distinction is critical. What is labeled as "noncompliance" may, in fact, be an intelligent boundary set in the face of accumulated medical mistrust.

Additionally, the frameworks many providers rely on to assess trauma are often shaped by White, middle-class norms. Standardized screening tools may fail to capture the embodied, relational, or spiritual dimensions of trauma experienced in racialized communities. For example, idioms of distress like somatic symptoms, spiritual visitations, or family-based guilt may be overlooked or misunderstood as culturally irrelevant. This gap in interpretation can result in underdiagnosis, misdiagnosis, or interventions that fail to resonate.

To move beyond these limitations, occupational therapists must reorient their lens not only to observe what is present, but to question what has been silenced. This involves recognizing how diagnostic systems and care pathways are built on cultural defaults that often exclude the lived experiences of marginalized women. Instead of relying solely on pre-scripted intake forms or symptom checklists, therapists should approach the therapeutic relationship as an act of witnessing, not just evaluating. Building trust may require slowing down, honoring nonlinear progress, and making space for complex emotions that resist tidy categorization. True healing work begins when providers are willing to step back from clinical authority and instead become skilled co-navigators of recovery, attuned to what is said, what is withheld, and what has never been safe to name.

Misrecognition in Clinical Spaces

Women of color are frequently misdiagnosed or underdiagnosed due to implicit bias in clinical care. For example, Black women's expressions of pain are more likely to be labeled as aggression or noncompliance, while Asian and Native women's symptoms may be dismissed as compliance or stoicism. These misinterpretations prevent the accurate identification of trauma-related conditions and delay intervention. Moreover, standard assessments often fail to account for culturally influenced expressions of distress, such as somatic complaints or spiritual language.

Implicit bias refers to unconscious attitudes or stereotypes that influence how we interpret behavior, assign value, and make decisions, often without conscious intent. In clinical settings, these biases can shape everything from diagnostic impressions to the perceived credibility of a client's narrative. Research shows that implicit bias can operate across a range of domains, including race, gender, age, disability, socioeconomic status, and body size. For example, older women of color may be infantilized or viewed as passive recipients of care, while younger women may be judged as emotionally unstable or "too sensitive." Gendered expectations also intersect—where assertiveness in men is interpreted as leadership, the same behavior in women may be pathologized as defiance or emotional dysregulation.

Fortunately, tools now exist to help clinicians assess and reflect on their own implicit bias. Instruments like the Implicit Association Test (IAT), Project Implicit, or Harvard's bias assessment platforms allow practitioners to examine automatic preferences that may otherwise go unnoticed. While these tools are not diagnostic, they offer a valuable starting point for self-awareness. For occupational therapists, engaging with these assessments can support ongoing professional development and inform supervision, case formulation, and interdisciplinary consultation. Regular bias reflection also aligns with ethical responsibilities outlined in occupational therapy practice frameworks that emphasize justice, client autonomy, and cultural responsiveness.

Occupational therapists can interrupt the downstream effects of bias by anchoring evaluation in function rather than assumption. Instead of focusing solely on symptomatology, they can explore how trauma is shaping the client's roles, routines, and engagement with the world. This functional lens helps reposition the client as expert while disrupting clinical gatekeeping. Interventions may include collaborative documentation that affirms the client's narrative, advocacy in interdisciplinary teams, or development of culturally attuned tools that allow women to define their distress in their own words. Ultimately, recognizing and addressing implicit bias is not a one-time act of awareness, it is a continuous, reflective process that safeguards the therapeutic relationship and enhances the integrity of trauma-informed care.

Cultural Silence and the Weight of Representation

In many communities of color, trauma is not easily named or disclosed. This silence is not avoidance but a historically informed strategy for survival. Legacies of forced institutionalization, coerced confession, and community surveillance have taught generations that to speak pain aloud is to invite harm. Disclosure may be perceived not only as a violation of family loyalty but also as an abandonment of cultural values such as endurance, modesty, or spiritual surrender.

For women shaped by these narratives, rest may feel unsafe, therapy may feel self-indulgent, and boundary-setting may be interpreted as disobedience rather than protection (Dmowska et al., 2024).

This burden becomes heavier for those who are navigating environments where representation is rare. Women of color who are the first in their families to enter academia, health care, or leadership often carry the dual responsibility of achievement and community preservation. In these contexts, strength is not a choice, it is an unspoken requirement. A first-generation physician may work through burnout rather than risk disappointing her family. A young professor may downplay the impact of microaggressions because her presence alone is seen as symbolic progress. The emotional cost of being visible while remaining silent is profound.

Occupational therapy offers a rare opportunity to interrupt these cycles not by asking clients to surrender their cultural frameworks, but by helping them translate them into sustainable practices. Therapists can introduce reflective tools that help clients differentiate between inherited obligations and chosen values. They can guide meaning-making through expressive mediums such as visual art, textile creation, or music composition, allowing women to externalize unspeakable experiences in culturally congruent ways. Clinicians might also support the adaptation of spiritual rituals into daily wellness routines, such as modifying prayer practices into grounding activities or integrating ancestral storytelling into memory work.

Moreover, occupational therapists are uniquely positioned to address the invisible labor of representation. This can involve role negotiation interventions that make space for authenticity within professional settings, support scripts for responding to cultural tokenism, or environmental modifications that create psychologically safe spaces for rest and recovery. The goal is not to pathologize resilience, but to decenter it as the only available mode of functioning. For many women of color, healing does not begin with disclosure. It begins with the experience of being witnessed, not as a symbol, but as a complex and fully human self.

Collective Memory and Intergenerational Load

Maria Clarke, a 56-year-old Afro-Caribbean woman, was admitted to inpatient rehabilitation after experiencing a left hemispheric stroke. On the surface, she was cooperative and independent, but her therapists noticed a persistent reluctance to use adaptive equipment or accept rest breaks. She avoided leisure-based tasks in therapy, insisting, "I'm not here to play—I have work to do." When the team recommended pacing strategies to conserve energy, she responded with visible irritation and refused to adjust her care goals. In conversation, she frequently referenced her grandmother, who worked as a midwife in rural Jamaica without formal training or rest. She also described her own role in raising her younger siblings after her mother's early death, noting that "tired is a luxury woman in my family do not have."

Over the course of therapy, Maria's emotional distancing, hyperfunctional behavior, and resistance to self-care revealed more than individual coping—it reflected the weight of collective memory and intergenerational role inheritance. Her family's narrative was steeped in survival through service: laboring through illness, caregiving as identity, and emotional endurance as expectation. In the clinical space, this legacy translated into overidentification with productivity, internalized pressure to remain the "strong one," and difficulty imagining a recovery process centered on her own needs. For Maria, healing was not only physical rehabilitation, but it was also a confrontation with long-standing narratives about worth, work, and womanhood.

Collective memory refers to the transmission of lived trauma, cultural grief, and adaptive survival strategies across generations. Unlike personal memory, which is formed through individual experience, collective memory is embedded in stories, rituals, social expectations, and bodily habits passed down within families and communities. These memories are often somatic, implicit, and emotionally charged, held in the way a grandmother folds laundry in silence or in a daughter's refusal to eat the last portion of food. For women of color, collective memory can include recollections of colonization, forced migration, systemic neglect, and survival under dehumanizing conditions. These histories shape how individuals experience roles, safety, authority, and deservingness of care, often unconsciously.

Intergenerational load is the psychological and occupational weight of inherited roles, traumas, and expectations. It is not simply about family history, but about the unspoken agreements many women carry: to protect others at their own expense, to endure without complaint, to perform competence even when unwell. In rehabilitation, these inherited roles can clash with clinical goals. A woman who sees herself as the family anchor may forgo needed rest or emotional processing to avoid appearing "weak." Without understanding this context, providers may misinterpret the client's behavior as resistance or noncompliance. Occupational therapists must instead recognize that recovery often requires navigating not only a healing body, but also a legacy of protective silence and duty.

The impact of collective memory and intergenerational load is rarely visible on intake forms, but it shapes everything from goal setting to discharge planning. It influences which tasks feel meaningful, which identities feel permissible, and which supports feel safe to accept. Without careful exploration, clinicians risk prescribing solutions that conflict with inherited values—pushing independence when interdependence is the norm or recommending rest in a family narrative where rest has always been denied. Understanding these forces allows occupational therapists to design care that is not only culturally responsive, but also historically aware and emotionally intelligent.

Historical Trauma in Family and Community Systems

In some families, expectations are handed down more reliably than genetics. A woman may enter inpatient rehabilitation with hemiparesis, but what shapes her recovery is not just the stroke. It is the unspoken rules passed down over generations: do not ask for help, do not show pain, do not be a burden. These rules are not written, but they are enforced, often with love, often with fear. Historical trauma in this context is not defined by a singular rupture—it is a lineage of protective adaptation.

What is often missing from clinical care plans is an analysis of how historical harms have reorganized family life. In communities impacted by colonization, slavery, displacement, or state surveillance, survival often meant restructuring emotional expression, labor division, and bodily autonomy. For instance, touch may have been reserved only for necessity, not comfort. Privacy may have been denied across generations, leading to a complex relationship with exposure and vulnerability. What might look like withdrawal in a client could be a deeply practiced form of self-preservation, shaped by generations who were not allowed to let their guard down.

Occupational therapists must move beyond surface-level intake questions and instead approach history-gathering with curiosity about inherited roles and unspoken rules. Rather than asking only, "What are your goals for therapy?" therapists might begin with, "What did rest look like in your home growing up?" or "Were there expectations in your family about who gives care and who receives it?" These kinds of questions surface the adaptive strategies shaped by generations of structural pressure—insight that is critical when evaluating participation in daily routines. If a client resists assistance with dressing, it may reflect not just a desire for independence but a family legacy of shaming vulnerability. When crafting goals, therapists should consider not only physical capacity but the emotional cost of certain occupations. An ideal goal may not be bathing independently by discharge, but bathing with support while maintaining agency and dignity.

Cultural scripts around caregiving, body exposure, and productivity are not just personal beliefs, they are inherited frameworks that dictate what feels acceptable, respectable, or shameful in clinical settings. Exploring these scripts in therapy is not about challenging culture but about giving clients the power to examine which inherited roles continue to support their healing and which quietly erode it. For example, a middle-aged Haitian woman recovering from a neurological injury may refuse to let her daughter help her bathe, not out of modesty alone, but because body exposure in her cultural upbringing was tightly guarded and associated with vulnerability or loss of status. Rather than labeling her as "resistant," the therapist might frame this as a protective value and shift the goal from independent bathing to partial assistance with adaptive garments that minimize exposure. Similarly, a first-generation Filipina client may insist on resuming homemaking tasks immediately, not realizing that her drive stems less from volition and more from a deeply internalized script that equates rest with laziness. Instead of simply redirecting her, the therapist might help her reframe recovery as a contribution to her family—such as creating a visual schedule to delegate tasks, which allows her to maintain leadership while honoring her healing. These conversations invite clients to author their own occupational narratives, rather than reenacting inherited ones by default. Through trauma-informed questioning and culturally attuned goal setting, occupational therapists can help women discern which roles affirm their agency and which ones were written for someone else's survival. This distinction can be the difference between compliance and empowerment, between participation and transformation.

Inherited Roles and the Suppression of Self

Some identities are chosen. Others are inherited long before a woman has the words to name them. In many families and cultural systems, roles like the caregiver, the emotional buffer, the peacekeeper, or the responsible one are passed down not through direct instruction, but through necessity. Women of color are often socialized into roles shaped by generations of structural inequality, migration stress, or survival under patriarchal norms. These roles may be protective in one season of life and imprisoning in another. What begins as a strength can eventually become a cage, especially when no space is left for self-discovery or internal permission to pause.

The result is a profound erosion of identity that often masquerades as competence. A woman may be praised for how much she manages but rarely asked what she wants. The suppression of self in these inherited roles does not always present as distress. It presents as high performance, meticulous caregiving, and the quiet abandonment of personal goals. In clinical settings, this can lead to occupational therapy plans that reinforce over-functioning rather than disrupt it. A woman who insists on returning to her caregiving duties immediately after a stroke may not be demonstrating volition—she may be reenacting an identity scripted before she had a choice.

Occupational therapy must approach this with a different lens. Instead of only building capacity for previously held roles, therapists can introduce structured space for role renegotiation. This may begin with a relational identity map or a tool used to explore which current responsibilities feel aligned and which feel inherited. Therapists can guide clients in examining their "occupational inheritance," identifying routines or obligations that have never been questioned. During goal setting, they might offer two versions of each goal: one that preserves an existing role and one that rewrites it. For example, instead of helping a woman return to preparing all family meals, the therapist might facilitate her transition into a shared planning role, where she oversees but does not execute all tasks, thus preserving meaning without reinforcing exhaustion.

Interventions can include guided nonproductive occupation trials—activities that are intentionally unstructured, enjoyable, and without outcome. These serve as both assessment and exposure, helping women tolerate unfamiliar states of pleasure, leisure, or uncertainty.

Therapists might also use sensory integration tasks not just to regulate the nervous system but to allow clients to experience body-based engagement without responsibility or oversight. Another approach involves legacy mapping, where women reflect on what legacies they want to pass on and which they are ready to release. This tool can be transformative for women who are mothers, community leaders, or first-generation professionals navigating inherited expectations. Importantly, the role of the occupational therapist is not to dismantle these inherited roles but to offer the client a mirror and the tools to decide what she wants to carry forward. Therapy in this context becomes a space for reclamation, where function is not only measured by what a woman can do but by what she chooses not to do any longer.

Occupation as Resistance and Recovery

Isabela Perez is a 24-year-old Colombian woman participating in an outpatient neurorehabilitation program after a mild traumatic brain injury sustained during a domestic altercation. Though her cognitive screening scores are within functional limits, she presents with low affect, difficulty initiating tasks, and chronic tension headaches. During one session, her occupational therapist noticed Isabela humming quietly while knotting colorful thread around her wrist. When asked about it, she shared that it was a traditional friendship bracelet, the kind her abuela taught her to make as a child in Bogotá. She had begun making them again each night—not to sell or gift, but to "keep her hands busy." This was not just a craft. It was a ritual. It was resistance to forgetting. And it was the beginning of recovery.

For women navigating both personal trauma and collective stress, occupation is often their first and most enduring form of language. Before diagnosis, before treatment plans, there is doing. Occupation as resistance involves choosing to engage in life-sustaining, identity-affirming actions that counteract systems of erasure. These are not always loud or revolutionary; they are frequently intimate and habitual. A woman who lights a candle for her ancestors before every meal is not performing a routine but is restoring a lineage.

Occupation as recovery asks not just what women are doing but what that doing restores. In trauma-informed care, it is essential to distinguish between coping that conceals pain and occupation that fosters integration. Isabela's bracelets were not only fine motor tasks. They were neuro-sensory anchors. They gave her structure, reclaimed cultural continuity, and offered tactile evidence that her body could still make beauty, even after violation. Occupational therapists should develop frameworks to help clients evaluate their everyday tasks for embedded meaning.

For example:

- Ask, "When do you feel most like yourself?" or "What do your hands know how to do that your mind might forget?"
- Document occupations that soothe versus those that numb. Braiding hair may connect generations; excessive hair-pulling may signal distress.
- Encourage clients to examine how certain occupations reflect inherited survival scripts. Is caregiving being used as a form of self-erasure? Is overworking masking avoidance?

This approach invites clients to move from reenactment to reinvention. Rather than stripping away their coping mechanisms, therapists can help them explore which occupations continue to serve them and which ones may be reenacting past harm. Recovery becomes less about stopping behaviors and more about shifting the intention behind them. A woman returning to traditional cooking may not be doing so from cultural obligation but as an act of reconnection to a grandmother who nurtured her when no one else did. A ritual once associated with silence may now be transformed into a site of storytelling. In this way, occupation becomes a vehicle for resisting invisibility, reclaiming agency, and rewriting inherited roles. Therapists can guide this process by helping clients discern which occupations are aligned with restoration and which may be preserving survival scripts that are no longer adaptive.

The Dark Side of Occupation

> At 25, Malia Heydari had spent nearly a decade navigating the unpredictable pain and fatigue of endometriosis. Her symptoms flared without warning, making everything from work deadlines to brunch plans feel like a gamble. But there was one thing she could control: food. At first, she started eliminating certain ingredients to reduce inflammation, such as gluten, dairy, and then sugar. When that didn't ease her symptoms, she tightened her diet further. By the time she sought occupational therapy, Malia was surviving on 500 calories a day, meticulously tracked and ritualized. "I'm not trying to be thin," she explained. "I just need something to feel manageable." Her days revolved around food planning, calorie counting, and solitary meals. Cooking had once been a shared joy with her sister, but now it was a private battleground. Despite appearing "disciplined," Malia's occupation of nourishment had become a coping mechanism for deeper sadness and a distorted sense of safety. The cost was high: weakened muscles, cognitive fog, social isolation, and a nervous system locked in survival mode.

The Invisible Toll of Dysfunctional Occupation

A 2022 study published in *Frontiers in Psychology* explored the pandemic's impact on eating behaviors, occupational patterns, and body perceptions in the general Canadian population. The authors identified three distinct profiles of "eaters" situated along a functional–dysfunctional continuum, highlighting how incongruent eating behaviors were closely tied to disrupted occupational balance, negative body image, and emotional strain. The findings emphasize that eating is not merely a biological act but is deeply embedded in our routines, identities, and sensory environments. For many, especially women, eating behaviors became distorted during the pandemic as a way to regain perceived control amid overwhelming uncertainty. These findings highlight a critical truth in occupational therapy: not all occupations support health. The line between a meaningful habit and a harmful compulsion is often drawn by context, emotional regulation, and underlying trauma. Malia's restrictive eating, while appearing health-motivated on the surface, reflected a breakdown in occupational adaptation. She wasn't eating less to nourish herself; she was eating less to regain a sense of control.

Trauma, chronic illness, and structural pressures can all distort the meaning and function of everyday activities. Occupations like cooking, grooming, organizing, or even exercise can shift from restorative to rigid, becoming vehicles for self-punishment or control when the broader system feels unsafe. In these cases, what appears to be productive engagement may actually signal nervous system dysregulation or covert distress. When a client devotes hours to perfectly arranging their meals but avoids all social interaction, or when a meticulously organized home hides a paralyzing fear of unpredictability, therapists must ask: is this truly meaningful occupation—or is it protective occupation masquerading as function?

Non-Restorative Patterns: When Occupation Masks Distress

Some occupations do not nourish the self; they deplete it. Yet they often go unnoticed in clinical settings because they present as discipline, motivation, or even wellness. A woman who maintains a rigorous gym schedule despite chronic fatigue may be praised for her consistency, even as she is using exercise to numb emotional pain. A client who insists on overdelivering at work after a miscarriage may be quietly reenacting a belief that productivity is the only shield against vulnerability. These are not maladaptive choices in the traditional sense. They are adaptations to environments where slowing down was never safe.

The danger is that non-restorative occupations frequently get mislabeled as resilience. Therapists may encourage routines without exploring their underlying function. For women of color in particular, many of whom have been conditioned to prove their worth through performance, activities that look "healthy" on the outside may serve a very different purpose internally. Interventions that focus on time use, without addressing trauma-informed meaning, risk reinforcing the very scripts that keep clients stuck.

Occupational therapy must develop a sharper lens for detecting these patterns. This means asking not just *what* a client does, but *why, when, and for whom.* A woman who restricts calories may not be trying to change her appearance but may be enacting control in an otherwise chaotic life. A caregiver who refuses respite may fear that rest is a betrayal of those who never had it.

Therapists can explore the energetic cost of occupations by integrating questions like:

- "How do you feel in your body before, during, and after this task?"
- "Does this occupation restore you, drain you, or numb you?"
- "Who taught you that this was the way to cope?"

These inquiries help distinguish between occupation that supports recovery and occupation that preserves reenactment. From an intervention standpoint, therapists can introduce body-based check-ins during routine activities, support re-engagement with abandoned leisure roles, or develop sensory profiles to help clients detect the line between regulation and compulsion. In Malia's case, therapy might involve shifting the goal from "planning meals" to exploring sensory-safe foods that evoke comfort rather than control. It could also mean practicing communal meals in supported environments to reconnect food with relationships instead of isolation.

Case Vignette and Reflections

For many women of color, trauma is not confined to a single moment in time. It often persists across settings, embedded in the institutions they must engage and the roles they are expected to uphold. The health system, in particular, can become a site where past harms are reactivated, not by overt violence, but through dismissal, misdiagnosis, and the failure to see the full context of a woman's life. Occupational therapy can play a transformative role in these moments by restoring function, recognizing invisible burdens, and reframing clinical narratives that have long excluded or misunderstood women of color.

Case Example 1: Carmen, Age 73—Compensatory Perfectionism After Critical Illness

Carmen, a 73-year-old Puerto Rican woman, was admitted to subacute rehabilitation following prolonged hospitalization for respiratory failure due to pneumonia. Though medically stabilized, she presented with profound muscle weakness, post-ICU fatigue, and low appetite. Despite her frailty, Carmen was deeply distressed by her perceived lack of productivity. She insisted on dressing independently, declined rest breaks, and became visibly agitated when offered assistance during basic tasks. During one session, she broke down in tears, stating, "If I am not useful, I am nothing."

Her occupational therapist learned that Carmen had been the primary caregiver in her multigenerational household for over four decades. She helped raise her grandchildren, translated during family medical appointments, and prepared daily meals for her husband with diabetes. Her caregiving role was never questioned; it was simply assumed. The sudden loss of function not only disrupted her physical routines, it destabilized her identity. Carmen's compulsion to do everything herself was not a sign of noncompliance, it was an attempt to reclaim meaning and belonging in a body she no longer trusted.

To respond to this layered presentation, the occupational therapist moved beyond rote ADL retraining. First, she introduced a **role-based functional interview**, asking questions such as, "What parts of your day made you feel most needed before you got sick?" and "What happens at home when you are not there to manage things?" These questions uncovered Carmen's fears of being replaced or forgotten within her family unit. Rather than immediately challenging her desire for independence, the therapist reframed functional goals to focus on *relational leadership*, not just physical capacity.

Next, the therapist implemented a **structured co-occupation planning tool**, mapping out which caregiving tasks Carmen valued most, which she could share, and which could be adapted. For instance, instead of preparing full meals, Carmen was supported in directing simple kitchen routines while seated, assigning tasks to others while still being "the head of the kitchen." To reinforce this shift, the therapist used **simulation-based sessions** with family members, during which Carmen practiced giving verbal instructions and managing pacing from a supported position. This helped preserve her identity as a caretaker while reducing the physical toll.

Because Carmen equated rest with weakness, the therapist also introduced **culturally anchored rest strategies** (Bovey et al., 2025). These included guided breathing layered with traditional prayer rhythms and using music from Carmen's childhood to create sensory anchors for relaxation. The therapist framed rest as an act of generational continuity: a way to preserve her strength so she could still "show up" for her family, even if differently. Energy conservation education was rebranded as legacy preservation.

Finally, the therapist supported Carmen in developing a **homecoming script**, which she could use with her family to explain her new routines and needs in her own voice. This was paired with visual handouts created in Spanish that identified fatigue signs and activity pacing cues. Carmen reported that having language to advocate for herself felt empowering, particularly in a household where emotions were rarely verbalized. These interventions went beyond restoring function. They affirmed Carmen's dignity, restructured her roles to fit her current capacity, and protected her from falling into a pattern of re-injury driven by internalized expectations. They also modeled how occupational therapy can honor cultural values without reinforcing harmful survival scripts.

Case Example 2: Tasha, Age 33—Trauma Reenactment Through Over-Functioning After Physical Injury

Tasha, a 33-year-old African American woman, was referred to outpatient occupational therapy following a motor vehicle collision that resulted in a fractured wrist and rotator cuff injury. Although her orthopedic healing was within expected timelines, her therapist noted persistent pain behaviors, emotional flatness, and an overwhelming urgency to resume her full caregiving responsibilities. Tasha was the legal guardian of her teenage nephew and managed care coordination for her mother, who lived with advanced diabetes and early-stage dementia. When asked about her pain during evaluation, she deflected: "Pain I can handle. What I can't handle is falling behind."

Over multiple sessions, her occupational therapist discovered that Tasha had taken on caregiving roles from adolescence, when her own mother's health began declining. As a child, she had balanced school with pharmacy pickups, meal prep, and medical translations. This role became central to her identity and sense of safety. The car accident, and the temporary loss of upper body function that followed, represented more than physical impairment; it triggered a profound sense of helplessness that echoed earlier life disruptions. This pattern of reenactment is not uncommon among women with intergenerational trauma histories, especially those shaped by early caregiving burdens and systemic inequities (Jones et al., 2023).

The occupational therapist implemented a dual-track approach: physical rehabilitation alongside trauma-informed occupational restructuring. Tasha was guided through a "role identity audit," a reflective tool that mapped her current responsibilities and helped identify which ones were essential, which could be delegated, and which were inherited scripts never revisited. This process illuminated that many of her tasks were driven by fear: of being seen as unreliable, of losing respect in her family, of being replaced.

The therapist introduced a modified co-occupation model. Instead of encouraging Tasha to "take a break" (which she rejected), they created shared routines with her nephew—such as prepping meals together with one-handed adaptations and teaching him to support her transfers safely. These sessions reframed caregiving as a collaborative process rather than a solitary burden.

Additionally, the therapist used expressive occupation through guided journaling and voice recording to help Tasha externalize the pressure she carried in silence. Rather than framing her behaviors as maladaptive, the OT acknowledged their origin in early survival and positioned the therapy plan as an evolution rather than a dismantling of who she had been. By session seven, Tasha reported feeling "less like I'm failing and more like I'm changing." She had begun allowing a family friend to support her with errands and had reinstated a previously abandoned goal: applying for part-time remote work in health administration, a field she had always wanted to pursue but postponed for family obligations.

Therapist Reflections on Clinical Decision Making

Carmen and Tasha's cases illustrate how occupational performance can become deeply intertwined with identity preservation, especially for women of color whose lives have been shaped by generational caregiving, systemic neglect, and cultural expectations of self-sacrifice (Abrams et al., 2019). What may appear in clinical settings as resistance or over-functioning is often a reenactment of survival roles that once protected the client emotionally or physically. In these moments, occupational therapy is not simply about regaining strength or restoring routines. It becomes a way to explore what a client believes about her worth, her body, and her role within her family or community.

For Carmen, the clinical goal was not to promote independence at any cost, but to reframe her occupational contributions in a way that preserved her sense of dignity without reinforcing exhaustion. Her therapist introduced collaborative caregiving routines, such as shared mealtime planning with visual recipe cards and activity pacing supported by adaptive kitchen tools. These strategies allowed Carmen to continue participating in meaningful roles while protecting her energy and respecting her need for rest. The goal was not to do less. It was to redefine how to do enough in a way that felt both safe and sustainable.

In Tasha's case, the therapeutic focus shifted away from orthopedic milestones and toward occupational discernment. A role identity audit allowed her to examine expectations that had never been questioned. Most importantly, integrating shared routines with her nephew helped her maintain relational connection while gently reducing isolation. Through voice journaling, expressive goal setting, and reengaging with long-postponed dreams, the therapist supported Tasha in reimagining her future not only through functional recovery but through restoration of purpose and possibility.

Across both cases, the core clinical lesson is clear: trauma recovery in occupational therapy cannot be measured only by visible improvements in function. Therapists must become fluent in recognizing when behaviors reflect reenactment rather than intention (Cerny et al., 2023; Dayo et al., 2023). They must learn to distinguish occupation as coping from occupation as healing. Tools such as values clarification interviews, culturally adapted sensory profiles, and relational role mapping can reveal how trauma is embedded within routines that appear functional but carry emotional cost.

Clinicians must also challenge the reflex to equate productivity, perfectionism, or stoicism with wellness (Jackson & Jewell, 2021). For many women, especially those who have survived cumulative stress and generational pressure, these traits are not signs of recovery. They are signals of a survival system still in motion (Crouch et al., 2024). Trauma-informed care calls us to slow down, listen differently, and make space for transformation of identity. Occupational therapy, at its best, becomes a space where survival can give way to self-authorship and where care is measured not only in outcomes but in the freedom to choose a different path forward.

Summary and Implications

Trauma in the lives of women of color often accumulates through relational dynamics, cultural roles, and systemic forces that remain unrecognized in traditional models of care (Johnson et al., 2024). These experiences shape not only how women survive, but how they show up in daily life, through routines, expectations, and coping mechanisms that can be misread as compliance or strength. What is often labeled as high functioning may in fact be reenactment. What looks like disengagement may be self-protection.

Occupational therapy holds the unique potential to meet these complexities with care that affirms identity, restores agency, and addresses the invisible labor that so many women carry (Khan, 2025). Function alone is never the full picture. Participation must be interpreted through the lens of safety, dignity, and choice. Therapists must learn to ask different questions, observe meaning behind routine, and support clients in separating what was inherited from what is truly chosen (Monthuy-Blanc et al., 2022). Values clarification, role mapping, sensory attunement, and co-authored goal planning are not just interventions—they are acts of justice that help women reclaim space within their bodies and lives. Healing is not about doing more. It is about having the right to decide what enough looks like (Patchen et al., 2024). When therapy becomes a place for that decision-making, it becomes more than a service. It becomes liberation in practice.

References

Abrams, J. A., Hill, A., & Maxwell, M. (2019). Underneath the mask of the strong Black woman schema: Disentangling influences of strength and self-silencing on depressive symptoms among U.S. Black women. *Sex Roles, 80*(9–10), 517–526. https://doi.org/10.1007/s11199-018-0956-y

Bovey, M., Hosny, N., Dutray, F., & Heim, E. (2025). Trauma-related cultural concepts of distress: A systematic review of qualitative literature from the Middle East and North Africa, and Sub-Saharan Africa. *SSM—Mental Health, 5*, 100402. https://doi.org/10.1016/j.ssmmh.2025.100402

Cerny, S., Berg-Poppe, P., Anis, M., Wesner, C., Merrigan, M., & LaPlante, K. (2023). Outcomes from an interprofessional curriculum on trauma-informed care among pediatric service providers. *Journal of Interprofessional Care, 37*(2), 288–299. https://doi.org/10.1080/13561820.2022.2070142

Crouch, M. C., Miller-Roenigk, B. D., Schrader, S. W., Griffith, F., Simmons, S., & Gordon, D. M. (2024). Potentially traumatic events of women of color in an urban adult basic education program. *Journal of Aggression, Maltreatment & Trauma, 33*(4), 432–450. https://doi.org/10.1080/10926771.2023.2231384 Epub 2023 July 5. PMID: 38798799; PMCID: PMC11114608.

Dayo, E., Christy, K., & Habte, R. (2023). Health in colour: Black women, racism, and maternal health. *Lancet Regional Health: Americas, 17*, 100408. https://doi.org/10.1016/j.lana.2022.100408

Dmowska, A., Fielding-Singh, P., Halpern, J., & Prata, N. (2024). The intersection of traumatic childbirth and obstetric racism: A qualitative study. *Birth (Berkeley, Calif.), 51*(1), 209–217. https://doi.org/10.1111/birt.12774

Jackson, M. L., & Jewell, V. D. (2021). Educational practices for providers of trauma-informed care: A scoping review. *Journal of Pediatric Nursing, 60*, 130–138. https://doi.org/10.1016/j.pedn.2021.04.029

Johnson, S., Konopasky, A., & Wyatt, T. (2024). In their own voices: A critical narrative review of Black women faculty members' first-person accounts of racial trauma across higher education. *Teaching and Learning in Medicine, 37*(2), 218–228. https://doi.org/10.1080/10401334.2024.2329680

Jones, A. A., Duncan, M. S., Perez-Brumer, A., Connell, C. M., Burrows, W. B., & Oser, C. B. (2023). Impacts of intergenerational substance use and trauma among black women involved in the criminal justice system: A longitudinal analysis. *Journal of*

Substance Use and Addiction Treatment, *153*, 208952. https://doi.org/10.1016/j. josat.2023.208952

Khan, S. (2025). *Occupational therapy and women's health: A practitioner guide*. Routledge.

Miljkovitch, R., Danner-Touati, C., Gery, I., Bernier, A., Sirparanta, A., & Deborde, A. S. (2022). The role of multiple attachments in intergenerational transmission of child sexual abuse among male victims. *Child Abuse & Neglect*, *128*, 104864. https://doi.org/10.1016/j.chiabu.2020.104864

Monthuy-Blanc, J., Corno, G., Bouchard, S., St-Pierre, M. J., Bourbeau, F., Mostefa-Kara, L., Therrien, É., & Rousseau, M. (2022). Body perceptions, occupations, eating attitudes, and behaviors emerged during the pandemic: An exploratory cluster analysis of eaters profiles. *Frontiers in Psychology*, *13*, 949373. https://doi.org/10.3389/fpsyg.2022.949373

Patchen, L., McCullers, A., Beach, C., Browning, M., Porter, S., Danielson, A., Asegieme, E., Richardson, S. R., Jost, A., Jensen, C. S., & Ahmed, N. (2024). Safe babies, safe moms: A multifaceted, trauma informed care initiative. *Maternal and Child Health Journal*, *28*(1), 31–37. https://doi.org/10.1007/s10995-023-03840-z

Chapter 9

Stress and Trauma in Women with Disabilities

Chapter Objectives

Upon completion of this chapter, the reader will be able to:

1. Critically examine the intersection of disability, gender, and trauma, identifying how dependence, stigma, and institutional power imbalances contribute to unique occupational vulnerabilities in women with disabilities.
2. Analyze the mechanisms of diagnostic overshadowing and recognize how trauma symptoms are frequently misattributed to pre-existing conditions, leading to fragmented care and missed opportunities for intervention.
3. Apply trauma-informed strategies to assessment and treatment planning, including the use of somatic safety frameworks, narrative-based tools, and co-regulated routines that honor autonomy and lived experience.
4. Evaluate the occupational consequences of cumulative stressors, such as systemic inaccessibility, surveillance, and emotional labor, and describe how these disrupt participation across life stages, including the postpartum period.
5. Demonstrate how occupational therapy can serve as a vehicle for both clinical recovery and structural advocacy, addressing not only individual needs but also the systems that sustain marginalization and trauma in the lives of disabled women.

After a fall caused by faulty wheelchair brakes, 36-year-old Miriam Katz was admitted to outpatient rehabilitation. Miriam, a Jewish woman with cerebral palsy, had recently ended a ten-year relationship marked by increasing emotional and financial control. Though polite and cooperative, she grew tense during sessions, especially

DOI: 10.4324/9781003658559-9

when discussing her home environment or support needs. Her therapist noted that Miriam avoided using adaptive devices she clearly qualified for, refused physical assistance even when fatigued, and often apologized for "taking up too much time." As trust built, Miriam shared that her former partner managed all her appointments, controlled access to her mobility equipment, and frequently undermined her autonomy while presenting as a caregiver to others. The injury that brought her to therapy was only the most visible wound but beneath it were years of erased preferences, conditional support, and internalized fear of being seen as incapable.

More than 250 million women around the world live with disabilities, yet their experiences with trauma remain among the most underrecognized in public health and rehabilitation discourse. The intersection of gender, disability, and violence is not merely additive; it is multiplicative, compounding vulnerability through social exclusion, economic marginalization, and power asymmetries that are often embedded in the very systems designed to provide care. These women face higher rates of every form of violence: physical, sexual, psychological, and financial. Yet the pathways to safety and healing are often obstructed by institutional barriers, diagnostic overshadowing, and assumptions that frame disability as the central problem rather than the context in which trauma unfolds.

A 2023 qualitative study from Sweden found that women with disabilities were nearly twice as likely to experience intimate partner violence as women without disabilities, and that psychological abuse, though deeply harmful, was often dismissed or difficult to prove. Participants described prolonged exposure to multiple forms of abuse, often continuing even after separation, and shared the emotional toll of navigating systems that failed to recognize their experiences as valid. These findings reflect broader global patterns: that trauma against women with disabilities is not only more common, but more likely to be silenced, misinterpreted, or medicalized without context.

What emerges is not just a higher prevalence of trauma, but a different shape of it—where dependence can be exploited, advocacy may be misread as defiance, and trauma lives in the body not only as memory but as constraint. Recovery, in this context, is not about returning to a baseline of function. It is about reclaiming access to meaningful participation in environments that have too often treated women with disabilities as both invisible and incapable. The work begins by understanding not only what has happened to these women, but what has been denied to them in the aftermath, and how clinical practices can either reinforce or disrupt that denial.

Compounded Vulnerabilities and Invisible Burdens

Women with disabilities live at the intersection of ableism, sexism, and structural neglect, with each compounding the other in ways that intensify vulnerability to trauma and violence. Research consistently shows that women with disabilities experience intimate partner violence at nearly double the rate of women without disabilities, with higher exposure to all forms of abuse: physical, emotional, financial, and sexual. But what is less often discussed is how these abuses manifest in settings shaped by dependence, stigma, and limited access to recourse.

Rather than isolated episodes, violence against women with disabilities is often sustained, cumulative, and entangled in the systems meant to provide care or support. The effects are not only physical but occupational—interfering with routines, access to services, relational autonomy, and the ability to seek safety without compromising basic needs. Functional dependence, whether for mobility, communication, or daily living tasks, can become a site of exploitation, particularly when caregivers are also perpetrators. In many cases, the threat is not dramatic but persistent: the fear of being left unattended, spoken over, or punished through neglect.

Even when women attempt to disclose abuse, they are frequently met with disbelief or misattribution. Symptoms of trauma are dismissed as part of the disability, or assumptions about cognitive capacity prevent full recognition of the harm endured. The result is a cycle in which the trauma is both magnified and rendered invisible—a double burden that occupational therapy is uniquely equipped to address. Occupational therapists must be attuned to these compounded dynamics. Trauma-informed care for women with disabilities cannot rely on generalized screening tools or surface-level rapport building. It requires a nuanced understanding of power, access, and systemic failure. It demands an approach that not only recognizes the trauma but actively works to dismantle the structures that allow it to persist in silence.

Dependency and Power Imbalances

Ruth Pesci, an 82-year-old woman with advanced multiple sclerosis, had been living at home with the support of a rotating team of home health aides. Paralyzed from the waist down and requiring assistance with toileting, transfers, and meal preparation, she had grown increasingly withdrawn during occupational therapy home visits. Her therapist noticed that Ruth's skin was often unwashed, her call bell was placed out of reach, and she seemed anxious when discussing her daily care. One afternoon, Ruth whispered, "She says if I complain, I'll be sent to a home." The "she" was a daytime aide who regularly left Ruth alone for hours, delayed meals, and refused to help with repositioning unless Ruth apologized first. Ruth had never disclosed the neglect to her case manager, fearing retaliation, disbelief, and the threat of institutionalization. Her body was technically safe, but her autonomy, dignity, and psychological safety were under siege.

Women with disabilities may rely on others for transportation, medication management, feeding, hygiene, or mobility. This dependence can be exploited to establish control and perpetuate harm. Perpetrators in these contexts may be partners, family members, paid aides, or institutional caregivers. Abuse may involve physical aggression but often takes subtler forms: withholding of assistive devices, overmedicating, sabotaging appointments, or enforcing rigid routines that limit autonomy. This type of coercive control is particularly insidious because it blends into the landscape of care. A woman denied her wheelchair for hours may not be viewed as a victim of violence but simply a patient awaiting assistance. A caregiver who manipulates medication schedules may not be questioned if their role is perceived as essential. These dynamics erode the boundary between support and domination, making it harder for women to name their experiences or to be believed when they do.

Occupational therapists must become fluent in identifying not only functional limitations but also the subtle manifestations of coercion and control that may appear as care. This requires a shift from asking solely about what a client can do to also exploring who controls when and how those activities occur. For example, therapists might include structured inquiry around access such as "Are there times when someone limits your ability to move freely, use your wheelchair, or complete hygiene routines?" and ask about patterns of missed appointments, changes in medication routines, or unexpected declines in participation. These questions should be framed with cultural humility and in accessible language, especially for women with communication or cognitive differences.

Research consistently shows that women with disabilities experience trauma at significantly higher rates than men. This disparity is shaped by gendered power dynamics, social isolation, and the reality that many women depend on others for assistance with intimate care. Their vulnerability is often compounded by societal tendencies to infantilize women with disabilities or dismiss their reports as confusion or exaggeration. Abuse may not be obvious—it may look like excessive "help," delayed access to basic needs, or rigid control over routines. These behaviors are often overlooked because women are viewed primarily through a medical or support lens, rather than as autonomous individuals whose rights can be violated.

To address this, occupational therapists must embed trauma awareness into both assessment and treatment planning. Clinical tools should include questions about choice, control, and daily interruptions. Therapists can document concerns about caregiver dynamics within the occupational profile, noting not just what the client does but under what conditions. Interventions may include scripting for assertive communication, using task checklists that reinforce the client's role in directing care, or collaborating with care teams to ensure backup plans are in place when the primary caregiver relationship becomes compromised. In cases where abuse or coercion is suspected, therapists may be the first to observe these signs and can play a vital role in reporting, advocacy, and supporting transitions to safer arrangements.

Diagnostic Overshadowing and Missed Screening

When women with disabilities present with symptoms that stem from trauma, such as autonomic instability, intrusive somatic sensations, or abrupt shifts in emotional tone, these signals are frequently subsumed under the framework of their existing diagnosis. This phenomenon, known as diagnostic overshadowing, distorts clinical interpretation and narrows the lens through which behavior and health are understood. Rather than being recognized as distinct indicators of possible violence or psychological injury, these symptoms are often reframed as manifestations of the disability itself.

For instance, a woman with a sensory processing disorder who begins avoiding touch or eye contact following an incident of sexual violence may be labeled as regressing or deteriorating without consideration for new trauma exposure. Similarly, a woman with a history of psychiatric hospitalization who shows increased irritability or somatic preoccupation may have her distress dismissed as baseline instability, rather than recognized as a shift requiring deeper contextual analysis. These interpretive errors are not merely clinical oversights—they represent epistemic injustice, wherein the survivor's testimony and embodied signals are systematically discredited due to her disability status.

In occupational therapy, where functional observation is central to care, practitioners are uniquely positioned to detect incongruities between baseline occupational performance and emerging patterns of dysregulation. However, trauma signals are often masked by the very strategies that have allowed the client to survive: scripted compliance, flattened affect, or hyper-functioning in high-demand tasks. Recognizing these as potential trauma adaptations, rather than indicators of functional stability, requires a clinical lens informed by both neuro-education and trauma-informed care.

Occupational therapists can mitigate diagnostic overshadowing by adopting trauma-aware assessment practices that attend to both verbal and nonverbal cues across multiple domains of function. For example, shifts in praxis, interoceptive awareness, or activity pacing may signal nervous system dysregulation, even in the absence of verbal disclosure. Practitioners should consider integrating observational tools that track micro-patterns in routine activities, such as hygiene, mobility, or communication initiation, as these often provide early indicators of trauma impact in populations who may not express distress in expected ways.

Documentation also becomes a critical site of advocacy. Rather than recording withdrawal or task refusal in pathologizing terms, occupational therapists can highlight discrepancies between prior and current occupational engagement, framing them within a trauma-responsive model. Language such as "client demonstrates occupational avoidance patterns inconsistent with previous levels of autonomy" or "emergent dysregulation during previously mastered tasks" invites further interdisciplinary evaluation without requiring the client to provide verbal confirmation of trauma. This approach maintains therapeutic alliance while signaling the need for integrated trauma-responsive care pathways.

Silencing, Surveillance, and Reporting Barriers

Klara Weiss, a fifty-two-year-old German woman with a mild intellectual disability, had been living in a skilled nursing facility for the past year following a fall at home. Known for her punctuality and love of gardening, Klara had recently begun refusing to attend group activities and was observed flinching during routine dressing assistance. When asked about her change in behavior, she looked down and said only, "I do not like Tuesdays." Her occupational therapist, attuned to the subtle shifts in Klara's engagement and affect, noted that her distress coincided with a particular staff rotation. Rather than confronting Klara with direct questions about possible harm, the therapist initiated a sensory-based life story activity and adjusted care routines to increase Klara's sense of control and predictability. Over time, Klara began to reengage with her morning walks and expressed preference for staff who helped her feel safe in her own room. Her story exemplifies how trauma in women with disabilities often communicates itself through occupation, not words, and how trust can be rebuilt when therapists create environments that center autonomy, observation, and gentle inquiry.

For many women with disabilities, the decision to disclose violence is shaped not only by fear of the perpetrator but by a broader system of surveillance that casts their behaviors, choices, and relationships under constant scrutiny. Disclosures of abuse are often met not with validation, but with disbelief, blame, or administrative consequences. Women who require assistance with daily living, for instance, may fear that reporting an abusive caregiver could result in institutionalization, withdrawal of services, or retaliation that threatens their autonomy (Anyango et al., 2023; McConnell & Phelan, 2022).

Surveillance is particularly acute in institutional settings, where residents are often monitored in ways that erode privacy and choice. Staff rotations, inconsistent communication, and hierarchical cultures can create an environment in which women feel watched, but not truly seen. In these contexts, silence becomes an adaptive strategy, used not out of passivity, but out of calculated self-protection. The cost of disclosure is weighed against the risk of losing housing, services, or perceived credibility, especially when previous reports have been dismissed or led to punitive interventions.

Communication barriers further compound the problem. Women with intellectual disabilities, cognitive impairments, or speech differences may struggle to articulate experiences of harm in ways that are considered credible by healthcare or legal systems (Njelesani et al., 2021; Mueller & Sutherland, 2023). Even when language is not a barrier, the expectation of linear, emotionally neutral recounting can disqualify narratives that are fragmented, emotionally charged, or somatically expressed. These expectations reflect a profound misunderstanding of how trauma lives in the body, nonlinear, sensory-based, and often accessible only through metaphor or occupation.

Occupational therapists are in a position to notice what others overlook: sudden disruptions in routine, loss of engagement in previously meaningful activities, or subtle signs of distress during hands-on care. In contexts where direct inquiry about abuse may be unsafe or unethical, therapists can instead use indirect strategies grounded in narrative-based and sensory-informed assessment. Questions such as "Are there parts of your day that feel unsafe or uncomfortable?" or "When do you feel most in control of your space?" can surface disclosures that are encoded in occupation rather than direct language.

Documentation and interdisciplinary communication must also reflect these subtleties. Rather than requiring a formal report of abuse, occupational therapists can flag unexplained functional decline, changes in affective tone during care routines, or environmental triggers that correlate with dysregulation. These observations can support further investigation by social work, nursing, or case management teams without pressuring the client to confirm trauma that they are not yet ready or able to verbalize.

Reframing Disability and Violence Through a Trauma-Informed Lens

Disability and violence are often treated as distinct clinical concerns. One is typically categorized as a functional limitation requiring rehabilitation, while the other is framed as a discrete social issue or psychological trauma. But this dichotomy is misleading. For many women, especially those with chronic conditions or acquired impairments, the two are intimately intertwined. Emerging research in neuropsychology and occupational science reveals that prolonged exposure to violence can alter motor planning, sensory integration, autonomic regulation, and neuroimmune function—blurring the boundaries between psychological trauma and physiological impairment.

For example, neuroendocrine disruptions from chronic abuse may impair pain modulation, leading to heightened sensitivity to stimuli and difficulty tolerating therapeutic touch. Muscle guarding patterns that were once protective during violence can calcify into long-term movement restrictions. What looks like fibromyalgia, postural instability, or executive dysfunction may, in fact, be somatic expressions of lived trauma. This means that some disabilities are not simply medical outcomes but are biologically shaped by prolonged survival in unsafe environments.

Occupational therapists are uniquely positioned to uncover these patterns. Rather than viewing disability through a fixed diagnosis, therapists can examine how tasks are performed, how environments are navigated, and how bodily cues are managed. When a woman hesitates to use adaptive equipment, avoids certain spaces, or becomes fatigued with tasks that were once manageable, it may not be due to motivation or capacity, but rather an unspoken history that has shaped her nervous system's calibration to risk (Gesi et al., 2021).

In this context, clinical objectivity must make space for narrative complexity. For example, consider a woman who delays toileting routines not because of incontinence but because of prior abuse in care settings where privacy was violated. Or a woman who avoids group rehabilitation because the presence of strangers elevates her startle reflex and limits concentration. These are not signs of behavioral resistance. They are neurobiological adaptations to environments that once demanded constant vigilance.

When these patterns are misinterpreted, women are often labeled nonadherent or overly sensitive. Their care plans become less effective, and their outcomes suffer. Trauma-informed occupational therapy requires not only awareness of past events but the capacity to identify their present-day imprint on occupation, regulation, and participation. This reframing allows therapists to see complexity where others see compliance, to honor adaptation where others see dysfunction, and to reconstruct care around what safety truly means to the individual, not just what performance metrics demand.

Diagnoses That Obscure Trauma

For women with disabilities, trauma often hides in plain sight. Not because the signs are absent, but because they are reframed through the lens of existing diagnoses. When a woman with multiple sclerosis reports chronic fatigue and emotional lability, her experience is often attributed solely to her neurological condition. When a woman with cerebral palsy exhibits hyperarousal, sleep disruption, or exaggerated startle responses, these are frequently interpreted as features of spasticity or autonomic dysregulation. This is not just diagnostic error. It is diagnostic compression, the narrowing of clinical interpretation until trauma disappears into the folds of a known condition.

The process is subtle but far-reaching. Standard clinical protocols prioritize primary diagnoses, especially those with visible or measurable pathology. This emphasis creates a hierarchy of explanation. Trauma, with its diffuse and context-dependent presentation, rarely takes precedence. As a result, women who live at the intersection of chronic disability and trauma often receive fragmented care. One provider manages bowel irregularities. Another addresses mood instability. A third attempts to adjust medications for pain or fatigue. No one asks about history. No one maps the pattern. And no one names what the body is trying to say.

This fragmentation is not unique to medicine. It is embedded in the systems that govern rehabilitation, education, and even therapeutic support. When trauma is obscured by a primary diagnosis, it becomes harder to identify the full impact on function, identity, and participation. Women are told they are noncompliant, emotionally unstable, or behaviorally difficult. Their coping strategies are labeled as symptoms. Their boundaries are viewed as resistance. And the trauma continues, unacknowledged, untreated, and often exacerbated by the very systems that were meant to help.

Occupational therapy has a distinct opportunity to break this pattern. Rather than defaulting to symptom management, therapists can approach each clinical presentation as a constellation, a set of signals that require interpretation, not just intervention. This requires fluency in both the clinical profile of the disability and the nuanced markers of unresolved trauma. It also requires a shift in therapeutic stance—from problem solving to pattern recognition. When we stop asking what is wrong and start asking what has been survived, our interventions change, and so do the functional outcomes. See Table 9.1 for examples of common diagnoses that may obscure trauma in women with disabilities and how occupational therapy can reframe these presentations through a trauma-informed lens.

Occupational therapists working with women with disabilities must move beyond symptom-based frameworks and into a model of pattern recognition and contextual inquiry. One of the most overlooked strategies is **dual coding**—the process of simultaneously interpreting a symptom through both the lens of the primary diagnosis and the possibility of trauma. For instance, when a woman with cerebral palsy reports worsening spasticity during medical visits, therapists might ask whether appointments evoke earlier experiences of coercion, bodily exposure, or loss of control (Aguillard et al., 2022; Piantedosi et al., 2023; Wint et al., 2016). By integrating trauma screening questions into functional assessments—such as asking when symptoms worsen, who is present, or what environments feel safest—clinicians gain insight into both the biology and biography of the response.

Another underutilized approach is **occupation-based backtracking**, where therapists trace an interrupted routine back to its point of breakdown and identify whether trauma cues or relational dynamics were involved. If a woman with MS discontinues community outings, it may not be due to fatigue alone. It could reflect anxiety after a recent public incident involving accessibility barriers or microaggressions. In these cases, the intervention is not simply energy conservation. It is about restoring choice, predictability, and environmental control.

Table 9.1 Diagnoses That May Obscure Trauma in Women with Disabilities

Primary Diagnoses	Overlapping Trauma-Related Symptoms	Common Misattributions	Trauma-Informed OT Considerations
Cerebral Palsy	Startle reflex, hypertonia, sleep disturbance	Attributed to neuromotor patterns	Assess for trauma-related hyperarousal or sleep avoidance
Multiple Sclerosis	Fatigue, numbness, depression	Seen as disease progression	Screen for loss triggers, trauma anniversaries, or emotional blunting
Autism Spectrum Disorder	Sensory avoidance, emotional shutdown	Misread as social withdrawal or rigidity	Explore past sensory trauma, medical trauma, or relational rupture
Chronic Pain Syndrome	Anxiety, withdrawal, mood changes	Labeled as catastrophizing	Integrate trauma narrative with somatic regulation goals
Intellectual Disability	Emotional dysregulation, behavioral shifts	Attributed to cognitive limitations	Investigate relational patterns and coercive environments
Traumatic Brain Injury	Memory issues, irritability, sensory sensitivity	Framed as neurological sequelae only	Differentiate between neurological and emotional triggers

Techniques such as graded exposure to previously avoided occupations, co-creating safety plans for public engagement, and using narrative tools to process past encounters can help re-establish agency where it was once lost. These strategies shift the focus from symptom containment to functional liberation, an outcome that centers dignity as much as it does participation.

Navigating Systems That Reinforce Disability

For many women with disabilities, trauma is not an isolated event but a condition sustained by the systems meant to provide support. Healthcare, education, housing, and even rehabilitation services often function in ways that inadvertently reinforce marginalization. When appointments are only available during standard work hours, when intake forms fail to capture accessible communication preferences, or when treatment goals prioritize independence over interdependence, the message is clear: the system was not designed with you in mind.

This misalignment is not simply an inconvenience. It is a structural barrier to safety, participation, and recovery. A woman who relies on paratransit cannot access urgent care if transportation must be scheduled days in advance

(Aguillard et al., 2022). A woman who uses a communication device may find herself excluded from shared decision making if her provider does not pause long enough to wait for her response. These are not clinical oversights. They are points of systemic friction that accumulate over time, diminishing self-efficacy and eroding trust in care (Aguillard et al., 2022).

Occupational therapy holds the tools to challenge these embedded inequities, but only if practice is expanded beyond the individual to include the systems that shape occupational opportunity. Therapists must ask not only what routines are disrupted, but what policies, protocols, or cultural norms are making participation harder than it needs to be. This means taking inventory of more than fine motor skills or ADL proficiency. It requires looking at referral patterns, physical environments, and reimbursement models that reward compliance over autonomy.

In practice, this might mean supporting a client not by optimizing her grooming routine, but by helping her negotiate with a personal care attendant agency to secure consistent, respectful support. It might mean writing documentation not to meet a productivity target, but to advocate for extended services when trauma complicates recovery timelines. Systems reinforcement is often invisible to those operating within them. Occupational therapists are uniquely positioned to make these patterns visible and to co-create new ones—that recognize that participation is not just a personal ability. It is also a political outcome.

Restoring Therapeutic Alliance Through Somatic Safety

For women with disabilities who have experienced trauma, the clinical encounter itself can become a site of dysregulation. Touch, evaluation, and even well-intended encouragement may register as intrusive if the nervous system is still scanning for threat. What looks like resistance or avoidance in therapy may, in fact, be a finely tuned survival response—one shaped not only by past trauma but by repeated exposure to clinical environments that were overstimulating, disempowering, or dismissive.

Therapeutic alliance in this context must begin at the level of the body. Before a woman can engage in goal planning or participate in structured intervention, her nervous system must receive signals of safety. This is not a passive state. It is created through attunement, pacing, and the predictable use of relational cues. Therapists must track not only progress but physiological shifts: breath holding, gaze aversion, muscle tension, flattened affect. These are the early indicators that trust is being challenged, even if the client remains verbally compliant.

This is where the concept of **somatic safety** becomes essential. Rather than focusing on what the therapist wants to teach or correct, the emphasis shifts to what the body can tolerate and integrate (Hashimoto et al., 2023). This means asking permission before initiating physical contact, allowing choice in posture or position during sessions, and offering a rhythm of predictability in how sessions are structured. But beyond these fundamentals, somatic safety involves building **interoceptive awareness**—helping women notice and name what is happening inside their bodies without shame or confusion.

Occupational therapy can draw from both neuroscience and trauma theory to operationalize this. Techniques such as co-regulated breathing, rhythmic movement, or grounding through tactile input are not supplemental; they are primary. They lay the physiological groundwork for cognitive and functional recovery. Without these anchors, even the most evidence-based interventions can feel invasive. See Table 9.2 for examples of strategies that promote somatic safety across the therapeutic process.

Creating somatic safety requires more than being gentle or friendly. It means building a session structure that consistently communicates predictability, control, and choice. One of the most effective ways to do this is by offering small but meaningful options throughout the session. For example, before beginning a

Table 9.2 Restoring Somatic Safety Across the Phases of Occupational Therapy for Women

Phase of Care	Common Risks to Somatic Safety	Trauma-Informed OT Strategies and Examples
Initial Evaluation	Sensory overload from clinical settings, rapid information gathering, power imbalances, and lack of preparation for hands-on assessments	Use calming environmental inputs (e.g., soft lighting, minimal noise). Begin with co-regulated breath or grounding. Narrate steps before starting. Ask, "Would it feel better to talk through options first?"
Intervention Planning	Feeling unheard in goal setting, pressure to agree with therapist recommendations, reactivation of past coercion related to authority or care planning	Offer choices and ask, "What matters most to you right now?" Validate ambivalence. Include reflective practices (e.g., draw your daily energy map) before deciding on activity focus.
Task Initiation	Activation of trauma responses (freeze, dissociation) when asked to perform tasks with uncertain outcomes or under perceived observation	Normalize pauses and allow opt-out points. Frame participation as experimentation, not testing. Say, "Let's try it and stop whenever your body says it's enough."
Physical Handling	Re-traumatization through unconsented touch, clinical posture positioning that mimics past immobilization or loss of control	Always ask permission before contact. Provide alternatives (e.g., verbal prompts, mirrors, adaptive equipment). Let the client choose the angle, pace, or location of physical support.

(Continued)

Table 9.2 (Continued)

Phase of Care	Common Risks to Somatic Safety	Trauma-Informed OT Strategies and Examples
Sensorimotor Work	Sensory tools or modalities may evoke discomfort, overwhelm, or flashbacks, particularly if linked to previous restraint, medical trauma, or neglect	Allow full autonomy in selecting textures, sounds, and proximity. Use layering (e.g., combine vestibular input with calming scent). Monitor shifts in breath or posture as cues of safety or distress.
Narrative-Based Work	Disclosure of past trauma can dysregulate the nervous system or lead to post-session shutdown	Frame processing as optional, not expected. Pair narrative work with grounding before and after (e.g., pressure input, bilateral movement). Anchor stories in strengths and current context.
Group Participation	Fear of exposure, loss of control over boundaries, comparison, or group-triggered dysregulation	Offer opt-in formats for all sharing. Create "quiet roles" within groups (e.g., timekeeper, note writer). Normalize co-regulation (e.g., synchronized breathing to begin).
Intervention Implementation	Loss of agency if protocols feel rigid, especially if routines mimic institutional care or past control dynamics	Embed routine flexibility: "You can lead today or follow along." Use co-occupation and mirroring. Adjust task steps based on moment-to-moment feedback ("Would pausing help here?").
Outcome Measurement	Re-experiencing performance pressure, fear of being judged, association of scoring with failure	Use collaborative reflection ("How does this feel in your body?"). Replace numerical goals with narrative ones (e.g., "What made this task easier today than last time?").
Discharge Planning	Feelings of abandonment, loss of structure or connection, prior experiences of unsupported transitions, reactivation of rejection trauma	Begin transition planning early. Offer co-created visual maps of routines or coping strategies. Use a "continuity anchor" such as a written letter to self, recorded message, or chosen object (Chitapi et al., 2024).

transfer or mobility task, the therapist might ask, "Would you like to try this from your chair or the mat?" or "Would you prefer to go through the steps together before doing anything?" These are not just courtesies. They are nervous system interventions. They give the client an opportunity to regulate before acting, which increases the likelihood of sustained engagement. This is especially important for women whose past trauma has involved physical helplessness or procedural violation. The ability to pause, redirect, or say no without penalty becomes part of the therapeutic process, not a disruption of it.

Another practical approach is to shift how we interpret and respond to non-verbal cues. If a client begins fidgeting, avoiding eye contact, or answering in short phrases, it may signal a stress response rather than disinterest. The therapist can respond by lowering the cognitive or sensory load without calling attention to it. This might include dimming lights, simplifying task steps, or shifting to a more rhythm-based or sensory-rich activity. When preparing for transitions such as discharge, it is equally important to avoid abrupt endings. Instead, therapists can co-create a written or visual tool that summarizes what helped the client feel regulated, what routines supported participation, and what signals might indicate that external support is needed again. These practices do not require special equipment or extra time. They require attention to how the body speaks—and a willingness to respond in real time with clinical skill and relational care.

Occupational Disruption Across the Continuum of Disability

Interruptions to daily life are not uncommon, but for women with disabilities, these interruptions are rarely temporary. They are sustained, cumulative, and deeply tied to how society structures participation. Occupational disruption in this context is not only about function. It reflects an ongoing negotiation with environments that restrict access, systems that delay care, and assumptions that limit what roles are available—or even imaginable.

The nature of this disruption varies. Some women grow up navigating barriers that others never have to see. Others face abrupt transitions after injury or illness that redraw the boundaries of independence overnight. Still others live with conditions that shift gradually, making each stage of adjustment feel both invisible and exhausting. What unites these experiences is the steady erosion of roles and routines that once gave structure to everyday life. When those roles begin to slip away, the loss is not just practical. It is personal. In these moments, occupational therapy is not simply a tool for recovery. It becomes a vehicle for meaning making. The work is not only about helping women regain skills but about helping them preserve identity in the face of change. It involves shaping routines that reflect current realities without diminishing the individual's value. It asks therapists to move beyond the task at hand and into a conversation about how participation is defined—and who gets to define it.

Chronicity, Unpredictability, and Erosion of Role Identity

Living with a chronic or episodic condition means navigating an ever-changing landscape of energy, function, and control. One week, a woman may manage her roles at work and home with ease. The next, she may struggle to move through daily tasks, sidelined by pain, fatigue, or cognitive fog. These fluctuations do not follow a linear trajectory. They disrupt routines without warning, often eroding confidence in one's ability to plan, participate, or be perceived as dependable.

This unpredictability places immense pressure on identity. Many women describe themselves not by what they can no longer do, but by who they can no longer be. The dependable employee. The present mother. The partner who could once be counted on. When these roles are interrupted repeatedly, they begin to feel fragile. Over time, the effort to protect them becomes another form of labor: emotional, cognitive, and often invisible. Occupational therapy in these contexts must move beyond surface-level adaptation. It is not enough to modify a task or offer energy conservation tips. What is needed is a reframing of how identity is supported when consistency is no longer guaranteed. Therapists can help women identify flexible versions of familiar roles, or entirely new ones that allow for expression, purpose, and social contribution on terms that match their current capacities. This is not about returning to a previous version of self. It is about creating continuity through change. See Table 9.3 for examples of how different disability trajectories can disrupt occupational identity and participation, along with trauma-informed strategies that support meaningful engagement across changing capacities.

Supporting women with disabilities through chronic or progressive change demands therapeutic presence, the ability to notice when an occupational loss

Table 9.3 Trauma-Informed Occupational Therapy in Episodic and Progressive Conditions

Condition Type	Common Disruption Pattern	Impact on Identity and Roles	Trauma-Informed OT Strategies
Episodic (e.g., lupus, MS)	Sudden loss of function during symptom flares	Perceived unreliability; reduced self-efficacy; social withdrawal	Design routines that accommodate unpredictability; use energy mapping and values clarification
Progressive (e.g., ALS, MD)	Gradual decline in motor or cognitive function	Anticipatory grief; loss of autonomy; fear of future dependency	Integrate legacy-building roles; support gradual role redefinition and future planning
Congenital (e.g., CP, spina bifida)	Lifelong environmental and social exclusion	Internalized stigma; limited exposure to meaningful occupations	Expand occupational repertoire; affirm identity outside of performance metrics

is not just functional but emotional, and the willingness to stay in conversation about what those losses mean. This is where trauma-informed care intersects with identity-centered practice. When therapists recognize that role erosion is not a failure of adjustment but a natural response to disruption, they can help clients reconstruct participation around what is possible today, rather than what was expected yesterday.

These reconstructed roles are not secondary versions of what once was. They are full and valid expressions of self, grounded in adaptability rather than consistency. A woman who cannot predict how she will feel tomorrow does not need a rigid routine. She needs a framework that allows her to opt in without fear of being seen as unreliable. Occupational therapy can help create those frameworks, including routines that shift with energy, social roles that flex with capacity, and personal narratives that make space for pride even in the face of change. In doing so, therapy becomes not only a means of recovery, but a way to restore participation as an act of self-respect. These disruptions are especially pronounced during major life transitions, when shifting roles intersect with heightened physical and emotional demands. One of the most vulnerable periods for women with disabilities is the postpartum stage, a time when occupational expectations increase, while structural support often decreases.

Postpartum Mental Health and the Impact of Cumulative Stress

By her thirty-fourth birthday, Tara Mendelson, a small business owner with spastic cerebral palsy, had long mastered the routines of daily life using adaptive strategies tailored to her limited upper extremity range of motion. But after the birth of her first child, she found herself unprepared for the physical and emotional toll of postpartum caregiving. Breastfeeding triggered intense frustration. Her shoulders burned from strain, and standard pillows failed to position her baby safely. Simple tasks like transferring her infant or reaching for supplies became stress-inducing puzzles that left her feeling inadequate and overwhelmed. With her occupational therapist, Tara explored alternate positioning techniques such as side-lying nursing, used adjustable forearm supports, and trialed adaptive baby carriers that provided hands-free closeness. Therapy also focused on reducing task demands, scheduling recovery periods, and validating the emotional weight of constantly adapting. The postpartum period, for Tara, was not just about learning a new role—it was about renegotiating her relationship with her body in a context that offered few built-in supports.

The postpartum period is often framed as a time of healing and bonding. But for women with disabilities, it is more often a period marked by isolation, under-supported transitions, and intensified vulnerability. These experiences are not just byproducts of new parenthood. They are amplified by systemic inattention to the structural and emotional demands placed on disabled mothers (Devkota et al., 2019). For women who enter the postpartum period already navigating chronic pain, energy depletion, or inaccessible environments, the addition of caregiving responsibilities can destabilize even well-established routines. What looks like depression may, in fact, be a nervous system overwhelmed by sustained effort with too few safety cues.

A 2021 study analyzing data from over 8,400 postpartum women found that 37.4 percent of women with disabilities experienced depressive symptoms after childbirth, compared to just 8.79 percent of nondisabled women (Booth et al., 2021). The disparity was most pronounced among those reporting multiple stressors, such as financial strain, relational conflict, and traumatic events were reported at significantly higher rates among women with disabilities. Among those who experienced six or more stressful events in the year before birth, the odds of developing postpartum depression were nearly four times higher. This is not a coincidence. It is a reflection of cumulative occupational injustice during a period when support is critical and often unavailable. See also Chapter 4 for a deeper exploration of trauma in the perinatal period.

For occupational therapists, postpartum care cannot focus solely on infant rou-tines or maternal self-care checklists. It must begin with an understanding of what the woman has carried into the postpartum period—both physically and emotion-ally. Therapists should assess not only daily functioning but also relational safety, history of medical trauma, and prior occupational losses that may be reactivated by new caregiving roles. When possible, care should include sensory regulation practices tailored to postpartum physiology, co-occupations that support mater-nal-infant bonding without overwhelming the mother's capacity, and flexible role planning that adjusts for fluctuating energy, mobility, and emotional state.

Perhaps most importantly, trauma-informed postpartum care must reject the notion that independence is the goal. For many disabled mothers, the pressure to appear self-sufficient can delay help-seeking and deepen shame. Occupational therapy offers a different frame—one in which participation can include delega-tion, co-regulation, and asking for support without penalty. When we understand postpartum depression as both a psychological and occupational outcome, we widen the possibilities for intervention. We create room for disabled mothers to define parenting on their own terms, and we help protect not only their mental health, but their sense of self in a season often shaped by invisible loss.

While the postpartum period reveals the acute consequences of unsupported participation, it is far from the only context where emotional strain accumulates. For many women with disabilities, simply engaging in everyday life requires continuous negotiation with inaccessible spaces, social stigma, and systems that demand more than they give back.

The Emotional Labor of Participation in Inaccessible Contexts

For many women with disabilities, the act of participating in daily life requires more than physical effort. It involves an ongoing expenditure of emotional and cognitive resources that often goes unacknowledged in clinical spaces. Every appointment, every workplace interaction, every public outing demands not only preparation but anticipation: of stares, of barriers, of questions that reduce identity to diagnosis. This kind of emotional labor is not incidental. It is cumulative. And it is deeply linked to how trauma is experienced and perpetuated in everyday environments.

Even routine activities can carry hidden costs. Entering a building without an accessible entrance requires strategizing, planning, and often a decision between speaking up or staying silent. Navigating a workplace without accommodations means constantly choosing between advocating for needs or risking being labeled difficult. Participating in therapy can require revisiting the language of progress in systems that have only ever measured productivity. Over time, these moments build into patterns of self-surveillance and emotional exhaustion. The body may move through the environment, but the nervous system remains on alert.

Occupational therapists are well positioned to recognize and respond to this burden, but doing so requires a shift in perspective. Rather than focusing solely on what a woman is able to do, therapists must consider what it costs her to do it. This includes evaluating the environmental, interpersonal, and sensory demands that surround participation. For example, a woman may have the physical skills to attend a community event, but if the space is overwhelming, the staff untrained, or the route uncertain, her participation comes at a cost that far exceeds the task itself. These are not issues of compliance. They are indicators of chronic adaptation to inaccessible systems.

Trauma-informed occupational therapy in these contexts begins with validation. It acknowledges that effort is not always visible, and that withdrawal is not the same as disengagement (Piantedosi et al., 2023). Clinicians can support women in identifying environments that are not only physically accessible but emotionally sustainable. They can work to co-create scripts for advocacy that do not rely on constant self-explanation. They can help reshape expectations so that success is defined not by how much is done, but by whether it is done on terms that protect well-being. In this model, participation becomes more than access. It becomes autonomy.

Relational Trauma and Intimate Partner Violence in Women with Intellectual Disabilities

Women with intellectual disabilities experience one of the highest known rates of intimate partner violence, yet their trauma is rarely named in disability or mental health services. Abuse often extends beyond the physical. It is deeply relational, unfolding in environments where communication is controlled, autonomy is diminished, and support systems are inconsistent or absent. Because of intersecting stigma and dependency, many women remain in abusive relationships longer than their nondisabled counterparts, often without ever being screened or believed.

A 2022 study by McConnell and Phelan introduced a relational framework for inclusive, trauma-informed care that centers **relational autonomy**—the ability to make choices and express needs within the context of supportive relationships. Drawing from interviews with social service professionals, the authors outlined four essential principles: reflexivity, recognition, solidarity, and safety. These principles inform approaches to safety planning, emotional regulation, social support, and the development of self-respect, self-efficacy, and self-trust. For occupational therapists, this means moving beyond traditional ADL training or resource referrals. It means building co-regulatory routines, helping women identify early warning signs in relationships, and reconstructing occupational roles that reflect not just survival, but dignity.

Intervention must be structured around **relational recovery**, not just individual skill building. This includes mapping safe versus unsafe relational patterns, co-creating scripts for setting boundaries, and practicing decision-making within trusted therapeutic alliances. Therapists may also support women in identifying community-based networks that reinforce agency without placing them in new forms of surveillance. IPV in the context of intellectual disability is not just a clinical issue, it is a structural one. Trauma-informed occupational therapy has the power to name it, disrupt it, and help women redefine safety on their own terms.

Beyond the Clinic: Advocacy, Access, and Structural Change

Therapeutic skill is not limited to the clinic. For women with disabilities who have experienced trauma, much of the harm occurs in systems that lie outside the treatment room but shape every aspect of daily life. These systems, including healthcare, housing, education, transportation, and employment often determine whether participation is possible at all. When occupational therapists ignore these structures, they risk reinforcing them. When they engage with them directly, they become agents of disruption and repair.

Access is often framed as a physical problem: ramps, elevators, door widths. But the deeper issue is relational and political. Who designs the spaces? Who decides what is reasonable? Who defines independence? These are not rhetorical questions. They are practice questions. A trauma-informed therapist must be prepared to see the built and procedural environment as a therapeutic target. When a woman repeatedly loses services because she misses appointments due to inaccessible transit, the intervention is not just a new scheduling strategy. It is advocacy for transportation reform and policy alignment.

This shift requires a redefinition of what counts as occupational therapy. Writing a support letter for housing access. Partnering with disability-led organizations to challenge institutional policies. Collaborating with social workers to document system failures that retraumatize. These are not extras. They are essential practices when working with women whose trauma is not only personal but structural. Therapists who recognize this are not stepping outside their scope. They are practicing in alignment with their ethical obligation to promote participation.

Every woman deserves access to care that is not only trauma aware, but structurally responsive. That means recognizing how policies restrict, how bias infiltrates service delivery, and how systems create the very conditions they claim to treat. Occupational therapy in this context is not neutral. It can either reproduce injustice or help dismantle it. The choice lies in how broadly we define our role and how deeply we are willing to act.

Case Vignette and Clinical Reflections

The following case vignettes illustrate how trauma-informed occupational therapy can be applied when working with women who live with disabilities and have experienced layered forms of harm. Each example highlights not just what was done, but why it mattered. These are not idealized scenarios. They reflect the messiness of real lives, shaped by systemic failure, cultural expectations, and fluctuating capacity. They remind us that trauma is never just about what happened. It is about what continues to be denied, and what must be rebuilt to move forward with safety, dignity, and authorship.

Case 1: Amina, Age 52—Reclaiming Occupational Identity After Years of Medical Dismissal

Amina is a 52-year-old Moroccan French woman with a long history of endometriosis, fibromyalgia, and pelvic floor dysfunction. She is a mother of three and was formerly employed as a literature teacher. Over the past decade, she gradually withdrew from her professional and community roles due to worsening pain and fatigue. She described herself as someone who was once "always prepared, always present." After multiple surgical interventions and inconsistent care, Amina entered outpatient occupational therapy at the suggestion of her urogynecologist. Her referral stated only, "functional decline due to chronic pain."

Rather than starting with standard energy-conservation protocols, her occupational therapist implemented a layered assessment model that integrated narrative mapping, trauma screening, and functional-rhythm profiling. This included a timeline of body memories linked to care experiences, identification of her peak energy times, and discussion of what participation had once felt like before chronic disruption. Amina initially hesitated to name goals, stating, "What would be the point? I will just lose them again." Her therapist did not rush her. Instead, they co-created a map of her daily occupations using values-based journaling and somatic-cue tracking. This highlighted hidden moments of regulation, such as pouring tea, lighting incense, listening to poetry, that had gone unnoticed as therapeutic anchors.

As therapy progressed, sessions incorporated dynamic-pacing routines using breath-led transitions between activities, sensory-modulation tools selected by Amina, and intentional co-regulation through mirrored seated movement. Instead of prescribing rigid goals such as "engage in a 30-minute walking program five days a week . . ." or ". . . resume previous homemaking tasks . . ." the therapist introduced flexible goals that honored Amina's energy variability and creative identity. These included facilitating a ten-minute storytelling session with her grandchildren once per week, writing a reflective journal entry on days when pain levels allowed, and practicing a guided breath and movement sequence each morning to anchor her attention and body awareness. Each goal was framed not as a task to complete but as an invitation to reconnect with herself through moments of meaning and rhythm. Amina began to facilitate her storytelling sessions using seated movement, breathwork, and poetic recitation as co-occupations that felt both expressive and sustainable. She also began documenting her medical experiences in a bilingual blog, stating that it was "the first time she had spoken without being interrupted."

By the end of her plan of care, Amina still lived with pain, but her relationship to it had shifted. She no longer measured her days by what she could push through, but by what felt worth doing. Her routines became acts of expression rather than obligation. Through occupational therapy, she reestablished a sense of rhythm and authorship; choosing when and how to engage, and on what terms. Her roles were no longer dictated by productivity. They were grounded in creativity, presence, and self-defined contribution. What emerged was not a return to a former identity, but the formation of a new one—built not around what had been lost, but around what still felt meaningful.

Case 2: Camila, Age 35—Cognitive Disruption, Institutional Trauma, and Navigating Invisible Injury

Camila is a 35-year-old Colombian American woman referred to outpatient occupational therapy following a workplace incident in which a coworker pushed her into industrial shelving during a dispute. Though the bruising appeared minor, Camila began experiencing cognitive fog, light sensitivity, difficulty concentrating, and episodes of emotional dysregulation. She had no previous therapy history and worked in a distribution warehouse as a shift lead, a role she had held for seven years without incident.

On evaluation, Camila appeared hyperalert. She avoided overhead lighting, scanned the environment repeatedly, and gave clipped responses. The therapist used a somatic-safety checklist developed in collaboration with clients from culturally diverse backgrounds. This included seating choice, permission cues before visual or auditory input, and co-created scripts to describe internal states. Rather than initiating a return-to-work protocol, the therapist spent the first several sessions building regulatory scaffolds: bilateral tapping with music selected by Camila, task-based cueing with low visual load, and structured silence as a co-occupation. This allowed her to remain present without verbal processing.

By week three, Camila disclosed that she had sustained a similar head injury as a teenager but had never been evaluated. The current incident had retriggered symptoms she had long masked. With this information, the therapist conducted a contextual cognitive assessment using dual-task sequencing and embedded feedback, revealing executive-function disruptions consistent with mild traumatic brain injury. More importantly, the therapist helped Camila articulate the emotional labor of navigating her job in a setting where physical intimidation had been normalized.

Rather than designing a generic work simulation, therapy centered on functional scripting, environmental modification, and advocacy planning. Camila practiced memory strategies using familiar workplace materials and co-wrote a communication plan with her therapist for human resources. The therapist documented the cognitive and emotional impacts in language that aligned with ADA protections, coordinated with her primary care provider to initiate a formal TBI evaluation, and connected her to a culturally affirming community center offering trauma recovery groups for Latina workers.

By discharge, Camila had not yet returned to her full duties, but she had reentered her workplace with a different posture. She advocated for modified shifts, negotiated protected lighting accommodations, and established a check-in routine that helped her regulate transitions. Her sense of competency was not measured by how much she could remember or how quickly she could work. It was measured by her ability to participate without hiding.

Therapist Reflections on Clinical Decision-Making

Working with women who live at the intersection of trauma and disability is not only a clinical responsibility but a personal reckoning. It requires the therapist to confront their own assumptions about progress, productivity, and participation. It means learning to recognize the moments when urgency to help may override the need to listen, or when well-meaning plans reflect professional goals more than the client's lived priorities.

What often emerges in this work is the discomfort of slowness. Progress does not always follow a measurable arc. Rapport may take weeks to form. Some goals remain undefined because safety has not yet been established. These delays are not setbacks. They are the work. For many women, therapy is one of the few spaces where they are allowed to pause without having to explain why. The therapist's willingness to stay in that pause—to resist the impulse to fix—can be more healing than any intervention.

The clinical tools used in these cases, such as narrative mapping, somatic-safety assessments, regulatory scaffolds, flexible role reconstruction, are not advanced because they are complex. They are advanced because they require restraint. They demand presence, curiosity, and the humility to accept that the client holds the most accurate version of her story, even when that story unfolds slowly or without words.

These cases also raise another reality: therapists work within systems that are often ill equipped to support this depth of care. Productivity requirements, documentation demands, and institutional expectations can all interfere with the values of trauma-informed practice. Therapists must constantly navigate these constraints while advocating for what is clinically and ethically necessary. Doing so requires both skill and courage. It also requires community—spaces where therapists can reflect, debrief, and stay grounded in their own regulation.

Ultimately, trauma-informed care is not about special protocols. It is a posture. A way of approaching human experience with respect, nuance, and the awareness that healing is not defined by doing more, but by being seen, understood, and supported in ways that feel safe. When therapists adopt this posture with intention, they do more than treat; they accompany.

Summary and Implications

Women with disabilities often carry trauma that is misrecognized or entirely overlooked, not because the signs are absent, but because they are reframed as symptoms of diagnosis or compliance failure. The disruption they face is not only biological, but occupational. It takes the form of roles that become unsustainable, environments that demand self-surveillance, and systems that measure progress in ways that ignore fluctuation, fatigue, and fear. Trauma, in this context, is not a single moment. It is the accumulation of interruptions to participation and the loss of safety in places where care is supposed to occur.

Occupational therapy offers a path forward, but only if practice expands beyond tasks and timelines. Evaluation must include emotional labor, occupational loss, and structural constraint. Interventions must reflect real-world complexity, where energy, regulation, and trust shift from day to day. The work involves pacing, presence, and co-creating routines that flex without penalty. Progress is measured not by how much a woman can do, but by whether her participation protects her dignity, supports her nervous system, and aligns with her values.

This kind of practice requires courage. It means documenting what systems have failed to provide, advocating beyond the clinic, and naming harm where it occurs. Trauma-informed care with women who have disabilities is not a special approach—it is a necessary one. When occupational therapy restores agency, honors grief, and creates safe conditions for becoming, it becomes not just a service but a source of repair.

References

Aguillard, K., Hughes, R. B., Schick, V. R., McCurdy, S. A., & Gemeinhardt, G. L. (2022). Mental healthcare: Experiences of rural women with disabilities following interpersonal violence. *Violence and Victims*, *37*(1), 26–43. https://doi.org/10.1891/VV-D-21-00045

Anyango, C., Goicolea, I., & Namatovu, F. (2023). Women with disabilities' experiences of intimate partner violence: A qualitative study from Sweden. *BMC Women's Health*, *23*(1), 381. https://doi.org/10.1186/s12905-023-02524-8

Booth, E. J., Kitsantas, P., Min, H., & Pollack, A. Z. (2021). Stressful life events and post-partum depressive symptoms among women with disabilities. *Women's Health (London, England)*, *17*, 17455065211066186. https://doi.org/10.1177/17455065211066186

Chitapi, U. M., van Niekerk, L., & Blank, A. (2024). Scoping review of women with disabilities' livelihood occupation experiences: An equity perspective. *Work (Reading, Mass.)*, *77*(3), 735–753. https://doi.org/10.3233/WOR-220348

Devkota, H. R., Kett, M., & Groce, N. (2019). Societal attitude and behaviours towards women with disabilities in rural Nepal: Pregnancy, childbirth and motherhood. *BMC Pregnancy and Childbirth*, *19*(1), 20. https://doi.org/10.1186/s12884-019-2171-4

Gesi, C., Migliarese, G., Torriero, S., Capellazzi, M., Omboni, A. C., Cerveri, G., & Mencacci, C. (2021). Gender differences in misdiagnosis and delayed diagnosis among adults with autism spectrum disorder with no language or intellectual disability. *Brain Sciences*, *11*(7), 912. https://doi.org/10.3390/brainsci11070912

Hashimoto, J., Izutsu, T., Sunagozaka, S., Iiyama, S., & Tsutsumi, A. (2023). A comparison of traumatic experiences and human rights violations of persons with mental health conditions or psychosocial disabilities and persons with other disabilities. *PLoS One*, *18*(11), e0292750. https://doi.org/10.1371/journal.pone.0292750

McConnell, D., & Phelan, S. K. (2022). Intimate partner violence against women with intellectual disability: A relational framework for inclusive, trauma-informed social services. *Health & Social Care in the Community*, *30*(6), e5156–e5166. https://doi.org/10.1111/hsc.13932

Mueller, S. D., & Sutherland, M. A. (2023). College women with a disability and interpersonal violence: A call to action. *Journal of the American Association of Nurse Practitioners*, *35*(12), 761–764. https://doi.org/10.1097/JXX.0000000000000969

Njelesani, J., Teachman, G., & Bangura, I. R. (2021). "The strength to leave": Women with disabilities navigating violent relationships and occupational identities. *The American Journal of Occupational Therapy: Official Publication of the American Occupational Therapy Association*, *75*(4), 7504180040. https://doi.org/10.5014/ajot.2021.045542

Piantedosi, D. K., Reed, K., & O'Shea, A. (2023). Supporting occupational therapists to initiate conversations about sexuality with people with intellectual disability: Co-design by deliberative dialogue. *Australian Occupational Therapy Journal*, *70*(5), 581–598. https://doi.org/10.1111/1440-1630.12888

Wint, A. J., Smith, D. L., & Iezzoni, L. I. (2016). Mothers with physical disability: Child care adaptations at home. *The American Journal of Occupational Therapy: Official Publication of the American Occupational Therapy Association*, *70*(6), 7006220060p1–7006220060p7. https://doi.org/10.5014/ajot.2016.021477

Chapter 10

Gender and Sexual Minority Women

Renee Cruz Santos, a 32-year-old queer Filipina woman, was referred to occupational therapy after a workplace injury left her with persistent lower back pain and difficulty with mobility. During the initial sessions, she appeared guarded and hesitant, deflecting personal questions and minimizing the impact of her injury on daily life. It was only after several weeks that Renee disclosed she had delayed seeking care because her last medical encounter involved a provider making

DOI: 10.4324/9781003658559-10

assumptions about her gender identity and relationship status. "They kept calling my partner my friend," she said, "and it just made me want to disappear." Renee described feeling hypervigilant in public spaces and exhausted by the constant effort to self-edit in both professional and clinical settings. Although her injury had physically healed, she struggled with sleep, avoided social outings, and reported a sense of disconnection from her body and routines. Her therapeutic needs extended far beyond musculoskeletal rehabilitation—they involved restoring a sense of safety in environments that had repeatedly rendered her invisible.

For many gender and sexual minority women, trauma is not the disruption of an otherwise stable life. It is the scaffolding around which identity is often built. From an early age, cues from family, media, school, and religion communicate that their existence is conditional—that safety is earned through silence, self-correction, and careful concealment. These messages do not only threaten emotional well-being but also shape the nervous system, the rhythm of daily routines, and the calculus of participation. The impact is not always visible, but it is persistent. It shows up in the hesitation to speak honestly with a physician, in the decision to use a different name at work, or in the exhaustion that comes from navigating spaces that demand constant self-monitoring.

Unlike trauma rooted in a single event, the experiences of queer and trans women are often relational and chronic. They involve repeated encounters with exclusion, rejection, and surveillance, forms of harm that accumulate and restructure the body's baseline for safety. A young woman may learn to dissociate not because of one specific incident, but because every environment she entered signaled that part of her had to be erased. When trauma is relational and identity-based, it does not end when the event ends. It continues through every subsequent interaction that echoes the original wound.

In a 2023 study of young adult sexual minority women in the United States, researchers found that higher PTSD symptom severity was associated with significantly lower levels of social support from family, friends, and intimate partners. The presence of recent sexual assault further intensified these effects, especially in romantic relationships (van Stolk-Cooke et al., 2023). The study emphasized what clinicians often miss: trauma in these women is not an isolated psychological response. It is a rupture in the systems that are meant to buffer distress, an erosion of the very relationships that could support recovery. This has consequences not only for healing but also for how time is structured, how roles are chosen or concealed, and how intimacy is navigated when trust has been fractured at the level of identity. Participation for these women is not simply about access or performance. It is about whether they are allowed to show up fully—and whether anyone is prepared to receive them when they do.

Prevalence, Risk, and Erasure in Health Systems

Gender and sexual minority women consistently face higher rates of trauma exposure across the lifespan, including childhood abuse, sexual assault, and intimate partner violence. Yet these patterns remain underrepresented in research and routinely overlooked in clinical care. Health systems often fail to capture data on sexual orientation or gender identity, and when this information is collected, it is rarely integrated into meaningful care pathways. The result is a system where risk is well-documented in literature but largely invisible in practice. Without structures that account for identity-based harm, trauma goes unrecognized, and participation in care becomes conditional—contingent on silence, conformity, or self-protection.

Elevated Risk Does Not Equal Elevated Visibility

Gender and sexual minority women face disproportionate exposure to trauma across multiple domains, including family rejection, sexual violence, institutional discrimination, and systemic neglect. Yet these patterns are consistently underrecognized in clinical care. Most healthcare systems lack integrated tools to collect or respond to data on sexual orientation or gender identity. When this information is collected, it is often siloed from the rest of the clinical reasoning process. Women who choose not to disclose their identities, whether due to prior harm or anticipated judgment, are frequently placed into default categories, resulting in risk profiles that do not reflect lived experience.

The gap between risk and recognition is more than a data failure. It is a systemic erasure with real psychological consequences. A 2023 study published in *Epidemiology and Psychiatric Sciences* reviewed data from nearly 32,000 LGBTQ participants and found that LGBTQ individuals were more than twice as likely to meet criteria for posttraumatic stress disorder compared to their cisgender and heterosexual peers (Marchi et al., 2023). The highest risk was observed among transgender and bisexual individuals. These findings confirm what many providers have witnessed but few systems acknowledge—trauma exposure among LGBTQ+ groups is not incidental or marginal. It is patterned, persistent, and too often invisible in health records, assessment protocols, and even research inclusion criteria.

This lack of visibility leads to missed opportunities for prevention and trauma-informed care. In occupational therapy, the absence of identity-aware assessments can result in the misattribution of trauma responses, such as avoidance, dissociation, or emotional blunting, to noncompliance or personality traits.

Clinical reasoning suffers when it is not informed by the broader context of marginalization. When identity is seen as peripheral rather than central to participation, the full picture of occupational disruption is lost (Ramos & Marr, 2023). Visibility is not simply about collecting more demographic boxes, it is about shifting the framework of care so that identity is seen as inseparable from safety, regulation, and participation.

Diagnostic Overshadowing and the Myth of Neutral Care

When LGBTQ+ women enter care environments, they do so carrying more than symptoms. They bring with them histories of relational harm, internalized stigma, and systems that have consistently failed to reflect their realities. And yet, the language of clinical reasoning often excludes these dimensions. Trauma-related behaviors, such as vigilance, boundary-setting, avoidance, or emotional flatness, are frequently misread. A client who hesitates to discuss her home life may be labeled avoidant. A trans woman who declines physical contact during an assessment may be marked as "nonparticipatory." These responses are not dysfunction. They are adaptive strategies developed in response to living in a world that has not offered safety.

This kind of misinterpretation is not simply a matter of oversight. It is a reflection of how normative expectations dominate clinical spaces. Providers may pride themselves on being neutral or inclusive, but neutrality is rarely experienced as safe by those who have never been centered. In systems designed around cisgender and heterosexual norms, neutrality often translates to invisibility. And when invisibility is compounded by trauma, the result is diagnostic overshadowing—where identity-based distress is interpreted as individual pathology rather than the outcome of accumulated structural violence.

In a 2023 study published in the *Journal of Traumatic Stress*, researchers examined how minority stress interacts with posttraumatic symptom severity among LGBTQ+ survivors of sexual assault. They found that experiences of victimization were significantly associated with higher posttraumatic stress, anxiety, and alcohol use, even after accounting for other risk factors. Internalized stigma was also linked to increased cannabis use, while community connectedness appeared to buffer anxiety symptoms (Bedford et al., 2023). These findings reinforce what trauma-informed clinicians have long observed: that LGBTQ+ trauma does not occur in isolation. It is shaped by the presence or absence of social support, the chronic stress of erasure, and the internal conflict of having to hide who you are in order to be treated.

For occupational therapists, this has direct implications. When we view symptoms only through a diagnostic lens, we risk ignoring the very systems that sustain trauma. A queer woman navigating both PTSD and identity-based discrimination may not need more behavioral strategies—she may need someone to name what has gone unnamed. Trauma-informed occupational therapy cannot rely on visual neutrality or well-intended documentation language. It must interrogate the assumptions embedded in our assessments, our definitions of progress, and our own comfort with identity disclosure. Otherwise, we risk becoming another source of harm cloaked in care.

From Health Avoidance to Participation Fatigue

Avoidance is often interpreted as a symptom of trauma. But for many sexual minority women, avoidance is not only psychological—it is strategic. It reflects years of navigating services that were not designed for them and surviving interactions that reinforced harm rather than repair. Opting out of medical visits, therapy sessions, or wellness programs is not necessarily a sign of disengagement. It is often an act of preservation. Over time, this pattern becomes more than avoidance. It becomes exhaustion, a slow depletion of the emotional and cognitive energy required to keep showing up in spaces that demand silence, code-switching, or constant explanation.

This exhaustion is not unfounded. In a 2023 scoping review published in *Trauma, Violence, & Abuse*, researchers synthesized findings from 42 studies examining the connection between adverse childhood experiences (ACEs) and long-term health outcomes among sexual minority women (SMW). The evidence was striking: SMW were significantly more likely than heterosexual women to report nearly every type of ACE, including childhood physical and sexual abuse, neglect, and household dysfunction. These early experiences were strongly associated with a range of negative adult outcomes, from chronic illness and depression to substance misuse and social isolation (Bochicchio et al., 2024). The review highlighted a pattern that occupational therapists must understand—many SMW enter adulthood already carrying an embedded occupational burden. They are not just managing trauma. They are navigating systems that have ignored it for decades.

This cumulative exposure, with ACEs layered with minority stress, medical dismissal, and fractured social support, alters how participation is experienced. Tasks that seem routine to others, such as scheduling an appointment or asking for accommodations, may carry significant emotional weight. Participation fatigue emerges when every act of engagement requires risk calculation. When entering a clinic could mean being misgendered, or disclosing a partner could derail the appointment, the cost of participation becomes too high. And when these costs are invisible to providers, the response is often pathologizing rather than empathic.

Occupational therapists working with sexual minority women must go beyond affirming language and commit to structurally inclusive practice. This includes integrating identity-informed assessments that explicitly ask about safety, cultural belonging, and prior harm in healthcare. Therapists can design intervention plans that reflect not only trauma history but also the energy cost of navigating invalidating systems. Concrete strategies may include scripting for medical appointments to reduce anticipatory anxiety, co-creating communication cards for disclosing identity or access needs, or facilitating peer-supported participation through group-based occupations. Environmental audits of clinical spaces can be conducted with LGBTQ+ clients to identify sensory or visual cues that enhance safety or perpetuate exclusion. By explicitly naming identity-based barriers during treatment planning and offering tools to navigate them, occupational therapy can reclaim its full scope as a healing profession that not only adapts tasks but dismantles the structures that have made participation unsafe.

Occupational Identity and Role Fragmentation

Occupational identity does not exist in isolation. It forms through interaction, through being seen, mirrored, and supported in meaningful roles across settings. For gender and sexual minority women, that process is routinely interrupted by environments that invalidate, surveil, or pathologize who they are. Over time, these women learn to edit themselves across contexts. They withhold personal details in health settings, adjust their appearance in professional spaces, and monitor how affection is displayed in public. These adaptations are not expressions of preference. They are strategic responses to harm. In a 2022 study published in *Frontiers in Public Health*, over half of Spanish LGBTQ adults reported experiences of harassment, with transgender women and nonbinary individuals reporting the highest rates—particularly in public, healthcare, and educational settings (Devís-Devís et al., 2022). These patterns were not isolated to youth. Even in adulthood, identity-based harassment persisted across daily environments that most people move through without fear. The cumulative effect is more than emotional. It fractures the continuity of identity, interrupting participation at the level of self-definition.

This kind of fragmentation is occupational at its core. When a woman cannot safely bring her whole self into a space, whether that is a clinic, a classroom, or a family gathering, her roles become compartmentalized. What may appear clinically as low engagement, social withdrawal, or difficulty sustaining routines is often the expression of a divided self. Occupational therapy has the tools to help women rebuild routines. But without first understanding the fracture of identity that often precedes disruption, those tools remain superficial. Recovery is not about helping women resume old roles. It is about making space for roles that have never been publicly supported—and allowing those roles to unfold without fear of retaliation or repair.

The Trauma of Nonrecognition

Rivka Klein, a 27-year-old woman raised in a conservative household, was referred to occupational therapy after experiencing significant burnout that disrupted her ability to manage basic daily routines. She had recently been cut off by her parents after disclosing her same-sex relationship. "They told me I could come home for dinner, but only if I came alone," she shared quietly. "It felt like they were choosing silence over me." In the weeks that followed, Rivka found herself increasingly detached from the rhythms of daily life. She stopped meal prepping, lost her sense of time, and avoided previously meaningful activities like Sunday hikes or community volunteering. Holidays and family-centered routines now brought a mix of grief and dread. Although she maintained a professional appearance at work, the cognitive load of masking and emotional suppression left her exhausted by midday. In therapy, it became evident that her struggles were not about executive dysfunction alone, but the cumulative toll of nonrecognition of being asked to fragment herself to remain acceptable. For Rivka, healing would not begin with routine retraining, but with reclaiming a sense of wholeness in spaces where her identity no longer had to be negotiated.

For many gender and sexual minority women, trauma is not always loud or acute. It is quiet, chronic, and cumulative. It takes the form of being excluded from family milestones, having a partner referred to as a "friend" in medical records, or never seeing someone like oneself represented on an intake form. These moments may seem minor when taken alone. But over time, they create a profound form of erasure: the trauma of nonrecognition. It is a trauma not rooted in one singular event, but in the steady denial of affirmation, visibility, and belonging.

Nonrecognition is especially damaging when it begins during development. A child whose gender expression is dismissed or punished may internalize shame before having language to describe it. A teen who is asked to conceal their identity at school may come to associate authenticity with risk. These early patterns shape not only emotion, but occupation. The way routines are established, the way relationships are managed, and the way self-care is practiced all reflect adaptations to invisible threats. By the time these individuals reach adulthood, many have structured their daily lives around avoidance—not because they lack capacity, but because safety has always depended on fragmentation.

In clinical settings, nonrecognition often hides behind the appearance of neutrality. Forms that list only binary gender options. Providers who steer away from discussions of identity "to stay on task." Therapists who write detailed notes on function and progress without ever referencing the client's chosen family, cultural expression, or experience of belonging. These omissions are not incidental. They communicate who is welcome to take up space in the therapeutic process and who must shrink to fit it (D'Angelo, 2024). For LGBTQ women with histories of trauma, this kind of invisibility can reinforce mistrust and reproduce patterns of silence (Bochicchio et al., 2024).

Occupational therapists are in a position to disrupt this cycle, not just through inclusive language, but through practices that embed recognition into the structure of care. This includes reflecting clients' chosen terms in documentation, acknowledging identity when it is central to participation, and being willing to name what has been systematically overlooked. For some women, the most meaningful therapeutic outcome is not the number of tasks completed. It is the ability to move through care without having to hide. Recognition is not just relational. It is regulatory. And for those who have never known what it means to feel visible in their bodies, their communities, or their roles, it can mark the beginning of something entirely new.

Navigating Split Roles

Many gender and sexual minority women live in a constant state of occupational division. They are one version of themselves at home, another in the workplace, and yet another in healthcare settings. These shifts are not expressions of preference or personality. They are adaptations to environments that have proven unsafe. Whether consciously or not, women learn to assess which parts of themselves can be revealed and which must be hidden in order to avoid harm. Over time, this role-splitting becomes so habitual that it is no longer noticed—by the client or by the clinician. But the emotional and physiological cost of constantly adjusting identity is profound.

A 2023 article in *Pastoral Psychology* introduced a critical concept that helps explain this burden: **queer allostatic load**. Allostatic load refers to the "wear and tear" on the body and brain that occurs when someone is exposed to repeated stress without adequate recovery (Menhinick & Sanders, 2023). For LGBTQ+ individuals, this stress is not just physical. It is deeply social. It comes from family rejection, religious exclusion, institutional silencing, and cultural messages that mark queer lives as deviant or disposable. The term queer allostatic load captures the unique toll of having to monitor language, posture, safety, and belonging across every setting. This is not just background stress. It is a trauma pattern with physiological and occupational consequences.

The same article also introduced the idea of **traumatic temporality**—a disruption in how time is experienced. Many LGBTQ+ people grow up with no visible future. They do not see themselves reflected in the lives of adults around them. Their histories are erased from textbooks, and their relationships are dismissed by legal and religious institutions. When there is no visible path forward and no affirmed lineage to look back on, participation becomes fragmented. Time itself becomes a source of disorientation. The future feels uncertain not because of personal instability, but because of societal refusal to imagine queer lives as sustainable or worthy.

In therapy, these effects may show up in subtle ways. A client may thrive in certain roles while disengaging in others. She may describe deep connection in queer community but remain cautious in clinical sessions. These are not contradictions. They are survival responses to environments that have required compartmentalization. Occupational therapy must move beyond surface-level role descriptions and begin to ask how roles have been constructed—and at what cost. Integration cannot happen in settings that continue to reward concealment. The work of healing is not simply about helping clients re-engage in life. It is about creating space where the whole self is allowed to exist without apology.

Affirming Identity as Occupation

Occupation is often defined by action: what people do, when they do it, and how they perform it. But for many gender and sexual minority women, occupation is also about who they are allowed to be while doing it. Identity is not background context. It is an active process shaped by safety, memory, and imagination. When a woman has had to suppress or fragment her identity in order to survive family, religious, or educational systems, expressing that identity later in life becomes both meaningful and restorative. In these cases, identity is not just about "being." It becomes a doing.

A 2024 study published in the *Journal of Homosexuality* explored this process among sexual minority adults who were formerly members of the Church of Jesus Christ of Latter-day Saints. These individuals described profound conflict between their religious and sexual identities, shaped by rigid gender roles and heteronormative doctrine. Many experienced identity foreclosure, meaning that their sense of self was shaped not through exploration but through submission to external expectations. For many, only after leaving the church did they begin to construct an integrated sense of identity (Shuler et al., 2024). The study highlights that sexual identity development does not always happen in adolescence. For some, it is delayed until adulthood, and for others, it is never safely explored without therapeutic support. What this tells us as clinicians is clear: identity is not a fixed background trait. It is an unfolding occupation, one that can be disrupted, delayed, or reclaimed.

In trauma-informed occupational therapy, affirming identity means more than offering acceptance. It means actively supporting the client in building routines, relationships, and roles that reflect who they are—not who they had to be. This might include facilitating clothing choices that align with gender expression, supporting rituals around name affirmation or cultural pride, or helping clients participate in communities that reflect their values and experiences. These acts are not small. They are neurologically and socially reparative. They foster regulation, volition, and a renewed sense of narrative agency.

When identity has been constrained by religious or familial systems, rebuilding participation becomes a layered process. Occupational therapists can help guide that process by naming identity formation as therapeutic, not peripheral. Creating space for women to explore and affirm who they are, without fear of surveillance or correction, is itself an act of clinical care. Identity affirmation is not a sidebar to trauma recovery. It is often the clearest sign that recovery is happening. See Table 10.1 for examples of identity-affirming occupations and their clinical relevance.

These examples are not meant to be prescriptive or universal. Rather, they illustrate the diverse ways in which identity work can show up in everyday occupations when therapists are attuned to their significance. What might seem like a small shift in routine, such as a new wardrobe choice, joining a community group, or reclaiming spiritual language, can carry deep therapeutic value for a woman who has spent years hiding or fragmenting who she is. When occupational therapists recognize these actions as legitimate and powerful forms

Table 10.1 Affirming Identity as Occupation

Occupational Area	Example Occupations	Clinical Significance
Self-Care and Expression	Choosing clothing, hair, or makeup aligned with identity	Supports agency, body autonomy, and nervous system regulation
Ritual and Routine	Celebrating name change anniversaries, journaling personal milestones	Creates rhythm, reinforces narrative identity, builds self-trust
Spiritual or Cultural Practice	Reclaiming spiritual practices in affirming settings, leaving non-affirming traditions	Restores meaning-making without retraumatization
Community Participation	Attending LGBTQ+ community groups, pride events, or cultural gatherings	Enhances belonging and social connection; addresses isolation and minority stress
Creative Occupation	Storytelling, art, poetry, or performance exploring identity	Facilitates emotional processing and reintegration of suppressed aspects of self
Digital and Media Engagement	Curating affirming online spaces or following queer content creators	Expands access to representation and mirrors identity exploration in low-risk environments

of participation, they expand the scope of what healing looks like. The goal is not simply to restore function but to create environments where self-definition becomes both possible and safe. In that space, even the most ordinary occupations can become sites of repair.

Trauma-Informed Intervention Through an Affirming Lens

Affirming trauma-informed care for sexual and gender minority women requires more than recognition; it demands structural and relational redesign. For many queer and trans women, traditional roles no longer fit or were never safe to begin with. Healing is not a return but a reconstruction of identity through occupations that reflect autonomy and truth. Occupational therapists can lead this process by shifting from task completion to identity anchored participation, co-creating care environments where disclosure is not penalized, safety is built not assumed, and role development is flexible, not prescriptive. This approach invites therapists to examine intake language, therapeutic pacing, and even documentation practices through the lens of inclusion, ensuring the full self is not only seen but integrated into the recovery process.

Centering Safety Beyond the Physical Environment

In most clinical settings, safety is measured through physical design. Doors are clearly marked, rooms are accessible, and therapists follow ethical boundaries with care. But for gender and sexual minority women, safety is not only physical. It is relational, cultural, and often conditional. Many clients enter care with a nervous system that has been trained to scan for subtle cues, such as tone, language, or silence that signal whether or not it is safe to be fully seen. When past trauma has been tied to identity, the perception of safety is fluid. It must be earned in each encounter, not assumed because a space appears neutral.

A 2023 article in *Pastoral Psychology* reframed this dynamic by describing the queer experience as one that often falls along a **stress-trauma continuum**, shaped not only by discrete events but by the accumulation of chronic social threat. Drawing on the concept of **queer allostatic load**, the authors argued that what many LGBTQ clients live with is not a single trauma history but a sustained pattern of being regulated, surveilled, and erased in everyday environments. This includes schools, religious communities, family systems, and healthcare. In such contexts, safety is not a stable backdrop. It is a shifting terrain that requires constant negotiation.

Occupational therapists working from a trauma-informed lens must recognize that what is safe for one client may feel dangerous for another. A group-based intervention may activate shame or visibility fatigue. An open-ended art prompt may resurface memories of being silenced or misunderstood. A hands-on technique may reawaken somatic memories of nonconsensual touch. These are not outliers. They are patterned responses that make perfect sense in the context of relational trauma. The mistake is not in the client's reaction. It is in the system's assumption that safety can be standardized.

Therapists can begin to repair this rupture by centering the client's definition of safety from the outset. This includes asking what support has looked like in the past, what settings have felt affirming, and what sensory, relational, or cultural conditions allow the client to remain present. It also means acknowledging missteps when they occur. A client correcting a misused pronoun or disclosing discomfort is not being oppositional. They are testing whether the space will hold their truth without penalty. When those moments are honored, something changes. The nervous system begins to rewire its expectations. Ultimately, safety is not a checkpoint to pass before the work begins. It is the work. For many clients who have spent years editing their voice, hiding their family, or shaping their participation to match what is acceptable, the experience of being safe while being fully themselves is the most powerful intervention available. Therapists who learn to recognize this not only deepen trust but begin to shift the clinical relationship into something reparative. That shift is not decorative. It is foundational. Without it, nothing else holds.

Co-Creating Affirming Goals and Participation Pathways

Traditional goal setting in occupational therapy often prioritizes measurable outcomes, such as getting dressed independently, returning to work, managing fatigue. These goals matter. But for many gender and sexual minority women, especially those with trauma histories, participation cannot be reduced to tasks completed or functions restored. It is about whether they can show up as themselves while engaging in those tasks. When identity has been a source of rejection, and when systems have reinforced the message that visibility carries risk, goal setting itself becomes vulnerable. It becomes another space where the client must weigh honesty against self-protection.

In trauma-informed practice, goals are not simply agreed upon. They are co-created. This process requires the therapist to recognize not only what the client wants to do, but who they are trying to become. This distinction is subtle but essential. A goal to resume social activity might reflect the desire to reconnect with affirming queer spaces, not to return to a family dynamic where identity was policed. A goal to establish a daily routine might be less about productivity and more about regulating the nervous system after years of hypervigilance. Without this lens, therapists risk reinforcing normative expectations that have already caused harm.

Clients may not arrive with clearly stated goals. Some may avoid naming what they want out of fear that it will be dismissed, spiritualized, or pathologized. Others may express ambivalence, having never seen their needs reflected in systems of care. In these moments, therapists can draw on alternative methods for goal exploration, such as narrative mapping, values-based journaling, identity timelines, or visual storyboards. These tools do more than generate ideas. They reveal themes of longing, loss, and possibility that have been shaped by both trauma and resilience. When these themes are honored, goals shift from performance to meaning.

The pathway to participation must also be flexible. A client who disengages from a session may not be resisting progress. They may be protecting themselves from yet another setting that centers external expectations over internal truth. Adjusting the pace of therapy, offering choices around intervention style, and validating the emotional labor of showing up are all part of building a safe participatory process. The goal is not to return someone to the life they had before trauma. It is to support them in creating a life where occupation reflects who they are, not just what they can do. See Table 10.2 for examples of affirming goals and their clinical applications.

Table 10.2 Examples of Affirming Goals and Clinical Strategies

Goal Theme	Example Goal	Clinical Strategy
Identity Expression	Client will wear clothing that reflects their gender identity during one community outing with minimal cues weekly	Use values clarification and sensory-based exploration to support comfort and agency
Relational Safety	Client will initiate one affirming social interaction per week with verbal prompting in a chosen safe setting	Support client in identifying safe people and environments using a social eco-map
Narrative Reconstruction	Client will complete a visual identity timeline including at least three milestones with guided support in 4 weeks	Use photo elicitation or narrative mapping to scaffold storytelling
Self-Regulation Through Routine	Client will engage in two sensory grounding activities per day with visual cues as part of a co-created routine plan	Co-design morning or evening rhythms with chosen sensory supports and flexible pacing
Community Reconnection	Client will attend two LGBTQ+ group events in the next month with therapist support in planning and debriefing	Identify low-pressure entry points and use role-play or scripting to support access
Spiritual Reclamation	Client will engage in one affirming spiritual or cultural practice per week independently over the next 3 weeks	Integrate ritual, music, or movement-based practices that reflect identity and meaning

Goal setting in trauma-informed care invites a deeper examination of how participation reflects identity, not just function. When gender and sexual minority women begin to name what they want to engage in, they are often navigating years of internalized constraint and external invalidation. Goals that may appear straightforward from a clinical perspective often require significant emotional labor to define and pursue. This is especially true when past experiences of erasure, surveillance, or punishment have shaped how desire and choice are expressed.

In practice, identity-affirming goals can activate complex psychological responses. Resuming a once-loved occupation, entering a new community, or re-engaging in spiritual or creative practices often brings up memory, grief, or self-doubt. These reactions are not barriers to progress; they are part of the process. Therapists must be prepared to recognize and support these layers without misinterpreting them as avoidance or disengagement. Affirming care means understanding that forward movement sometimes includes stillness, recalibration, or deliberate retreat. Clinical success is not defined only by completion but by whether the process remains aligned with safety, autonomy, and self-trust.

Restoring Regulation Through Authentic Occupation

Nervous system regulation does not emerge from standard routines applied across all clients. It arises from sustained engagement in occupations that are experienced as safe, chosen, and identity-affirming. For gender and sexual minority women with trauma histories, dysregulation often results from years of identity-based discrimination and chronic relational threat. Authentic occupation offers a neurologically informed and culturally grounded way to reestablish equilibrium. It allows the body and brain to relearn safety through meaningful action, not scripted compliance.

A 2023 study published in *Child and Adolescent Psychiatric Clinics of North America* provides insight into how toxic stress and trauma affect neurophysiology in transgender and gender diverse youth. The authors describe how chronic identity-based stress disrupts the body's ability to maintain allostasis, leading to what is termed allostatic overload. This includes dysregulation of the hypothalamic-pituitary-adrenal axis and the sympathetic adrenomedullary system, both of which are implicated in trauma-related changes in brain structure and function. Key regions such as the hippocampus and amygdala are especially vulnerable, contributing to hypervigilance, emotional dysregulation, and altered memory encoding. These same processes affect adults who have experienced sustained trauma, especially when trauma is compounded by systemic marginalization.

Occupational therapy that centers authentic occupation supports the restoration of physiologic balance by creating new patterns of engagement that are not mediated by fear or concealment. These occupations are chosen for their resonance, not their familiarity. A morning ritual that involves affirming touch, sound, or movement can create coherence in a system that has learned to fragment.

A creative task that reflects cultural or sexual identity can activate regions of the brain associated with reward, integration, and emotional clarity. These shifts are not incidental. They are central to the long-term restoration of regulation.

Therapists must be prepared to evaluate not only the task but also the relational and symbolic context in which it occurs. What feels grounding for one client may provoke vigilance in another. What restores attention in one setting may feel inaccessible in a space where the client does not feel seen. Regulation strategies should never be extracted from context. They should be discovered in collaboration and shaped by narrative, not protocol. When clients experience occupation as a source of both meaning and safety, they begin to reconnect not just to tasks, but to themselves.

Queer Time and Disrupted Developmental Pathways

Development does not follow a singular timeline. For many gender and sexual minority women, particularly those navigating trauma, identity, or chronic marginalization, development unfolds through nonlinear, interrupted, or postponed stages. Occupations that are typically associated with adolescent or early adult milestones—such as self-expression, autonomy, intimacy, and goal exploration—are often delayed, reframed, or inaccessible altogether. These disruptions are not indicative of pathology. They reflect adaptation to conditions that deprioritize safety, suppress identity, and limit agency.

A 2024 study published in *Health Education & Behavior* highlight how LGBTQ+ youth and young adults experienced pronounced developmental interference during the COVID-19 pandemic. Interview data revealed that identity formation, autonomy seeking, and access to affirming community were all significantly disrupted by isolation, stigma, and the reassertion of social norms in unsupportive home environments. Participants described this period as a time when the passage of time itself felt distorted. Days were marked less by progression and more by survival. For many, this compounded pre-existing delays in developmental processes already shaped by concealment, rejection, or trauma (Ruprecht et al., 2024).

Occupational therapists working with LGBTQ+ clients must be attuned to the concept of "queer time", a term used in gender and sexuality studies to describe temporalities that diverge from normative life stages. Delayed identity disclosure, postponed role experimentation, or interrupted educational or vocational trajectories are not uncommon. These shifts often reflect efforts to navigate unsafe environments or to avoid retraumatization. When clients present with what appear to be age-incongruent occupations or goals, the therapist's task is not to reimpose linear timelines but to understand how those patterns emerged, and what they continue to protect.

Trauma-informed care in this context involves recognizing that many clients are not returning to developmental milestones; they are arriving at them for the first time. The role of occupational therapy becomes one of scaffolding reentry into identity formation, social participation, and meaningful risk taking, even when those occupations would typically be expected in adolescence or early adulthood. Progress may involve reclaiming roles or routines that were once denied. It may also include stepping into occupations that reflect who the client is now, not who they were expected to become.

Delayed Autonomy and Role Exploration

Autonomy and role exploration are foundational processes in adolescent development. Yet for many gender and sexual minority women, these experiences are postponed or fragmented due to early environments where identity-based safety was not available. The process of forming and testing roles across relationships, occupations, self-expression, and community engagement often occurs later than typical developmental timelines would predict. This delay is not a failure of insight or maturity. It reflects adaptive strategies shaped by threat, surveillance, and systemic invalidation.

Some clients enter adulthood without ever having experienced identity-affirming autonomy. They may not have explored their sexual orientation or gender identity in the context of safety. They may have avoided certain roles altogether due to fear of rejection, violence, or cultural invisibility. When these individuals seek care in occupational therapy, they are not returning to old roles but constructing new ones from a baseline of interruption. These clinical presentations may resemble role confusion or occupational instability, but they often signify a late arrival to experiences others encountered much earlier in life.

This developmental reality highlights the ethical importance of therapeutic approaches that support critical self-exploration, not premature action or conformity. A 2023 article in the *Journal of Medical Ethics* emphasized that psychotherapy, when conducted without presumption or restriction, can help clients differentiate between external pressures and internal needs. It promotes reflective capacity and agency, allowing individuals to clarify whether their distress is rooted in identity suppression, environmental adversity, or a broader matrix of psychological and social factors. Exploratory therapy becomes essential when autonomy has been denied or delayed. It creates a space where new directions can be imagined without coercion or defense.

Occupational therapists can contribute to this work by helping clients map their timelines of role suppression and identity delay. This may involve narrative life charts, values clarification, or future role envisioning exercises that do not rely on normative age expectations. For a woman in her thirties who is navigating her first intimate relationship or discovering affirming clothing styles, the task is not to explain the delay. The task is to scaffold choice, participation, and trust in one's own preferences. Clinical outcomes improve not when roles are achieved quickly, but when they emerge through sustained, consensual engagement with self and context.

Rethinking Milestone Through an Affirming Lens

Milestones are often treated as universal markers of maturity, independence, or success. Graduating from school, entering romantic partnerships, establishing careers, or becoming parents are framed as benchmarks that define a well-lived adult life. But for gender and sexual minority women, these milestones are often deferred, disrupted, or replaced altogether. The assumption that everyone moves through life stages in predictable sequences fails to account for those who have had to delay visibility, postpone safety, or navigate institutional barriers to full participation.

Clinicians who rely on age-based developmental expectations may misinterpret adaptive decisions as signs of immaturity or dysfunction. A woman who returns to higher education in her forties, or who explores gender-affirming healthcare after years of concealment, is not regressing. She is reclaiming opportunities that were once structurally or psychologically inaccessible. Similarly, clients who reject traditional family structures or career models may not be disengaged; they may be choosing roles that reflect autonomy, sustainability, and coherence with lived identity.

Occupational therapy offers a powerful framework for redefining milestones in terms of personal meaning rather than external timelines. This includes acknowledging less visible but deeply significant achievements: establishing boundaries with unsupportive family, initiating hormone therapy, joining a queer community group, or simply maintaining presence in environments where erasure once felt inevitable. These are occupational transitions that reflect profound developmental work, even if they do not align with cultural scripts about adulthood or success.

By supporting clients in identifying their own markers of progress, therapists help reorient the clinical relationship toward affirmation rather than normalization. Participation becomes a process of authorship, not assimilation. Therapists must remain attuned to the social, cultural, and historical forces that shape which milestones are celebrated and which are pathologized. In doing so, they uphold a model of care that centers equity, self-determination, and the right to move through life at a pace and in a direction that reflects who a person truly is.

Occupational Therapy Across Nonlinear Transitions

Life transitions are rarely linear for women whose identities have been shaped by marginalization and survival. Gender and sexual minority women often revisit, repeat, or bypass expected life stages entirely. These transitions may not follow the familiar arc from dependence to autonomy, or from education to career, but instead reflect complex negotiations with safety, access, and identity. Occupational therapy must be prepared to work across these nonlinear trajectories without assuming pathology, failure, or delay.

Clients may enter therapy at inflection points that defy traditional models. A woman may initiate care while divorcing a partner she married under family pressure. Another may be transitioning gender while entering higher education after a decades-long gap. Some may be exploring intimacy or body-based occupations for the first time after years of dissociation. These are not simply moments of adaptation; they are sites of reinvention, often accompanied by grief, liberation, and profound uncertainty. Therapists must approach them with humility, curiosity, and a clear departure from normative benchmarks.

Occupational interventions in these contexts must emphasize rhythm over sequence and regulation over performance. This includes tracking what feels accessible, tolerable, and meaningful at any given moment, not just what aligns with age, diagnosis, or function. Standard goal structures may need to be reimagined. Progress may look like establishing routines that restore bodily trust, reengaging in spiritual practice after religious trauma, or participating in queer-affirming spaces that foster relational safety. These transitions are layered with emotional labor that should be recognized and scaffolded, not minimized.

When practiced with attunement to these complexities, occupational therapy becomes a framework for integration. It can help clients move between fragmented roles and emerging identities with greater coherence. It affirms that healing is not always about restoration but about constructing a life that was never given room to fully emerge. In nonlinear transitions, occupational therapy is not just a support, it is a practice of witnessing and resourcing the profound work of becoming.

Occupational Futurity and the Right to Imagine

The ability to envision oneself in the future is not just a sign of motivation, it is a neurologically grounded and socially mediated function of identity. Neuroscience research has shown that imagining the future recruits many of the same brain regions involved in autobiographical memory, including the medial prefrontal cortex and the hippocampus. This process, known as "episodic future thinking," allows people to construct detailed mental simulations of what could be. It is fundamental to volition, and it requires both a stable sense of self and a repertoire of possibilities that feel emotionally and socially attainable.

For gender and sexual minority women, access to this internal capacity is often compromised. Trauma, marginalization, and historical erasure restrict not only behavioral participation, but the cognitive architecture needed for imagining future occupations. A woman who has never seen herself reflected in positions of leadership, family structures, or public life may not simply fear the future—she may lack the narrative raw materials to build it. This is not due to cognitive limitation but to sociocultural deprivation. The absence of occupational futurity is not a symptom. It is a consequence.

Clinically, these constraints can manifest in patterns that are easily overlooked. A client may avoid future planning not because she lacks goals, but because future-oriented thinking has been a source of distress. Others may deflect discussions about aging or long-term relationships because such conversations activate histories of invalidation or loss. Research on future self-continuity suggests that when individuals cannot see a meaningful connection between who they are now and who they might become, they are less likely to take action toward future goals. For clients who have survived identity suppression, the future can feel both irrelevant and unreachable.

Occupational therapy is one of the few professions equipped to intervene at this intersection of volition, trauma, and time. Therapists can begin by explicitly naming futurity as an occupational capacity and by assessing the client's relationship to future self-concept, not just task-based goal setting. Interventions might involve narrative reconstruction, expressive occupation, or guided visualization, but only when offered in environments that affirm identity and restore agency. Participation in community, creativity, and chosen kinship are not optional for this work—they are the scaffolding on which possibility is built. This is not a call to impose developmental timelines or aspirational frameworks. It is an invitation to ask: What does thriving look like on this client's terms? What roles, rituals, or dreams were once abandoned because survival came first? When occupational therapy centers imagination as a form of rehabilitation, it does more than restore function. It restores access to a future that includes the self.

Volition and Visibility in Clinical Practice

Volition is not just a trait or a mindset. It is a developmental capacity shaped by experience, safety, and access to identity-affirming environments. For gender and sexual minority women, volition is often constrained by the absence of social recognition. When the future has never reflected someone's identity back to them, making meaningful decisions about what to pursue, where to live, or who to become becomes an act of tremendous uncertainty.

A young adult who has never seen an openly queer woman in leadership may hesitate to consider a promotion. A client who has spent years navigating healthcare systems that invalidated her gender identity may avoid setting long-term goals related to wellness or aging. A middle-aged woman exploring same-gender relationships for the first time may feel reluctant to articulate desires that have never been treated as legitimate. These are not examples of avoidance or ambivalence. They are expressions of caution shaped by lived history.

Therapists sometimes mistake this hesitation for poor insight or weak motivation. In reality, many clients have learned that forward movement comes with risk. Pursuing a meaningful role can lead to exposure. Expressing an authentic goal can invite scrutiny. Volition becomes an internal negotiation between desire and the cost of visibility. Without visible models of who they can become, clients may unconsciously limit their future to what feels emotionally survivable.

Occupational therapy can intervene by making volition visible again. This begins with asking what possibilities were denied, what roles were abandoned, and what forms of expression felt unsafe. Therapy might involve building visual timelines of when certain goals first emerged and when they were suppressed. It might include exploring photographs or digital media that show real people living in ways that reflect the client's potential. In some cases, the work may involve role-playing new occupations or trying them out in low-pressure environments. When identity and safety are no longer in conflict, volition expands. The therapist's role is not to direct that expansion, but to make room for it—and to witness its return without judgment.

Imagination as a Clinical Tool

Imagination is not an escape from reality. It is a vital therapeutic function that allows individuals to explore possibility, rehearse change, and regulate emotional overwhelm in the face of uncertainty. For gender and sexual minority women, whose identities are often invalidated or erased, imagination becomes a powerful way to reclaim agency and test the boundaries of what has felt off limits (Rubinstein et al., 2023). It is through imagined futures that clients begin to disrupt internalized narratives of exclusion and begin to craft new trajectories for themselves.

Recent research on fantastic reality ability has begun to validate this function of imagination in clinical settings. A 2023 study published in *Frontiers in Psychology* introduced the Fantastic Reality Ability Measurement Scale, which assesses how people use imagination in response to stress and trauma. The study found that imagination operates across several dimensions—coping, control, transcendence, and playfulness—and contributes meaningfully to psychological resilience. These findings suggest that therapeutic work which activates imaginative processes is not simply creative or expressive. It is neuropsychologically grounded and clinically impactful.

Occupational therapy can incorporate this insight into everyday practice. For instance, a client working toward independent living might be asked to describe a typical week in a future that aligns with her values, even if the logistics are not yet in place. A client recovering from identity-based trauma might create a narrative of what it would have looked like to grow up in a supportive environment, then use that story to identify unmet needs and desired roles. Group sessions might include vision boards, future casting, or storytelling prompts designed to elicit alternative identities and roles that were previously considered inaccessible.

These techniques are not fantasy. They are exercises in psychological flexibility, grounded in the idea that the mind can practice outcomes before the body achieves them. The Fantastic Reality Ability Measurement (FRAME) study highlights that individuals who are able to engage in imaginative coping report higher levels of emotional regulation, problem solving, and sense of control during periods of uncertainty. In occupational therapy, this translates into the capacity to scaffold new routines, test new roles, and eventually step into occupations that were once foreclosed. Imagination is not a luxury but a clinical resource. See Table 10.3 for examples of imagination-based strategies that support occupational engagement across diverse contexts.

Table 10.3 Imagination-Based Strategies to Support Occupational Engagement in LGBTQ and Sexual Minority Women

Clinical Goal	Imagination Strategy	Clinical Rationale	Example for LGBTQ or Sexual Minority Women
Expand future-oriented thinking	Visioning a week in the future that reflects the client's values	Supports volition by allowing clients to mentally rehearse possible identities and routines	A lesbian client envisions a week where she lives with a partner, attends an LGBTQ book club, and co-leads a support group.
Reclaim suppressed roles or desires	Storytelling prompt: "What would life have looked like if you had grown up affirmed?"	Helps surface internalized barriers and initiate emotional processing of unmet developmental needs	A bisexual woman raised in a conservative religious home narrates a version of her adolescence with affirming mentors and community.
Build tolerance for identity exploration	Occupation-based play or expressive art tied to future roles	Uses safe symbolic expression to reintroduce flexibility and creativity into goal setting	A transgender woman explores gender expression by designing collages of work outfits for future career settings.
Process loss or stalled development	Narrative mapping of a "parallel life" where environmental barriers were absent	Creates emotional distance while allowing grief, hope, and insight into identity evolution	A queer client creates a parallel timeline where she joined an affirming college program instead of deferring due to fear of rejection.
Reduce fear of rejection in planning	Future casting in third person (e.g., "Imagine someone like you ten years from now . . .")	Externalizes future identity to lower emotional threat and increase cognitive engagement	A pansexual woman imagines "a woman like her" opening a queer-owned wellness business, gaining confidence through narrative distancing.
Encourage participation in new routines	Guided imagery tied to daily occupations (e.g., commuting, caregiving, activism)	Activates motor planning, sensory awareness, and emotional forecasting to prepare for role reentry	A gender diverse client visualizes taking the subway to a Pride event without fear, anchoring safety strategies and self-expression.
Explore personal meaning of thriving	Creating a values collage or multimedia board showing "what thriving could look like"	Reorients goals around identity and meaning rather than productivity or social conformity	A queer woman in midlife includes images of chosen family, spiritual rituals, and queer elders on her collage of meaningful life.
Normalize uncertain futures	Timeline drawing with alternate endings and branching paths	Reinforces that nonlinear progress is valid and fosters comfort with ambiguity in life planning	A bisexual woman maps out three possible futures: cohabiting with a partner, solo travel and writing, or parenting through adoption.

These strategies do more than foster creativity. They activate psychological resilience and reintroduce possibility in clients who have historically been denied it. For LGBTQ and sexual minority women, chronic exposure to trauma, rejection, and invisibility often narrows the ability to envision a livable future. Imagination becomes both a mirror and a doorway, reflecting what has been lost and opening space for what could be. The FRAME study (Rubinstein et al., 2023) validates this clinical insight, showing that imagination used intentionally in times of stress supports coping, self-regulation, and emotional repair. By incorporating structured imaginative tasks into therapy, occupational therapists are not only encouraging expression but are restoring the client's capacity to build futures on their own terms, where their identities are not hidden, negotiated, or erased, but centered as sources of strength and direction.

Case Vignette and Clinical Reflections

The following case vignettes illustrate how occupational therapy can engage trauma-informed, identity-affirming approaches with LGBTQ and sexual minority women. These examples are not templates for care. Instead, they reflect nuanced, individualized processes rooted in relational trust, cultural humility, and collaborative exploration. Each case demonstrates how clinical reasoning shifts when therapists move beyond symptom management toward deeper engagement with identity, meaning, and possibility.

Case 1: Teyah, Age 29—Rebuilding Identity and Reengaging with Community After Complex Trauma

Teyah is a 29-year-old Two-Spirit (Navajo) woman who presented to occupational therapy through a tribal health clinic following a recent period of incarceration, substance use recovery, and family estrangement. She reported chronic fatigue, sleep disruption, difficulty with focus, and a loss of direction in daily life. While her referral diagnosis focused on functional reentry support, Teyah's own concerns centered on deeper questions of identity, disconnection from culture, and a desire to "figure out how to live in this body."

In the early phase of intervention, her occupational therapist prioritized therapeutic alliance and nervous system regulation. Sessions began with co-regulated breathing, grounding protocols, and body scans that Teyah was invited to name using her own cultural metaphors. A layered occupational profile was developed using visual timelines, storytelling, and somatic mapping to help Teyah surface moments of both rupture and resilience. Her therapist avoided immediate goal setting, instead inviting Teyah to identify felt-sense indicators of safety in everyday occupations—pouring coffee, lighting sage, sketching in the margins of her journal.

Intervention strategies moved beyond traditional ADL or IADL retraining. Together, they used narrative mapping to document Teyah's disconnection from land-based roles after relocation and incarceration. Drawing from Indigenous frameworks of relationality, her therapist supported reconnection with cultural occupations by introducing eco-mapping and kinship role inventories. One key shift occurred when Teyah identified a desire to resume participation in seasonal ceremonies, not as a return to the past, but as a way to anchor future intentions. This insight was scaffolded through logistical planning tasks, including sensory preparation, pacing strategies, and bridging scripts for reentry into formerly triggering spaces.

To support future-oriented thinking, the therapist used guided imagery sessions where Teyah envisioned herself five years from now—not in a fixed career but actively contributing to her community in ways that felt meaningful. These sessions included drawing speculative futures and constructing a "daily life forecast" aligned with her values of care, sovereignty, and collective well-being. A personalized set of coping anchors, including visual icons, breath prompts, and audio affirmations recorded in her own voice, was integrated into her phone as a self-regulation toolkit. Over time, Teyah reengaged in community gardening efforts, began facilitating a weekly storytelling circle for other Two-Spirit individuals, and expressed interest in applying for a cultural leadership fellowship. While trauma, grief, and systemic barriers remained present, her occupational identity had begun to take shape again, now defined not by loss, but by agency, cultural continuity, and chosen contribution.

Case 2: Maëlle, Age 41—Reclaiming Occupational Identity After Institutional Betrayal

Maëlle is a 41-year-old queer woman from Brittany, France, who was referred to occupational therapy by her primary care provider for support with post-traumatic stress, burnout, and occupational withdrawal following workplace harassment and retaliation. A former humanitarian program director fluent in five languages, Maëlle described a collapse in both her routines and her sense of professional identity after being forced out of her position by colleagues who discredited her queer identity and mental health history. She also disclosed a history of conversion therapy as a teenager, which had never been addressed in clinical care.

The therapist began by building rapport through narrative practice, using a semi-structured storytelling protocol that invited Maëlle to share episodes of occupational strength, disruption, and reinvention. Rather than asking for symptom tracking or performance goals, the therapist created space for Maëlle to externalize the language of failure and self-blame that had become embedded in her narrative. Sessions integrated structured sensory regulation routines, including bilateral movement, tactile exploration through calligraphy, and low demand co-occupations such as collaborative playlist building and poetry reading aloud.

To reintroduce volition, the therapist implemented a future visualization series where Maëlle was guided to describe what a meaningful week could look like three years from now, without logistical constraints. These sessions included drawing alternative timelines, writing letters from her imagined future self, and constructing a role collage using images sourced from feminist publications and queer archives. This process uncovered dormant aspirations that had been buried under fear and identity invalidation, including mentoring others and documenting her lived experience through creative nonfiction.

As therapy progressed, Maëlle's re-engagement was scaffolded through the development of a values-based occupational map. Together, they identified a constellation of micro-occupations—preparing herbal infusions, editing personal essays, organizing mutual aid events—that supported her regulation and restored a sense of contribution. Her therapist also used a social role diversification inventory to challenge the binary of professional success versus collapse, encouraging Maëlle to reframe roles such as neighbor, writer, and caregiver as equally valid forms of legacy.

By the end of her course of care, Maëlle had launched an online platform for LGBTQ professionals recovering from workplace trauma, resumed a weekly writing circle at her local library, and negotiated a flexible consulting role that allowed her to maintain boundaries without retreating from impact. Occupational therapy did not provide a formula for healing. It created a structure in which Maëlle could explore, revise, and reclaim her occupational life with clarity, agency, and dignity.

Therapist Reflections on Clinical Decision Making

Working with LGBTQ and sexual minority women through a trauma-informed lens calls for more than compassion or technical skill. It requires critical reflection on the clinical models, assumptions, and treatment norms that have historically overlooked or misrepresented these clients. In both cases above, the therapist moved away from a prescriptive approach and instead followed the client's timing, cultural identity, and occupational values as the organizing principles for care.

Therapists can begin by expanding their assessment practices to include identity mapping, narrative exploration, and future visioning tools. These approaches surface information that may not emerge through standard intake forms or performance-based measures. They also help build trust in populations that may have experienced clinical harm. Interventions should be guided by client-defined indicators of safety and engagement, not just symptom reduction or functional gain.

Effective strategies often include small but intentional shifts—inviting a client to design a routine around chosen values, using speculative storytelling to reimagine roles, or co-creating environments that reflect cultural belonging. These are not superficial adjustments. They are clinical practices rooted in occupational justice. When therapy becomes a space for reclaiming agency and redefining possibility, it moves beyond function and into authorship. The goal is not to restore what was lost, but to support what is becoming. This demands flexibility, cultural humility, and a deep respect for the many ways that healing can unfold.

Summary and Implications

Gender and sexual minority women experience trauma not only through acute events but through chronic identity-based exclusion that restructures their access to participation, safety, and visibility. Their occupational lives are shaped by environments that demand concealment and reward compliance over authenticity. As a result, trauma often manifests as role fragmentation, participation fatigue, or dissociation not due to dysfunction, but as strategic adaptations to survive relational and systemic harm. These women are not only managing symptoms but navigating the fallout of erasure, diagnostic overshadowing, and institutional nonrecognition.

Occupational therapy has a critical role to play in rewriting this trajectory. Clinicians must move beyond performance-based metrics and symptom management to create therapeutic spaces where identity exploration is central, not peripheral. This requires developing fluency in structural competence, using identity-affirming tools like narrative timelines and values based occupational maps, and approaching participation as a dynamic expression of safety, meaning, and belonging.

Strategies such as guided future visualization, symbolic role collage, and community participation planning are not simply expressive techniques—they are therapeutic interventions that restore agency and coherence in clients whose identities have been repeatedly silenced.

Ultimately, affirming care is not about doing more, it is about doing differently. The measure of success is not just what tasks are completed, but whether clients can show up fully, without apology or fragmentation. This is where occupational therapy becomes a reparative practice, one that supports both recovery and redefinition. In this work, therapists are not only treating trauma, they are helping build futures that were once unimaginable.

References

Bedford, C. E., Trotter, A. M., Potter, M., & Schmidt, N. B. (2023). Minority stress and mental health in lesbian, gay, bisexual, transgender, and queer survivors of sexual assault. *Journal of Traumatic Stress*, *36*(6), 1031–1043. https://doi.org/10.1002/jts.22970

Bochicchio, L., Porsch, L., Zollweg, S., Matthews, A. K., & Hughes, T. L. (2024). Health outcomes of sexual minority women who have experienced adverse childhood experiences: A scoping review. *Trauma, Violence & Abuse*, *25*(1), 764–794. https://doi.org/10.1177/15248380231162973

D'Angelo, R. (2024). Supporting autonomy in young people with gender dysphoria: Psychotherapy is not conversion therapy. *Journal of Medical Ethics*, *51*(1). https://doi.org/10.1136/jme-2023-109282

Devís-Devís, J., Pereira-García, S., Valencia-Peris, A., Vilanova, A., & Gil-Quintana, J. (2022). Harassment disparities and risk profile within lesbian, gay, bisexual and transgender Spanish adult population: Comparisons by age, gender identity, sexual orientation, and perpetration context. *Frontiers in Public Health*, *10*, 1045714. https://doi.org/10.3389/fpubh.2022.1045714

Marchi, M., Travascio, A., Uberti, D., De Micheli, E., Grenzi, P., Arcolin, E., Pingani, L., Ferrari, S., & Galeazzi, G. M. (2023). Post-traumatic stress disorder among LGBTQ people: A systematic review and meta-analysis. *Epidemiology and Psychiatric Sciences*, *32*, e44. https://doi.org/10.1017/S2045796023000586

Menhinick, K. A., & Sanders, C. J. (2023). LGBTQ+ stress, trauma, time, and care. *Pastoral Psychology*, *72*(3), 367–384. https://doi.org/10.1007/s11089-023-01073-z

Ramos, N., & Marr, M. C. (2023). Traumatic stress and resilience among transgender and gender diverse youth. *Child and Adolescent Psychiatric Clinics of North America*, *32*(4), 667–682. https://doi.org/10.1016/j.chc.2023.04.001

Rubinstein, D., O'Rourke, N., & Lahad, M. (2023). Using imagination in response to stress and uncertainty in the time of COVID-19: Further validation of the Fantastic Reality Ability Measurement (FRAME) scale. *Frontiers in Psychology*, *14*, 1115233. https://doi.org/10.3389/fpsyg.2023.1115233

Ruprecht, M. M., Floresca, Y., Narla, S., Felt, D., Phillips, G., 2nd, Macapagal, K., & Philbin, M. M. (2024). "Being queer, it was really isolating": Stigma and mental health among lesbian, gay, bisexual, transgender, and queer (LGBTQ+) young people during COVID-19. *Health Education & Behavior: The Official Publication of the Society for Public Health Education*, *51*(4), 521–532. https://doi.org/10.1177/10901981241249973

Shuler, S. L., Klimczak, K., & Pollitt, A. M. (2024). Queer in the latter days: An integrated model of sexual and religious identity development among former mormon sexual minority adults. *Journal of Homosexuality*, *71*(5), 1201–1230. https://doi.org/10.1080/00918369.2023.2169087

van Stolk-Cooke, K., Price, M., Dyar, C., Zimmerman, L., & Kaysen, D. (2023). Associations of past-year overall trauma, sexual assault and PTSD with social support for young adult sexual minority women. *European Journal of Psychotraumatology*, *15*(1), 2287911. https://doi.org/10.1080/20008066.2023.2287911

Chapter 11

Tools for Trauma-Informed Practice Across the Continuum of Care

---

Chapter Objectives

Upon completion of this chapter, the reader will be able to:

1. Differentiate trauma-informed evaluation practices from traditional assessment models by identifying how attunement to client cues and relational safety shapes data gathering and early engagement.
2. Apply reflective intake tools and narrative-based assessments to support collaborative goal setting that prioritizes safety, identity, and lived experience over standardized benchmarks.
3. Match intervention strategies to trauma recovery phases (stabilization, processing, reintegration) using clinical reasoning grounded in nervous system regulation and occupational identity.
4. Design trauma-informed discharge plans that integrate continuity, autonomy, and relational closure, with practical tools that support sustainable transitions and community re-engagement.
5. Utilize occupation-centered frameworks to address participation fatigue, diagnostic overshadowing, and systemic harm in ways that reinforce agency, cultural context, and interdependence throughout the therapeutic process.

Trauma responsive occupational therapy is grounded in the clinician's capacity to perceive subtle patterns of engagement as meaningful data. Rather than focusing solely on task initiation or observable behavior, it requires therapists to interpret bodily cues, pacing preferences, and relational dynamics as reflections of a client's nervous system state and lived experience. A client's physical orientation in the room, the cadence of their speech, or their response to open-ended questions can offer insight into prior encounters with power, safety, and trust. When therapeutic encounters are structured with this level of attunement, participation becomes an invitation rather than a demand. Sessions can then be crafted to

DOI: 10.4324/9781003658559-11

reflect the client's internal timing, support self-definition, and reinforce occupational identity through co-constructed routines and emotionally congruent activities. The goal is not simply to reduce barriers, but to create a therapeutic structure that reinforces dignity, agency, and relational safety at every stage of care.

Trauma-Informed Evaluation and Intake

Traditional evaluation models in occupational therapy often prioritize independence metrics, task performance, and standardized functional benchmarks. While useful in many contexts, these frameworks can obscure the adaptive responses women develop when navigating chronic threat, invalidation, or systems of oppression. The cumulative impact of racism, ableism, classism, heterosexism, and gender-based violence is not peripheral to clinical care. It directly shapes occupational participation and reflects the interdependent systems of disadvantage that must be addressed through intersectional practice (King-Mullins et al., 2023). Trauma often shows up not in discrete symptoms but in patterns of disengagement, difficulty articulating goals, or ambivalence toward intervention, which are frequently misinterpreted as noncompliance.

A trauma-informed evaluation recognizes that trust is not presumed but earned. The initial session is not just a site for data gathering but a relational entry point, where the therapist's ability to attune to verbal and nonverbal communication helps shape the client's sense of safety. Observing how a client negotiates space, responds to transitions, or tolerates uncertainty provides clinically relevant information that may not be captured in formal assessments. This approach enables the therapist to develop a responsive plan of care that reflects both occupational needs and the emotional architecture that surrounds them. It also repositions the client as a co-author in the therapeutic process, making space for collaboration grounded in readiness, voice, and lived complexity.

Clinical Pitfalls to Avoid

Before applying a trauma-informed approach to evaluation, therapists must identify and address common clinical habits that can unintentionally reinforce harm. Standard intake processes often emphasize efficiency, objectivity, and performance-based data collection. For women who have experienced trauma, disability, or systemic discrimination, these same processes may feel intrusive, invalidating, or disconnected from their lived realities (Grossman et al., 2021).

Asking directly about trauma history in the first session may seem clinically appropriate, but doing so before safety has been established can lead to emotional shutdown, incomplete disclosure, or perceived threat. Likewise, relying on language that centers independence, productivity, or symptom reduction may obscure the ways clients have adapted for survival. A woman who hesitates to answer, avoids eye contact, or seems unsure about her goals may not be disengaged. She may be assessing whether this space is safe enough to be honest.

Another common misstep is interpreting emotion regulation challenges, lack of goal clarity, or missed appointments as resistance. In reality, these may be protective strategies shaped by past invalidation, unmet needs, or distrust of medical systems. Trauma-informed evaluation requires that therapists resist the impulse to diagnose and instead cultivate curiosity (Han et al., 2021). When we interpret responses as information rather than obstruction, we shift from pathologizing behavior to understanding the story behind it. See Table 11.1 for a reflective intake tool designed to support early sessions with clients who may not yet have words for what they carry.

When therapists approach the intake process as a chance to perform assessment rather than establish relationship, clients may sense that they are being evaluated rather than supported. The Reflective Intake Map is not designed to

Table 11.1 Reflective Intake Map

Domain	Reflective Questions	Purpose	Clinical Application
Values and Identity	What helps you feel most like yourself? Are there parts of your life that reflect who you are most fully?	Surfaces core identity anchors and emotional grounding points	Use these themes to shape early occupations that feel familiar and reinforcing
Relational Safety	Who in your life helps you feel understood? Are there past experiences in care where you felt dismissed?	Clarifies relational wounds and protective boundaries	Helps guide how rapport is built and how much relational scaffolding may be needed
Somatic Cues	How does your body tell you when something is off? Are there times when you feel more settled?	Identifies somatic signals of stress and safety	Guides pacing of session and helps anticipate moments of dysregulation
Environmental Triggers	Are there spaces, sounds, or types of touch that feel uncomfortable? Is anything about this space hard?	Reveals hidden sensory or emotional triggers	Use responses to adapt the sensory and relational environment of treatment
Role Disruption	Have you lost any roles or routines that mattered to you? What part of your day feels furthest from how you want to live?	Surfaces grief and misalignment between current life and core values	Helps prioritize meaningful goals that honor identity while addressing occupational loss

replace standardized tools, but to complement them with depth, nuance, and human context. Each question is an opportunity to reframe the intake as a collaborative exploration rather than a data extraction process.

Using this map also encourages therapists to remain responsive to what is not said. Pauses, shifts in body language, and hesitations may hold more clinical relevance than polished answers. When clients are not ready to name their experiences, it is not a sign of withholding. It is often a sign of wisdom. Offering open-ended prompts that prioritize emotional safety over diagnostic precision allows for a deeper kind of rapport to emerge—one that forms the foundation of effective and ethical intervention.

Gathering Trauma History Without Asking for It

Traditional approaches to trauma screening often begin with a checklist of events. While efficient, these tools can bypass the layered ways that trauma shows up in behavior, identity, and occupational engagement. For many

Table 11.2 Therapeutic Exercise: Mapping the Story Without the Label

---

Therapeutic Exercise: Mapping the Story Without the Labels

This reflective prompt can be introduced conversationally or in written form, depending on the client's preference and emotional state. The therapist may say:

"Sometimes, it can be hard to describe what brings us here in just one sentence. So I often ask people to tell me the story in a way that feels most true to them—not as a list of symptoms or events, but as a timeline of change. We can go at your pace."

Then guide the client through these four prompts, either aloud or in a journal format:

1. **"Think about a time when your life felt most steady. What was happening then? Who were you around? What were your days filled with?"**

Purpose: Surfaces moments of regulation, safety, or identity alignment that can anchor future intervention.

2. **"Now think about a time when something shifted. When did that steadiness start to change? What began to feel harder?"**

Purpose: Opens space for discussing trauma-related disruption without naming the trauma directly.

3. **"What has helped you get through hard times since then—even if it was messy or imperfect?"**

Purpose: Identifies coping patterns and protective strategies, including those not typically named in clinical models.

4. **"If there are parts of the story that feel too big or unclear right now, that is completely okay. We can circle back whenever you are ready."**

Purpose: Reinforces agency, pace, and permission to withhold or defer content that feels unsafe.

---

women, especially those with a history of medical invalidation, systemic discrimination, or chronic health conditions, trauma is not a single incident to be named. It is an ongoing undercurrent that shapes how they move through the world.

Rather than ask "what happened to you?" trauma-informed therapists invite story indirectly. They attend to metaphors, patterns, and moments of silence. They ask about loss, change, and resilience. A woman may not say "I was abused," but she might describe never feeling safe in her home. She may not identify a traumatic event, but she may recount needing to disappear in social situations or freezing when someone raises their voice. These moments of story often emerge not through direct questioning but through careful presence and thoughtfully framed invitations. Table 11.2 provides an example of a clinical exercise that can be used during the intake phase or early sessions to help clients share meaningful context- without pressure, labeling or diagnostic framing.

Decision Making Flow in Trauma-Informed Evaluation

In trauma-informed care, evaluation is not a static event. It is a dynamic process that evolves alongside trust, insight, and readiness. Therapists often find themselves balancing the need to gather information with the responsibility to protect emotional safety. A decision-making framework can guide this process by helping clinicians determine when to pause, when to probe, and when to pivot toward regulation or support. This clinical skill set is emphasized in trauma-informed care education models shown to improve provider responsiveness and outcomes (Chin et al., 2024). This flow is not meant to be linear. It is iterative and adaptable, shaped by the client's cues, language, and engagement style (Goldstein et al., 2024). It encourages therapists to move beyond binary decisions like "ask or do not ask" and instead recognize trauma signals as opportunities for clinical attunement. Table 11.3 outlines this framework.

This framework reinforces the principle that trauma-informed evaluation is not about extracting information but about co-creating a safe context where meaningful information can emerge over time (Hanson et al., 2024). By responding to nonverbal cues and patterns of engagement, therapists can adapt their approach in real time, ensuring that the evaluation process itself does not replicate dynamics of control, invalidation, or overwhelm. The goal is not simply to collect data but to establish a therapeutic flow that invites trust, autonomy, and shared authorship from the start

Trauma-Informed Goal Setting and Collaborative Planning

In trauma-informed occupational therapy, goal setting is not just a procedural step. It is a relational process. For many clients who have lived through chronic invalidation, coercion, or systemic marginalization, being asked to identify goals can trigger confusion or distress. Some may pause, deflect, or express indifference not because they lack volition, but because they have rarely been invited to imagine a future they could shape for themselves.

Table 11.3 Trauma-Informed Decision-Making During Evaluation

Client Presentation	Therapist Observation	Recommended Response	Clinical Rationale
Client provides detailed history without distress	Appears grounded, consistent eye contact, steady affect	Proceed with semi-structured narrative mapping	Indicates capacity for integration and reflective discussion
Client becomes withdrawn or vague	Body turns away, flat tone, delays in response	Shift to regulation activity or sensory grounding	Signals neurophysiological overwhelm; prioritize safety and nervous system reset
Client shares concrete events but avoids emotional tone	Describes facts without affect, avoids subjective language	Validate content and invite metaphors or occupational framing	May indicate dissociation; metaphors offer safer pathways for emotional processing
Client uses humor, sarcasm, or redirection	Laughs or changes topic after difficult disclosures	Reflect gently and explore story indirectly	Defense mechanisms may signal past invalidation; gentle curiosity builds trust
Client asks if they "are doing it right" or seeks reassurance	Repeatedly asks for validation or feedback	Slow the pace, reinforce choice and autonomy	May reflect past control, surveillance, or gaslighting experiences (Thang et al., 2024).

Rather than treating goals as fixed outcomes, therapists can co-create them through shared dialogue. This begins by shifting the focus from what a client should accomplish to what they need in order to feel more regulated, connected, or expressed. For example, instead of asking "what do you want to achieve," a therapist might ask "what would make your day feel less heavy" or "what feels worth protecting right now." These reframes invite goals that prioritize emotional safety, identity development, or re-engagement in occupations that were once abandoned for survival. For clients with trauma histories, progress often comes in layers. Goals must be allowed to evolve. What matters most is not how quickly someone reaches a milestone, but whether they feel safe enough to take the next step. See Table 11.4 for sample goal alignment and adaptation matrix.

Table 11.4 Goal Alignment and Adaptation Matrix

Client Challenge (Trauma Lens)	Occupational Domain or Theme	Collaborative Exploration Questions	Sample Trauma-Informed Goals
Avoids naming goals or says "I don't know"	Volition and Identity	What feels most important to you right now, even if it feels small?	Client will identify one personally meaningful activity to include weekly, using journaling or photo prompts.
Struggles with future planning due to fear or overwhelm	Time Use and Role Exploration	If you could imagine a peaceful day, what would be happening?	Client will describe one future-oriented role or activity they are curious about in a reflective session.
Expresses goals that mirror others' expectations, not personal desires	Autonomy and Boundaries	How do you know when something feels like yours and not someone else's idea?	Client will explore three occupational choices and practice naming their own preferences in sessions.
Minimizes needs or insists on total independence	Interdependence and Self-advocacy	What helps you feel supported without feeling controlled?	Client will co-create a daily task-sharing plan with support persons that feels sustainable and not overwhelming.
States desire to "go back to normal" without reflection	Integration of Past and Present Roles	What parts of your old routine still feel like they belong to you?	Client will reconstruct a valued routine from pre-trauma life, integrating one adapted strategy for current capacity.

This matrix is designed to shift goal setting from a task-focused checklist to a relational and trauma-informed process. Rather than pressuring clients to articulate ideal futures or standardized objectives, therapists can use the domain themes and exploration questions as scaffolds to co-create goals that are grounded in lived experience, emotional readiness, and evolving identity (Hart et al., 2024). Each goal is an opening, not a directive. Clinicians are encouraged to return to these prompts throughout the plan of care, adjusting for new insights, setbacks, or changes in context. When used flexibly, this matrix allows occupational therapy to function not just as rehabilitation, but as restoration of authorship over one's time, choices, and possibilities.

Intervention Planning and Implementation
Across Trauma Recovery Phases

Trauma recovery is not linear, and neither is intervention. Effective planning requires more than selecting the right modality. It demands attunement to the client's nervous system, meaning making process, and readiness for participation. While traditional models of care often assume a stable baseline from which to build, trauma-informed occupational therapy recognizes that clients may enter treatment in a state of distress, avoidance, or fragmented identity. The role of the therapist is to match the intervention approach to the client's phase of recovery, adjusting pace and complexity as safety and capacity increase.

Occupational therapy can support trauma recovery across three fluid phases: stabilization, processing, and reintegration. These phases are not rigid stages but reference points for organizing care. Stabilization focuses on emotional and physiological safety. Processing includes narrative reconstruction and meaning making. Reintegration supports the return to or reimagining of roles, routines, and participation. A mismatch between intervention and recovery phase, for example, introducing trauma narratives before building regulation, can undermine safety and trust.

Therapists can use recovery phases not to label clients but to shape their clinical decisions. For instance, during stabilization, a client who experiences persistent hypervigilance may benefit from structured co-occupations that restore predictability and sensory control. In processing, the focus may shift to reflective work that connects body-based sensations to memory and meaning. During reintegration, therapists may help clients scaffold reentry into valued occupations, rebuild social roles, or create new expressions of identity. The interventions must evolve as the client's inner stability grows. See Table 11.5 for a clinical planning tool that connects recovery phase, presentation, and suggested occupational therapy strategies.

This tool is designed to support clinical reasoning by aligning the recovery phase with observable client presentation and matching it with appropriate therapeutic focus and interventions (Huo et al., 2023). Rather than prescribing a rigid sequence, it offers a flexible framework that can be adapted based on the client's readiness, environment, and evolving goals. Clinicians can use it as a dynamic reference during team meetings, supervision, or documentation to ensure their approach remains both trauma responsive and functionally relevant.

In practice, this means evaluating not just what the client can do, but where they are emotionally and physiologically. A client presenting with shutdown or hypervigilance may require stabilization strategies before any reflective work can begin. On the other hand, a client who is expressing interest in community roles or advocacy may benefit from interventions that support reintegration and future planning. This tool helps therapists move with the client rather than ahead of them, promoting attuned and effective care.

Table 11.5 Recovery Phase Framework for Trauma-Informed Occupational Therapy

Recovery Phase	Client Presentation	Primary Clinical Focus	Trauma-Informed OT Strategies
Stabilization	Heightened arousal, hypervigilance, dissociation, limited trust or engagement	Establishing psychological safety, nervous system regulation, environmental predictability	• Sensory-based self-regulation tools (e.g., weighted items, breathwork kits) • Co-regulation strategies through mirrored movement or parallel activities • Structuring sessions with clear, predictable routines • Safety and sensory mapping for occupational environments
Processing	Emotional variability, beginning to verbalize past events, increased self-awareness, emergence of grief or identity disruption	Meaning-making, narrative integration, validating adaptive responses	• Guided timeline construction or occupational life-mapping • Symbolic and metaphor-driven occupations (e.g., collage, storytelling, guided drawing) • Role negotiation exercises (e.g., re-examining caregiving or worker roles) • Use of expressive media (e.g., music, movement) to support nonverbal integration
Reintegration	Greater self-regulation, interest in future planning, increased participation and interpersonal engagement	Role resumption, community participation, identity expansion and resilience-building	• Graded reentry into meaningful occupations (e.g., volunteering, part-time work, caregiving) • Advocacy-based activities to reclaim voice and agency • Peer-led co-occupations or support group facilitation • Narrative goal setting using values clarification and occupational storytelling

Although aligning interventions to recovery phases is essential, the language therapists use when initiating conversation can determine whether a client feels safe or exposed. For individuals who have internalized shame, survived systems of control, or learned to suppress their own preferences, being asked what they want may not feel empowering. It can feel disorienting or even unsafe. Standard goal setting prompts often assume that clarity, motivation, and planning are readily accessible. In reality, many clients need time and support to reconnect with those capacities. This requires prompts that are layered, invitational, and responsive to the emotional climate of the session.

Although aligning interventions to recovery phases is essential, the language therapists use when initiating conversation can determine whether a client feels safe or exposed. For individuals who have internalized shame, survived systems of control, or learned to suppress their own preferences, being asked what they want may not feel empowering. It can feel disorienting or even unsafe. Standard goal setting prompts often assume that clarity, motivation, and planning are readily accessible. In reality, many clients need time and support to reconnect with those capacities. This requires prompts that are layered, invitational, and responsive to the emotional climate of the session. See Table 11.6 for examples

Table 11.6 Prompt Bank for Trauma-Informed Goal Setting

Clinical Theme	Traditional Prompt	Reframed Prompt	Clinical Intention
Volition and identity	"What do you want to work on?"	"What feels most important to you today, even if it is not easy to name?"	Reduces pressure to have a concrete goal; invites authentic starting point.
Emotional regulation	"What helps you calm down?"	"When things feel overwhelming, what helps you stay connected to yourself or your environment?"	Encourages reflection beyond coping to include embodiment and self-awareness.
Role disruption	"What roles do you want to get back to?"	"Are there parts of your life you miss, or parts you never got to explore?"	Opens space for grief, missed experiences, or emerging desires.
Interpersonal boundaries	"Do you need help with relationships?"	"What helps you feel respected in your space or conversations?"	Shifts from pathology to self-protection and boundary awareness.

(Continued)

Table 11.6 (Continued)

Clinical Theme	Traditional Prompt	Reframed Prompt	Clinical Intention
Time use and daily rhythm	"What does your routine look like?"	"Are there any moments in your day that feel like they belong to you?"	Highlights small but meaningful anchors to build on.
Future planning and possibility	"Where do you see yourself in five years?"	"Is there something you hope to feel more of in the next season of your life?"	Reframes future orientation in terms of feeling and vision, not productivity.
Self-advocacy and autonomy	"What do you need from others?"	"When do you feel most able to speak for yourself, even in small ways?"	Builds empowerment through reflection on everyday micro-acts of voice and agency.

of exploratory questions that reframe goal setting as a collaborative and emotionally attuned process.

This prompt bank is not meant to be a checklist. It is a clinical posture. The way a question is asked can either invite safety or reinforce self-doubt. For clients with trauma histories, especially those whose autonomy has been disrupted by systems or relationships, the act of setting goals can feel exposing. These prompts are designed to reduce that threat (Liu et al., 2024). They allow therapists to move with the client's readiness, gently surfacing what matters most, even if what matters cannot yet be named.

In practice, therapists might introduce one or two of these prompts during early rapport-building sessions, embedding them into casual conversation or reflective journaling. Over time, the same question might take on new meaning as the client's sense of agency strengthens. The goal is not to extract definitive answers but to support a process of emergence. Some clients may respond in metaphor, others with practical ideas, and others still with silence that carries its own significance. These responses, however small, can shape a plan of care that feels aligned, possible, and anchored in lived experience.

Discharge Planning and Sustainable Transitions

Discharge is often treated as an administrative milestone, the moment when services conclude and documentation is finalized. But for women whose engagement in occupational therapy has involved trauma processing, identity reconstruction, and nervous system regulation, discharge can feel like another rupture. It may evoke earlier experiences of abandonment, sudden transitions, or the withdrawal of care before trust was fully established. Clinicians must approach discharge not as a single endpoint but as a carefully supported transition that honors continuity, autonomy, and emotional safety.

Trauma-informed discharge planning begins early. From the first phase of care, therapists can begin planting the idea that therapy is not about permanent dependence but about building the internal and external scaffolds needed to move forward. This might sound like, "Part of our work together will be identifying when you feel ready to take more of this into your own rhythm" or "We will check in regularly to see what supports you want in place for when our work winds down." These early messages lay the groundwork for empowerment and co-ownership of the process.

As discharge approaches, clients may show signs of anxiety, regression, or resistance. These are not failures of treatment but reflections of attachment and vulnerability. Rather than rushing to reassure, therapists can validate these responses and collaboratively explore what feels unresolved. This process can uncover lingering fears about navigating systems without advocacy, managing symptoms independently, or sustaining progress without structured support.

A sustainable discharge plan integrates relational closure, identity reinforcement, and accessible next steps. This may include creating a values-based summary of gains, co-authoring a transition letter that outlines what was learned and what matters most moving forward, or mapping post-discharge resources that align with the client's identity and goals. Some clients may benefit from gradual step-down models such as reduced frequency visits or virtual check-ins, while others may need support accessing community-based programs, peer networks, or ongoing creative outlets (Nagle-Yang et al., 2022). Ultimately, a trauma-informed discharge process is not about a clean break. It is about helping clients internalize safety, agency, and vision so they carry the work with them into the spaces they choose next. The goal is not independence in isolation, but interdependence rooted in awareness, capacity, and choice. See Table 11.7

Table 11.7 Trauma-Informed Discharge Planning Checklist for Occupational Therapy

Checklist: Trauma-Informed Discharge Planning

- Initiate discharge discussions early using gentle, collaborative language
- Validate and explore emotional responses related to transition and ending
- Review progress in language that centers identity, not just function
- Co-create a values-based summary or transition letter
- Identify specific supports needed after discharge (e.g., routines, people, tools)
- Connect to community resources aligned with the client's cultural and occupational identity
- Offer a gradual step down or check in option when appropriate
- Ensure the client knows how to re-access care if needed
- End with intention (e.g., shared closure ritual, reflection, or future visioning)

for a trauma-informed discharge planning checklist designed to support clinical decision making, client collaboration, and sustainable transitions beyond therapy.

This checklist is not meant to be a rigid protocol but a reflective tool to support intentional discharge planning. Clinicians are encouraged to review it collaboratively with the client, adapting each item based on individual readiness, cultural context, and support systems. When used flexibly, it can reduce the risk of abrupt endings and promote a more empowered transition, where the client's sense of safety, authorship, and continuity of care are actively preserved.

Sustaining Change After Discharge

Discharge is not the end of therapeutic work. It is the beginning of life without the structure of weekly sessions and without the familiar rituals of reflection and guidance. For many women whose trauma recovery has unfolded inside the therapeutic relationship, this transition can feel destabilizing. What sustains healing when the therapy room is no longer available? What anchors volition, regulation, or belonging once the safety of the clinical container dissolves?

Occupational therapy has a unique role to play in this passage. It can help clients create not just a plan for the next appointment or the next month, but a scaffold for continuity. This requires looking beyond clinical goals to the broader ecology of support. The client's rhythms, relationships, and resources become part of the discharge map. Therapists can help clients identify what structures already exist and what needs to be built—rituals that center identity, people who reflect worth, occupations that tether meaning. The goal is not independence in the sense of disconnection. It is sustainable interdependence shaped by awareness and choice.

One way to support this is through the use of a "Sustained Occupation Plan." This tool helps clients reflect on what supports will hold them across four domains: relationships, routines, resources, and reminders. See Table 11.8 for an example of how this plan can be used to create a living map of post-discharge scaffolding.

This plan can be filled out collaboratively in the final sessions and revisited periodically to build ownership. Therapists are encouraged to help clients identify tangible strategies in each domain and explore how these anchors can evolve as needs change. When integrated thoughtfully, this plan allows discharge to feel less like a rupture and more like a handoff into a life the client continues to author.

Not every client will feel ready for discharge, even when goals have technically been met. For many women and gender-expansive clients, therapy was the first space where their story was not minimized, their symptoms were not misinterpreted, and their sense of self was allowed to unfold without correction.

Table 11.8 Sustained Occupation Plan

Domain	Reflection Questions	Client Responses or Plan Components	Example for Practice
Relationships	Who helps you feel seen, grounded, or encouraged? Who can you reach out to when you feel disconnected?	List of trusted people, support groups, or mentors	Weekly phone check-in with a close friend or peer support network
Routines	What parts of your day help you feel most like yourself? What small rituals offer structure or calm?	Anchoring routines, restorative practices, meaningful occupations	Morning tea and journaling before work three days per week
Resources	What tools, practices, or spaces help you regulate or reset? What has helped you in the past?	Sensory tools, therapy notes, access to nature, grounding strategies	Use of calming app, art materials, or safe place visualization
Reminders	What helps you remember your own progress, strength, or values? What do you want to carry with you?	Notes, affirmations, meaningful objects, values-based reflections	Personalized quote in planner or framed note from therapy session

Leaving that space can feel less like an ending and more like a loss of belonging. Clinicians must recognize that emotional readiness for discharge may not align with administrative timelines and support the client in naming what they want to carry with them, not just what they are leaving behind.

Reflection is not a luxury at this stage of care. It is essential. Clients may have forgotten how much they have changed since the first session. They may be unaware of how their regulation strategies, self-advocacy skills, or engagement in daily life have shifted. A structured reflective process allows them to witness their own evolution, to locate the anchors they have built, and to create a resource that feels both honest and empowering. This reflection also reinforces continuity by inviting clients to articulate what support structures they will rely on next.

Rather than focusing on outcomes alone, this reflection is about narrative ownership. It gives clients the opportunity to write their own transition story, to identify what they want to sustain, what they need to release, and what still feels unknown. When shared collaboratively with the therapist, this reflection

Table 11.9 Reflective Transition Mapping Exercise

Reflective Exercise: Transition Mapping for Sustainable Closure		
This guided reflection can be introduced in the final few sessions, either as a written worksheet or through dialogue. It can be completed alone, with the therapist, or shared with a trusted support person after therapy ends.		
Reflective Domain	*Prompt*	*Purpose*
Then and Now	What felt most overwhelming when we started? What feels different now?	Helps the client track change and build insight into their own growth.
Anchors and Resources	What are the people, practices, or routines that help you feel most grounded?	Identifies external and internal supports that can sustain progress.
Identity and Values	What parts of you feel more visible or affirmed than they did before?	Reinforces identity development and therapeutic gains.
Still in Progress	What are you still figuring out? What questions feel alive for you?	Normalizes ongoing growth and ambiguity.
Carrying Forward	What do you want to take with you from this experience?	Supports intentional closure and future orientation.
Reentry Plan	If you need support again, how will you know? Where can you go?	Builds awareness of red flags and clear routes back to care or community-based support.

can become a bridge not only from therapy to post-therapy life, but from dependency to agency. See Table 11.9 for a reflective discharge planning exercise that supports this process.

This reflective exercise is not meant to be a closing formality but a therapeutic tool that affirms the client's agency. Therapists are encouraged to introduce it gradually in the final sessions, framing it as an opportunity to honor the client's work and clarify what they wish to carry forward. It can be completed verbally in conversation, written in a journal, or even structured as a creative project depending on the client's preferred mode of expression. The goal is not to summarize treatment through clinical metrics, but to help the client articulate their growth in a way that feels emotionally true and personally meaningful.

When used with care, this exercise becomes more than a review; it becomes an act of narrative integration. Therapists should allow space for ambivalence, grief, and pride to coexist. Clients may not have language for their evolution at first, and that is okay. Pausing after each section, validating what emerges, and reflecting back key phrases can reinforce the idea that their voice matters. Over time, this document or dialogue can serve as a compass for post-therapy life, one that reminds them of who they are becoming, what supports they value, and how they want to meet the next chapter.

Sustaining Trauma-Informed Gains Through Community and Role Re-engagement

Trauma recovery research increasingly points to a critical but often overlooked stage: the period after formal services end. This phase is where therapeutic gains must be practiced without the weekly scaffolding of clinical support. Yet despite growing recognition of this need, the post-discharge phase is rarely standardized in TIC implementation models, leading to inconsistent follow-up and systemic gaps in care (Berring et al., 2024). Integration requires more than symptom stability, it demands environments, relationships, and occupations that affirm the client's evolving self.

Occupational therapists can help bridge this phase by collaboratively identifying roles that reflect the client's post-therapy identity. This might involve returning to roles once put on hold, such as parenting or creative expression, or initiating new ones like community advocacy, peer mentorship, or culturally grounded healing practices. Some roles may need to be relinquished if they were shaped by survival rather than authenticity. For midlife women, these transitions often coincide with identity shifts brought on by hormonal changes, life-stage transitions, and evolving priorities, which occupational therapists must integrate into planning (El Khoudary et al., 2019). These choices must be approached with curiosity and flexibility, not as performance metrics but as reflections of internal readiness.

Reengagement after discharge should center around occupational identity. This is not limited to what clients do, but how they feel while doing it, and whether those experiences align with their values. Instead of prescribing reintegration, therapists can invite dialogue: "What roles feel nourishing now?" or "Who makes it easier for you to show up as yourself?" These inquiries shift the focus from independence to interdependence, helping clients build lives where safety and selfhood can be sustained. See Table 11.10 for a collaborative mapping tool that supports this reflective process.

This tool is most effective when used as a collaborative exercise in the final phase of therapy. Clinicians can introduce each question in session, offering space for reflection, journaling, or dialogue. Mapping responses visually (e.g., drawing or using post-it notes) can also help clients externalize and organize their evolving narrative. The responses can inform a personalized transition plan or be integrated into a closure summary to reinforce continuity and self-authorship.

Table 11.10 Collaborative Mapping Tool for Post-Discharge Role Integration

Reflection Area	Guiding Questions	Client Response Examples	Clinical Use/ Application
Current Anchors	What routines or relationships help you feel steady right now?	Morning walks, texting a friend, spiritual rituals	Reinforce existing supports and use them as stability points in planning
Evolving Identity	What parts of yourself feel stronger or more clear since starting therapy?	"I speak up more," "I am not ashamed of my past"	Shape future roles or activities that align with reclaimed self-perceptions
Occupational Loss or Release	Are there any roles or routines you want to leave behind?	Caregiver role that felt like a burden, job that erased identity	Support healthy boundary-setting and grieving of unaligned roles
Values-Based Reengagement	What kind of environments or people make it easier for you to be yourself?	Spaces with other survivors, nature, affirming peer circles	Prioritize role and community selection based on alignment with safety and authenticity
Future-Oriented Curiosity	What is one role or activity you would like to try, even if it feels uncertain?	Volunteering, taking a class, joining a creative group	Introduce scaffolded reentry with flexibility and affirm growth over perfection

Summary and Implications

Trauma-informed care becomes meaningful only when it translates into everyday practice. While often described as a mindset or guiding philosophy, it must ultimately take form through the specific choices therapists make during the course of care. From the first session to the final transition, every clinical decision becomes an opportunity to uphold or disrupt safety, agency, and equity. This chapter offers practical tools and frameworks to ensure that trauma-informed principles are not just understood but embodied in the structure and flow of occupational therapy.

The tools included here are not rigid protocols. They are scaffolds designed to support clients as they regain control over their time, choices, and occupational identity. Therapists are encouraged to tailor these strategies to the lived realities of the people they serve, taking into account culture, access, power dynamics, and history. Whether the client is navigating reentry into daily roles, adapting to new routines after loss, or building new expressions of self after trauma, these clinical tools can provide structure without constraint.

Trauma-informed occupational therapy is not about perfect answers. It is about attuned presence, responsive practice, and respect for complexity. Its success is not measured by how quickly someone returns to function but by how fully they are seen, heard, and supported in their healing. When clinicians adopt this approach with humility and skill, occupational therapy becomes more than a service. It becomes a relational act of repair.

References

Berring, L. L., Holm, T., Hansen, J. P., Delcomyn, C. L., Søndergaard, R., & Hvidhjelm, J. (2024). Implementing trauma-informed care-settings, definitions, interventions, measures, and implementation across settings: A scoping review. *Healthcare (Basel, Switzerland)*, *12*(9), 908. https://doi.org/10.3390/healthcare12090908

Chin, B., Amin, Q., Hernandez, N., Wright, D. D., Awan, M. U., Plumley, D., Zito, T., & Elkbuli, A. (2024). Evaluating the effectiveness of trauma-informed care frameworks in provider education and the care of traumatized patients. *The Journal of Surgical Research*, *296*, 621–635. https://doi.org/10.1016/j.jss.2024.01.042

El Khoudary, S. R., Greendale, G., Crawford, S. L., Avis, N. E., Brooks, M. M., Thurston, R. C., Karvonen-Gutierrez, C., Waetjen, L. E., & Matthews, K. (2019). The menopause transition and women's health at midlife: A progress report from the Study of Women's Health Across the Nation (SWAN). *Menopause (New York, N.Y.)*, *26*(10), 1213–1227. https://doi.org/10.1097/GME.0000000000001424

Goldstein, E., Chokshi, B., Melendez-Torres, G. J., Rios, A., Jelley, M., & Lewis-O'Connor, A. (2024). Effectiveness of trauma-informed care implementation in health care settings: Systematic review of reviews and realist synthesis. *The Permanente Journal*, *28*(1), 135–150. https://doi.org/10.7812/TPP/23.127

Grossman, S., Cooper, Z., Buxton, H., Hendrickson, S., Lewis-O'Connor, A., Stevens, J., Wong, L. Y., & Bonne, S. (2021). Trauma-informed care: Recognizing and resisting re-traumatization in health care. *Trauma Surgery & Acute Care Open*, *6*(1), e000815. https://doi.org/10.1136/tsaco-2021-000815

Han, H. R., Miller, H. N., Nkimbeng, M., Budhathoki, C., Mikhael, T., Rivers, E., Gray, J., Trimble, K., Chow, S., & Wilson, P. (2021). Trauma informed interventions: A systematic review. *PLoS One*, *16*(6), e0252747. https://doi.org/10.1371/journal.pone.0252747

Hanson, C. L., Crandall, A., Novilla, M. L. B., & Bird, K. T. (2024). Psychometric evaluation of the trauma-informed care provider assessment tool. *Health Services Research and Managerial Epidemiology*, *11*, 23333928241258083. https://doi.org/10.1177/23333928241258083

Hart, L., Bliton, J. N., Castater, C., Beard, J. H., & Smith, R. N. (2024). Trauma-informed language as a tool for health equity. *Trauma Surgery & Acute Care Open*, *9*(1), e001558. https://doi.org/10.1136/tsaco-2024-001558

Huo, Y., Couzner, L., Windsor, T., Laver, K., Dissanayaka, N. N., & Cations, M. (2023). Barriers and enablers for the implementation of trauma-informed care in healthcare settings: A systematic review. *Implementation Science Communications*, *4*(1), 49. https://doi.org/10.1186/s43058-023-00428-0

King-Mullins, E., Maccou, E., & Miller, P. (2023). Intersectionality: Understanding the Interdependent Systems of Discrimination and Disadvantage. *Clinics in colon and rectal surgery, 36*(5), 356–364. https://doi.org/10.1055/s-0043-1764343

Liu, V. C., Nelson, L. E., & Shorey, S. (2024). Experiences of women receiving trauma-informed care: A qualitative systematic review. *Trauma, Violence & Abuse, 25*(4), 3054–3065. https://doi.org/10.1177/15248380241234346

Nagle-Yang, S., Sachdeva, J., Zhao, L. X., Shenai, N., Shirvani, N., Worley, L. L. M., Gopalan, P., Albertini, E. S., Spada, M., Mittal, L., Moore Simas, T. A., & Byatt, N. (2022). Trauma-informed care for obstetric and gynecologic settings. *Maternal and Child Health Journal, 26*(12), 2362–2369. https://doi.org/10.1007/s10995-022-03518-y

Thang, C. K., Kucaj, S., Garell, C. L., Masood, K. M., Calhoun, A. W., Lay, K., Lee, J., Wilhalme, H., & Szilagyi, M. A. (2024). Development and validation of a trauma-informed care communication skills assessment tool. *Academic Pediatrics, 24*(8), 1333–1342. https://doi.org/10.1016/j.acap.2024.07.008

Chapter 12

Innovative Strategies in Trauma Care

Alyssa Broussard, a 32-year-old woman with a history of childhood sexual trauma and a recent pregnancy loss, was referred to occupational therapy for difficulty managing daily routines and emotional regulation. Since her miscarriage, she had struggled to return to work, maintain regular sleep, and engage in basic self-care. Repeated efforts to connect her with traditional mental health services had failed as she missed appointments, declined phone calls, and described therapy

DOI: 10.4324/9781003658559-12

offices as "too close, too fast." When her OT offered a hybrid care model that included a trauma-sensitive digital app, Alyssa agreed to try. Through the app, she could log sensory triggers, practice guided grounding exercises, and message her therapist between sessions without needing to speak aloud. Gradually, Alyssa began using wearable biofeedback data to notice when stress spiked during meals or transitions and modified her routine accordingly. This digital entry point became her bridge to healing and a safer path into it.

Innovation in trauma care is often associated with digital tools, emerging technologies, and novel clinical interventions. But in women's health, true innovation begins with reimagining how care is delivered, especially for those whose histories of trauma have shaped their relationship to healthcare. Technology alone cannot repair mistrust or reduce harm. It must be integrated into systems that prioritize agency, consent, and relational safety. Whether through wearable biosensors that track dysregulation or AI enhanced decision tools that support individualized planning, innovation must be anchored in the realities of trauma and tailored to the needs of those most at risk of retraumatization.

This need for adaptive, patient led innovation is not theoretical. A 2015 case report by Parker described how a woman with rape trauma syndrome experienced acute distress during obstetric care because of routine procedures that mirrored earlier violations. The report emphasized that even standard actions, such as cervical exams, anesthesia, or unannounced touch, can act as trauma triggers without appropriate clinical awareness. The absence of trauma-informed strategy is not neutral. It can replicate harm. As we explore digital tools, interdisciplinary models, and new modes of service delivery, the measure of innovation will be its ability to protect, empower, and restore dignity in care.

Technology as a Bridge, Not a Barrier

Technology is often characterized as impersonal, mechanistic, or emotionally distant, traits that may seem fundamentally misaligned with the relational depth required in trauma-informed care. Yet when developed with ethical foresight and clinical insight, digital tools can become powerful facilitators of access, continuity, and agency. For women impacted by trauma, especially those contending with identity-based marginalization, physical immobility, or geographic isolation, traditional models of care are frequently inaccessible or retraumatizing. In this context, trauma-informed technology is not a matter of convenience, it is a matter of equity, safety, and cultural relevance.

Rather than displacing human connection, well integrated technological solutions can amplify the therapeutic alliance. Mobile applications that support emotional regulation, telehealth platforms that eliminate transportation and stigma barriers, and asynchronous interventions that respect clients' temporal rhythms are not ancillary innovations—they are structural correctives. The critical challenge lies in ensuring these tools are not merely efficient, but also relationally attuned and rooted in occupational engagement. This section examines how thoughtfully designed technology can extend trauma responsive care to women historically excluded by mainstream systems, offering not just new modalities, but more just and responsive paradigms of healing.

Trauma-Informed Telehealth Practices

The shift toward telehealth during the COVID-19 pandemic created new possibilities for reaching women who may never have felt safe entering a clinic. For those living with trauma, the physical act of attending an appointment, navigating transportation, entering unfamiliar spaces, or facing institutional environments, can be a barrier in itself. Virtual care can reduce these stressors, but it must be intentionally adapted to meet the needs of clients who carry histories of invalidation, surveillance, or medical harm. Poor lighting, unclear privacy boundaries, or rushed pacing can trigger distress or recreate relational dynamics that feel unsafe.

Key strategies for trauma-informed telehealth include:

- Establishing shared rituals for session openings and closings, such as breath check-ins or naming visual grounding objects in the client's environment.
- Discussing digital boundaries early in care, including how clients can pause, disconnect, or choose to keep their camera off when needed.
- Using secure and simple platforms that allow clients to control their sensory surroundings, such as attending from a familiar room, adjusting lighting, or setting the pace of interaction.
- Pausing to check for regulation cues, watching for signs of screen fatigue, and offering moments of silence or co-regulation when emotional intensity arises.

When these strategies are integrated, telehealth shifts from a transactional format into a relational and supportive process. The screen becomes a portal for grounded presence, flexible care, and authentic therapeutic connection rather than just a clinical interface. Far from being a lesser alternative, trauma responsive virtual care can expand the reach of healing relationships, particularly for women who have been historically excluded or retraumatized in traditional medical settings.

Mobile Apps and Self-Guided Tools for Regulation and Reflection

The rise of mobile health applications has expanded access to mental health and wellness supports, particularly for women who are navigating trauma outside of traditional care systems. These tools offer privacy, portability, and autonomy—three elements that are essential for trauma survivors who may struggle with help seeking due to prior invalidation, fear of exposure, or distrust in clinical systems. However, not all digital resources are created with trauma responsiveness in mind.

Trauma-informed mobile tools must center agency. This includes allowing users to control what they engage with, how often, and in what format. Apps that deliver rigid behavior tracking or unsolicited reminders may feel intrusive rather than supportive. In contrast, platforms that offer options for journaling, body scans, creative expression, or guided sensory breaks can scaffold regulation without replicating systems of control.

Design also matters. Color palettes, language tone, and even font size can affect emotional accessibility. Tools that avoid clinical jargon, use affirming language, and include identity-congruent content (such as gender inclusive avatars or cultural references) help users feel seen. Some applications now allow users to customize their interface, create safety plans, or record self-soothing strategies that can be accessed during acute distress.

Clinicians can introduce these tools in session, co-navigate setup, or even co-create personalized protocols for when and how they are used. For clients transitioning out of care, a curated toolkit of self-guided apps can serve as a bridge to independence, reinforcing the work done in therapy and sustaining regulation across daily life. See Table 12.1 for a selection rubric clinicians can use when evaluating mobile apps through a trauma-informed lens.

This rubric is a clinical reasoning tool that helps occupational therapists evaluate the emotional, cultural, and relational safety of digital interventions. In practice, clinicians can use it in session when introducing a mobile app to support a client's self-regulation, journaling, or sleep hygiene. Rather than recommending an app based solely on ratings or popularity, therapists can walk through each rubric domain with the client, co-reviewing features and language to assess emotional fit and autonomy. This process itself can be a therapeutic opportunity, modeling collaborative decision-making and restoring a sense of control that trauma may have disrupted.

Importantly, the rubric supports clinicians in identifying potential misalignments before harm occurs. For example, a well-meaning app that sends daily motivational texts may overwhelm a survivor who is still navigating shame or dissociation. By previewing content tone and notification style, therapists can anticipate unintended impacts and adjust recommendations accordingly. The rubric also encourages critical awareness of design bias—inviting clinicians

Table 12.1 Trauma-Informed App Selection Rubric for Women's Health and Trauma Recovery

Evaluation Domain	Key Questions	Why It Matters	Example Indicators
User Autonomy	Does the app allow users to choose features, pace, and level of engagement?	Supports agency and reduces risk of re-triggering through forced tasks or notifications	Customizable reminders, optional modules, non-sequential content
Sensory and Aesthetic Design	Are visual and auditory elements calming, inclusive, and culturally sensitive?	Design can influence safety or distress, especially for trauma survivors	Soft color schemes, low-stimulation layout, identity-affirming visuals
Language and Framing	Is the tone empowering, non-judgmental, and free from clinical jargon?	Trauma-informed language reduces shame and promotes self-compassion	"Check in with yourself" vs. "Log your symptoms"; no deficit-based phrasing
Privacy and Safety	Does the app prioritize user privacy and offer clear data protection policies?	Survivors often fear surveillance or misuse of personal information	Password protection, anonymous mode, clear data use terms
Regulation Tools	Does it offer grounding, breathing, or body-based exercises tailored to women?	Regulation support is central to trauma recovery	Guided imagery, tactile prompts, or culturally attuned body scan practices
Cultural and Identity Inclusion	Are diverse lived experiences represented and affirmed?	Clients are more likely to engage with tools that reflect their identity	BIPOC representation, gender-expansive options, trauma-informed affirmations
Offline Functionality	Can tools be used without WiFi or data?	Ensures access in underserved areas and reduces reliance on digital infrastructure	Journals or exercises that save locally, offline mindfulness audio

to question whose bodies, voices, and experiences are centered in the app and whose are absent. In doing so, the tool supports a deeper level of trauma responsiveness, one that bridges digital convenience with relational care.

Augmenting Embodied Safety in Virtual Settings

Virtual care introduces both opportunities and limitations in how clients experience bodily safety. In face-to-face sessions, therapists rely on spatial proximity, tone, and shared physical cues to help clients regulate. Online, those cues are often truncated or distorted. Clients may struggle to feel grounded or embodied when confined to a screen. For those with histories of disassociation, medical trauma, or disrupted body image, virtual care may unintentionally disembody rather than anchor. Augmenting embodied safety is not just a workaround, it is a therapeutic imperative.

Occupational therapists can design sessions that intentionally reorient clients to their bodies, environments, and internal cues. This includes inviting clients to adjust physical positioning to feel more settled, such as placing their feet on the floor, holding a grounding object, or leaning into a weighted pillow. Naming small body-based anchors out loud, like breath, posture, or warmth, can serve as regulation cues. Some therapists create "body check-in" rituals at the start and end of each session, not to screen for symptoms, but to promote somatic attunement and self-recognition.

Technology can also be leveraged creatively. Therapists might use shared screens to display visual anchors, body scans, or co-create digital regulation maps. Clients can be invited to personalize their space with scents, textures, or lighting that signal safety. One innovative strategy involves offering clients two-minute offline embodiment breaks during emotionally heavy sessions, with the option to mute, pause video, and return after movement, breathwork, or simply rest. These small modifications counter the disembodied nature of virtual care and empower clients to reclaim agency over their sensory environment.

Virtual reality tools are also being explored as a means of reintroducing the body to therapeutic settings through immersive graded exposure. For example, trauma-informed VR environments can simulate calming natural spaces or replicate social scenarios, allowing clients to gradually reengage with feared stimuli while maintaining control over intensity and duration. When designed with consent and sensory regulation in mind, VR can support clients in rebuilding tolerance to bodily and relational presence in a way that feels scaffolded rather than overwhelming.

When clients are supported in reconnecting to their physical presence during virtual therapy, the screen no longer serves as a barrier. Instead, it becomes a flexible tool through which safety, presence, and bodily knowing can be restored. These micro-interventions are especially vital for women and gender-expansive clients whose histories may include bodily violation or objectification

(El Khoudary et al., 2019). Creating virtual rituals of embodiment signals that therapy is not just about what is said, but about how the body is allowed to feel during the saying.

Digital Storytelling and Expressive Technology for Trauma Integration

Emerging technologies such as wearables and biofeedback tools are reshaping how occupational therapists support nervous system regulation and client self-awareness. These tools offer real-time insight into physiological states, allowing clients to better recognize patterns in stress, calm, and recovery. For women and gender-expansive clients with trauma histories, this kind of visibility can be empowering. It makes nervous system literacy an active skill, not a theoretical concept, and invites clients to see their bodies as sources of wisdom rather than dysfunction.

Devices that track heart rate variability, skin conductance, or respiration can help clients notice how different environments or activities affect their emotional state. For instance, a smartwatch might reveal that a client's stress peaks before school pickup, linking parenting demands with trauma-related hypervigilance. Another client might track improvements in physiological recovery after expressive movement, illustrating that progress is not just cognitive but embodied. These insights allow therapists and clients to collaboratively explore how regulation shows up, or breaks down, across real-world occupations.

This is also where smart tools and storytelling can converge. In a recent scoping review, researchers found that digital storytelling interventions not only elevated underrepresented voices but also improved health literacy, shifted attitudes, and supported behavior change in marginalized populations. This has powerful implications for occupational therapy. Wearables and biofeedback data can become part of a client's personal health narrative—one that invites agency, reflection, and a deeper sense of coherence. When used alongside journaling or visual storytelling, these tools allow clients to create meaning from patterns and name what helps them return to a sense of safety.

Clinicians can integrate biofeedback into therapy by using guided sessions with pulse oximeters or simple breathing sensors and helping clients connect data to sensation. For example, a client might see that her stress response activates in crowded public spaces, and together, she and her therapist might co-design occupational strategies or sensory supports. The purpose is not performance optimization but physiological affirmation. This builds a foundation of trust between body and self. Clients learn to recognize that their responses make sense, that they can be tracked, and that they can be supported. These tools are most powerful when they are embedded in meaningful routines and paired with reflective practice. See Table 12.2 for examples of biofeedback-integrated interventions that support nervous system literacy and client-led regulation.

Table 12.2 Biofeedback-Supported Strategies for Trauma-Informed Occupational Therapy

Therapeutic Context	Biofeedback Tool Used	Client Application	Clinical Benefit
Regulation skill building	Pulse oximeter or wearable HR monitor	Client tracks heart rate during daily transitions (e.g., waking, commuting, bedtime)	Identifies patterns of dysregulation and anchors awareness to concrete metrics
Sensory-based intervention	Skin temperature sensor	Client compares baseline and post-activity readings after calming or alerting input	Reinforces effectiveness of sensory modulation strategies
Exposure work or community reentry	Portable EDA (electrodermal activity) tool	Client monitors arousal levels during gradual reintroduction to anxiety-provoking settings	Increases client agency in setting pace and recognizing thresholds
Sleep and rest routines	Wearable sleep trackers with HRV feedback	Client reviews sleep cycles and morning HRV to adjust wind-down rituals and routines	Links rest patterns to trauma-informed self-care practices
Creative or expressive occupation	Real-time visual HR/HRV display	Client uses art or music while viewing biofeedback display to notice impact	Builds somatic-emotional connection in low-pressure, creative environments

When used thoughtfully, biofeedback technologies can deepen the therapeutic alliance by shifting the focus from performance to embodied awareness. Rather than positioning physiological data as a measure of success, therapists can frame it as a mirror reflecting the client's internal state and creating a shared language around stress, comfort, or activation. This approach supports clients who struggle to name emotions or identify patterns of dysregulation. For example, a woman who has learned to mask her distress may not initially recognize when she is moving into a state of sympathetic arousal. Biofeedback can gently surface that shift without judgment, inviting curiosity and co-regulation rather than correction.

Therapists should introduce these tools with transparency and consent, explaining not just what the technology does but why it is being integrated. Clients should retain full autonomy to pause, decline, or modify the use of biofeedback at any point. Over time, the goal is not dependency on the tool but increased interoceptive trust—where clients begin to notice and respond to their own signals with more confidence. When integrated into trauma-informed occupational therapy, biofeedback does not replace therapeutic presence. It amplifies it, helping clients translate the invisible into the understandable and the overwhelming into something that can be met with choice.

Community-Driven Innovation and Co-Creation in Women's Health

Some of the most forward-thinking developments in trauma care are not happening in hospitals or universities. They are emerging in living rooms, community gardens, online forums, and peer-run collectives. When women and gender-expansive people shape their own health solutions, they surface forms of expertise that rarely appear in clinical research. These are not workarounds or stopgaps. They are grounded strategies that challenge who gets to innovate and why.

In occupational therapy, traditional models often rely on professional authority to define best practice. But in marginalized communities, innovation happens through necessity, not institutional planning. A survivor-run art studio might develop a safer way to engage in body-based expression. A neighborhood maternal support group might create culturally matched postpartum recovery kits. These are not alternative methods; they are frontline interventions forged in response to chronic gaps in care, and they deserve to be studied, resourced, and refined.

Occupational therapists have an opportunity to move from implementers to collaborators. This means asking different questions—ones that do not start with "what should we bring in?" but rather "what is already working here, and how can we support it?" Therapists can play a catalytic role by identifying points of friction in existing systems, offering clinical insight without overriding lived experience, and building infrastructure that sustains grassroots ideas over time.

This shift has implications beyond practice. When clinicians co-create with communities, they access new pathways for problem solving, service delivery, and advocacy. These approaches often prioritize dignity, mutuality, and cultural grounding in ways that top-down models miss. The goal is not to translate community knowledge into clinical language, but to let community knowledge expand what we consider valid, effective, and ethical care. See Table 12.3 for concrete examples of community-embedded innovations and their application in trauma-informed occupational therapy.

Community-driven innovation challenges therapists to rethink where authority lives in the care process. Rather than positioning the clinician as the sole expert, this model shifts focus to shared authorship and reciprocal learning. When supporting women and gender-expansive individuals, this shift is more

Table 12.3 Community-Driven Innovations and Applications for Occupational Therapy Practice

Community Innovation	Originating Context	Clinical Application	Therapist Role
Postpartum care circles facilitated by immigrant doulas	Created by refugee and immigrant women to address cultural mismatch in perinatal care	Supports culturally grounded recovery, reduces isolation, and promotes role continuity	Partner as a guest facilitator, advocate for institutional recognition, refer clients for peer-based support
Mobile van offering sensory-informed care kits at public housing complexes	Developed by a disability justice collective	Offers proactive regulation tools for women who avoid clinical settings	Collaborate on kit content, provide feedback on adaptive strategies, conduct follow-ups in safe locations
Storytelling circles for intergenerational healing in LGBTQ+ communities	Designed by queer elders and youth advocates	Promotes identity validation, emotional processing, and shared resilience	Co-create structured prompts, ensure safety protocols, use insights to inform intervention goals
Peer-designed zines on trauma and daily survival routines	Created by young adult survivors of gender-based violence	Acts as an accessible tool for psychoeducation, self-reflection, and occupational strategy sharing	Distribute with permission, integrate content into treatment plans, offer clients space to create their own zines
Community-run body movement classes for trauma survivors	Emerged from mutual aid networks during pandemic	Enhances body agency, rhythm, and safe expression	Observe or co-facilitate sessions, offer occupational framing, adapt strategies for home carryover

than a philosophy; it is a safeguard. Many have experienced care systems that pathologize, silence, or overlook them. Co-creating interventions with clients and community members can restore a sense of agency and reduce the risk of reenacting power imbalances. Practically, this might involve hosting story-sharing circles with peer facilitators, inviting clients to audit or redesign clinic materials, or embedding a feedback loop into program delivery that allows participants to shape ongoing services in real time.

Applying the aforementioned strategies begins with asking better questions. Clinicians can start by mapping out who is missing from decision-making spaces and identifying which parts of their work could benefit from lived experience input. This may feel unfamiliar or even uncomfortable at first—but that discomfort often signals where the most growth can occur. Community-driven innovation is not about perfect implementation. It is about fostering environments where clients feel they have a stake in the process and where their insight informs more than just individual care plans. Over time, these practices do not just improve outcomes, they help rebuild trust in systems that have historically failed to listen.

Reimagining Evidence and Impact in Women's Health

Sahara Paul, a 26-year-old woman with a history of complex developmental trauma, was referred to occupational therapy after repeated disruptions in school and work. Her chart noted fatigue, difficulty concentrating, and "low follow-through with recommendations." In early sessions, Sahara offered little detail about her goals and often completed tasks in silence. Traditional assessment tools failed to capture the nuance of her disengagement. However, the therapist began documenting nontraditional indicators, such as Sahara removing her coat during sessions, initiating a shared playlist for creative tasks, and later, naming specific boundaries she wanted to maintain in relationships. These shifts were subtle but significant. Sahara's ability to reflect on her energy, voice limits, and revise therapeutic goals were not visible on a symptom checklist, but they revealed the gradual restoration of agency. Her case exemplified how healing cannot always be measured by standardized outcomes, and how therapeutic progress often lives in moments that fall outside conventional definitions of evidence.

For decades, evidence in health care has been defined through narrow parameters—randomized control trials, symptom-based scales, and standardized metrics that often overlook the lived complexity of trauma. While these tools offer valuable data, they rarely account for the relational, embodied, and culturally shaped realities of recovery. In trauma-informed occupational therapy with women and gender-expansive individuals, progress may not look like symptom reduction. It may look like showing up to a session on time, making eye contact for the first time, or choosing rest without guilt. These moments are not incidental. They are indicators of healing that often escape traditional measurement.

Reframing evidence requires moving away from fixed benchmarks and instead honoring the diverse ways that healing can manifest. Rather than measuring change by productivity or task duration, therapists can observe subtle shifts in regulation, boundary-setting, or identity expression. These outcomes may not align with traditional metrics, but they reflect internal integration and restored agency. Practitioners must learn to document what cannot always be quantified—emotional pacing, choice making, or sustained engagement in meaningful roles. This broader lens not only validates progress that is often invisible but also supports clinical reasoning that centers the client's lived priorities.

Recognizing Indicators of Healing Beyond Function

Traditional outcomes in occupational therapy often emphasize skill acquisition, independence, and task mastery. While these metrics serve a purpose, they can inadvertently pathologize clients who move at a nonlinear pace or whose healing does not follow expected milestones. In trauma-informed practice, healing may first appear not as improved function, but as the capacity to tolerate slowness, to express dissent, or to remain present during discomfort. These signs are not peripheral; they are central indicators that the nervous system is beginning to find safety in engagement.

For women with complex trauma histories, progress might show up as increased awareness of needs, willingness to set limits, or choosing rest without guilt. A client who previously dissociated during sessions may begin to voice preferences or redirect the pace of an activity. Another might arrive to therapy with a clearer sense of what they do not want—an equally valuable insight. These shifts reflect a recalibration of agency and a restructuring of relational templates. They signal that the therapeutic space is no longer one of performance, but one of participation on the client's terms.

Recognizing these indicators requires therapists to expand their clinical gaze. Instead of looking only for improvements in time use or task completion, they must attend to the client's presence, language, posture, and self-directed choices. Does the client advocate for breaks? Do they reject goals that no longer align with their values? Have their occupational choices shifted toward alignment rather than obligation? These are markers of growth that are often missed when therapists rely solely on standard measures.

Therapists can begin to track these subtler outcomes through reflective documentation practices. This might include noting emotional pacing, instances of voice and agency, or moments when the client pauses to assess internal cues before acting. These forms of observation provide rich data that, while not numeric, offer insight into how trauma recovery is unfolding. By naming these changes as evidence, clinicians validate the client's labor and ensure their progress is neither minimized nor misunderstood. See Table 12.4 for examples of nontraditional indicators of healing that can be integrated into treatment notes and care planning.

Table 12.4 Examples of Nontraditional Indicators of Healing in Trauma-informed Occupational Therapy

Clinical Theme	Observable Indicator	Interpretation	Application in Documentation or Planning
Self-advocacy	Client requests a break or modifies a session activity	Reflects awareness of internal state and capacity for boundaries	Note as increased agency and co-regulation capacity
Emotional regulation	Client remains present during a triggering topic	Signals nervous system tolerance and relational safety	Document as resilience in emotional processing
Identity expression	Client challenges a previously set goal or reframes priorities	Suggests deeper connection to authentic values	Use to collaboratively revise treatment goals
Relational healing	Client uses "we" language or acknowledges therapeutic alliance	Indicates emerging trust and integration of relational experiences	Note as engagement in reparative relational dynamics
Shame resilience	Client shares a story of vulnerability without shutting down	Demonstrates decreased self-censorship and embodied courage	Reflect in narrative progress and therapeutic readiness
Occupation reintegration	Client returns to a previously avoided role or task	Shows reengagement with meaningful but once-threatening occupation	Plan graded support or celebrate as readiness milestone
Body-based awareness	Client notices or names body cues in session	Reveals somatic reconnection and trauma recovery progress	Integrate into co-regulation strategies and pacing plans

Clinicians often look for progress through standardized metrics, such as increased task performance or symptom reduction. While those data points can be helpful, they do not always capture the nuanced shifts that occur during trauma recovery. The indicators in this table offer a more expansive view of healing, one that recognizes subtle but meaningful changes in relational capacity, emotional expression, and occupational identity. These signs often precede larger behavioral shifts and can serve as early markers of progress even when outward performance remains unchanged.

To apply these indicators in practice, therapists can incorporate them into session notes, team discussions, and care planning conversations. Rather than framing progress solely through compliance or productivity, they can note moments when a client makes eye contact during a difficult story, modifies a plan to better fit their needs, or expresses a new sense of agency. These behaviors are not just observations, they are evidence of therapeutic integration. When reflected back to clients, they can also reinforce internal motivation and support narrative reconstruction. Using these indicators helps clinicians make more attuned, ethical decisions and validates the lived, often invisible, labor of healing.

Expanding Metrics of Success in Trauma-Informed Care

While occupational therapy has traditionally relied on standardized outcome measures, these tools often fail to capture the depth of transformation experienced by women and gender-expansive clients navigating trauma recovery. Many existing assessments focus on physical independence, symptom reduction, or return to baseline. Yet for clients whose trauma disrupted their sense of identity, safety, or belonging, success may look entirely different. It may be found in the ability to set a boundary, to speak about themselves with pride, or to reimagine roles they once abandoned. These outcomes hold equal clinical value, even if they resist easy quantification.

To address this gap, trauma-informed practitioners are turning toward participatory, narrative, and values-aligned measures that reflect what matters most to each client. For example, a client might create a personal success map that includes milestones like "I can rest without guilt" or "I can ask for help without fear." Therapists can document changes in affect, self-talk, and role satisfaction alongside traditional indicators. This reframing not only honors diverse definitions of progress but reduces the risk of retraumatizing clients by implying that healing must follow a predetermined path. Success becomes self-defined and relationally affirmed—an approach more congruent with trauma recovery itself.

Even as therapists expand how success is defined; they must still operate within systems that demand measurable outcomes. Insurance reimbursement often hinges on documentation that shows functional gains, reductions in symptoms, or improved performance on standardized assessments. This tension can leave clinicians wondering how to honor a trauma-informed lens while still meeting external requirements. The good news is that when care is truly aligned with client values and paced according to nervous system readiness, traditional outcomes often improve as a secondary effect. Clients who feel seen and safe are more likely to engage consistently, regulate more effectively, and demonstrate gains in occupational performance, even if those outcomes were not the initial focus.

Rather than abandoning standard assessments, trauma-informed therapists can use them strategically. For instance, a client who begins to tolerate discomfort in a grocery store after working through social hypervigilance may show improvements in community mobility or role satisfaction scores. Similarly, a client who reengages in caregiving after reframing her trauma history may report higher performance and satisfaction on the Canadian Occupational Performance Measure. When therapists document the connection between trauma-responsive goals and functional change, they generate a more complete clinical narrative—one that satisfies funders while preserving the dignity of client-defined success.

Bridging Clinical Innovation with Policy and Advocacy

Trauma-informed care often begins in the therapy room, but its most lasting impact is realized when it reshapes the systems around it. Occupational therapists who support women and gender-expansive clients know that trauma recovery does not occur in isolation. It unfolds within institutions, documentation practices, and funding models that can either reinforce or reduce harm. Therapists are uniquely positioned to become advocates not only for individual clients but for more humane and responsive care structures.

Bridging innovation with policy means translating clinical wisdom into institutional language. This might include updating intake forms to reflect inclusive gender identity and trauma-sensitive language, revising productivity expectations that prioritize depth over volume, or training interdisciplinary teams on sensory regulation and narrative safety. Small changes in documentation and environment can significantly affect whether clients feel safe enough to stay engaged (Jallo et al., 2024). These shifts also offer therapists a way to practice advocacy from within their everyday roles, without needing formal titles or legislative expertise.

Trauma-informed clinicians can also help shape the metrics that justify their care. By documenting shifts in regulation, role clarity, or self-advocacy as precursors to traditional gains, therapists can help redefine what success looks like in the eyes of funders and administrators. When therapists speak about clinical outcomes using terms like emotional regulation, self-determined pacing, or identity congruence, they expand what is considered billable, essential, and evidence worthy (Lumley et al., 2022; Meston et al., 2013). This is not just documentation but a cultural change through clinical practice. See Table 12.5 for a checklist of micro to macro strategies occupational therapists can use to advocate for trauma-informed systems across different levels of care.

Table 12.5 Advocacy Strategies for Trauma-Informed Systems Change

Level of Influence	Actionable Strategy	Example
Clinical (Individual)	Use trauma-informed terminology and strengths-based rephrasing in documentation to validate client experience	Use terms like "developing capacity for regulation" or "engaging in self-directed roles"
Departmental	Recommend concrete revisions to intake forms that allow for identity expression, safety preferences, and pacing	Replace binary gender fields, add prompts for sensory sensitivities and support needs
Interdisciplinary	Develop or lead an in-service training that introduces trauma recovery phases and nervous system literacy	Use a case study to illustrate pacing, emotional attunement, and co-regulation strategies
Institutional	Advocate for formal integration of trauma-informed principles in care protocols, supervision models, or QI plans	Propose reflective debrief tools and checklists for emotionally complex sessions
Policy/Systems	Partner with advocacy groups or professional boards to shape legislation or reimbursement policies	Submit a white paper or testimony on the need for trauma-responsive maternal care models (Parker, 2015).

These strategies can be implemented by therapists across settings, regardless of formal leadership roles. For example, rewriting documentation language to reflect client agency rather than pathology can reduce the risk of misinterpretation across care teams. Proposing changes to intake questions or discharge protocols can improve how safety and identity are addressed from the start. Even in shared decision-making meetings, clinicians can model trauma-responsive approaches that shift the tone and structure of team-based care.

Each advocacy action is designed to bring trauma-informed values into operational focus. This includes changing how forms are worded, rethinking how progress is measured, or challenging restrictive policies that limit access to care. By embedding advocacy into daily clinical decisions, therapists can influence both immediate care environments and broader systems. These efforts help reimagine occupational therapy not only as a treatment model, but as a vehicle for equity, choice, and lasting change.

Future Directions for Trauma-Informed Innovation

Trauma-informed care has evolved from a theoretical framework into a clinical necessity, but its full potential has yet to be realized. As occupational therapy continues to redefine its role in women's health, the next frontier lies in innovation that integrates neuroscience, design thinking, community engagement, and health technology. The future will not be shaped solely by tools or protocols. It will be shaped by how we listen, adapt, and respond to complexity with precision and compassion.

One promising direction is the advancement of AI-driven tools that personalize care based on nervous system patterns, identity context, and real-time feedback. These technologies could eventually help therapists detect early signs of dysregulation, adjust pacing dynamically, or offer personalized regulation strategies between sessions (Pennou et al., 2023). But as these systems evolve, ethical safeguards must keep pace. Client autonomy, data security, and bias prevention must be at the forefront of every design decision. Innovation that ignores these principles risks replicating the very systems that trauma-informed care seeks to transform (Moltrecht et al., 2022; Morison et al., 2022).

Another direction involves deepening cross-sector collaboration. Trauma recovery does not belong solely within mental health or rehabilitation. It intersects with education, housing, justice, and public policy. Occupational therapists are uniquely positioned to serve as boundary spanners—professionals who can translate between clinical realities and systemic change. Embedding therapists in community design teams, tech development labs, or policy think tanks can accelerate solutions that are both innovative and grounded in lived experience (Cikuru et al., 2021).

Lastly, future progress depends on how the profession invests in reflective practice and workforce development. Trauma-informed care is not a static skill set. It demands continuous unlearning, mentorship, and accountability. Building communities of practice that foster co-learning, story sharing, and interdisciplinary exchange will help ensure that innovation stays responsive, not performative (Glass et al., 2019). The goal is not to arrive at a perfect model, but to remain in active dialogue with the people and systems we serve.

Case Vignettes and Clinical Reflections

Innovation in trauma care gains meaning only when it improves the lived experience of clients. It is not the tool itself that creates impact, but how it is adapted to restore agency, safety, and participation in daily life. The following vignettes illustrate how emerging strategies in occupational therapy such as digital storytelling, community-based technology, and relational use of virtual platforms can be tailored to support women and gender-expansive individuals navigating trauma recovery. These examples do not present linear progress or fixed outcomes. Instead, they highlight how clinical creativity, cultural responsiveness, and attuned pacing can allow technology to serve as a vehicle for connection and transformation. Each vignette reflects real challenges and subtle shifts that define healing in complex lives.

Case 1: Imani-Rosa, Age 34—Reclaiming Voice Through Digital Storytelling

Imani-Rosa is a 34-year-old community health worker and mother of two who experienced childhood abuse and systemic discrimination throughout her education and healthcare encounters. Although she presents as highly functional and composed, Imani-Rosa reports chronic fatigue, difficulty setting boundaries, and recurring intrusive memories. She rarely speaks about her trauma and prefers to focus on caregiving roles and advocacy in her neighborhood. When occupational therapy was first introduced, she expressed skepticism, stating, "I am not broken. I do not need to be fixed."

In early sessions, the therapist observed that Imani-Rosa was articulate when discussing community issues but deflected when asked about her own needs. To support emotional safety, the therapist introduced a project-based approach using digital storytelling. Instead of framing it as therapy, the therapist invited Imani-Rosa to create a short story or video reflecting on a moment of resilience in her life, with the option to use images, music, or metaphors rather than direct narration.

Over six weeks, Imani-Rosa slowly constructed a three-minute story about planting a garden with her grandmother, weaving in themes of grief, cultural memory, and belonging. The process helped her access memories without retraumatization and allowed her to narrate identity from a strength-based lens. She reported sleeping better, setting clearer boundaries at work, and feeling less burdened by unresolved emotion. Sharing the story in a local women's health workshop became a turning point, as she realized her voice could hold meaning without explanation or justification.

Digital storytelling, in this context, was not used as a product but as a reflective occupation that allowed for emotional processing, cultural affirmation, and role exploration. The therapist's role was not to interpret the story but to witness it with care and invite integration into future-focused goals. This case illustrates how occupational therapy can transform digital tools into safe containers for agency and expression, especially for those who have spent years silencing their own narrative.

Case 2: Alessandra, Age 28—Building Regulation Through Virtual Co-Occupation

Alessandra is a 28-year-old Italian American graduate student who recently relocated for school and lives alone. She identifies as queer and has a history of intimate partner violence that was never formally addressed. Alessandra initially sought occupational therapy through a virtual clinic after experiencing sleep disruptions, disordered eating patterns, and a sense of isolation that worsened during high-stress academic periods. Though she rarely named her trauma directly, she disclosed feeling "on edge all the time" and expressed frustration about being "stuck in survival mode."

During the first few telehealth sessions, Alessandra kept her video off and participated with minimal eye contact or body engagement. Rather than push for traditional rapport-building, the therapist introduced options for shared virtual co-occupations. Alessandra was invited to choose a quiet, parallel activity she could engage in during sessions, such as stretching, doodling, or preparing tea. This removed the pressure to perform and helped reduce screen-based tension.

As trust developed, Alessandra began joining sessions from her kitchen and slowly opened up about her disrupted routines and sleep avoidance. Together, she and the therapist co-designed a digital regulation plan that included a "wind down" protocol with audio-guided breath work, sensory-based transitions before bed, and a weekly virtual "body check-in" using a simple template she could complete independently or with the therapist's support.

Over time, Alessandra reported improved sleep quality, reduced emotional volatility, and greater ease in initiating boundaries with peers. What made the intervention effective was not the format, but the therapist's ability to adapt it to Alessandra's regulation needs, sensory profile, and cultural context. Virtual care was not simply a delivery method, it became the medium for reconstructing a sense of choice, presence, and internal safety.

Therapist Reflections on Clinical Decision Making

Working at the intersection of trauma, identity, and innovation requires a recalibration of what it means to hold space. In both cases above, the therapist was not led by protocol but by presence. The interventions were not driven by diagnosis or standardized sequences. They were shaped by the client's nervous system, language, and way of relating. Whether through digital co-occupation, narrative processing, or community-based tools, the therapist's role was to create conditions in which self-expression and regulation could reemerge.

A critical takeaway is that innovation is not just about using new tools. It is about using familiar tools in new ways, ways that center agency, cultural congruence, and emotional pacing (Qian et al., 2020). For some clients, this might mean using asynchronous storytelling rather than live disclosure. For others, it might involve co-designing routines that include both digital and physical anchors for safety. What matters is not the novelty of the method but its attunement to the client's internal landscape and external constraints.

Therapists can also reflect on their own comfort with less structured formats. Virtual and community-based tools often require the therapist to trust emergence, to notice the micro shifts in posture, tone, or timing that signal readiness or overwhelm. Success in these models depends less on fixing and more on witnessing, less on outcome tracking and more on co-regulation. These case examples remind us that technology does not replace relationship—it repositions it. And when that relationship is approached with intention, even the most distant platform can become a site of transformation.

Summary and Implications

Innovation in trauma care is not defined by the novelty of tools but by their ability to respond to lived complexity. As occupational therapy expands into digital spaces, community partnerships, and participatory design, the opportunity arises to rethink how care is delivered, measured, and sustained. This chapter has illustrated how technology, when applied with clinical attunement and cultural humility, can extend the reach of trauma-informed care and deepen its relevance for women and gender-expansive clients. From telehealth rituals to digital storytelling and zine creation, these approaches are not accessories to therapy. They are essential expansions of what therapy can be (Heijman et al., 2024).

The clinical implications are clear. Therapists must be equipped not only with the technical skills to use emerging tools, but with the reflective capacity to ask: does this support safety, authorship, and meaningful engagement? Innovation should not widen disparities or reinforce clinical detachment. It should democratize care. This requires thoughtful implementation, ongoing feedback from clients, and a willingness to evolve beyond traditional models. Whether a client is narrating their story through images, navigating discharge with a digital roadmap, or building community in a virtual group, the role of the therapist remains constant: to listen closely, scaffold possibility, and make healing feel reachable, even in new and unfamiliar formats.

References

Cikuru, J., Bitenga, A., Balegamire, J. B. M., Salama, P. M., Hood, M. M., Mukherjee, B., Mukwege, A., & Harlow, S. D. (2021). Impact of the healing in harmony program on women's mental health in a rural area in South Kivu province, Democratic Republic of Congo. *Global Mental Health (Cambridge, England)*, 8, e13. https://doi.org/10.1017/gmh.2021.11

El Khoudary, S. R., Greendale, G., Crawford, S. L., Avis, N. E., Brooks, M. M., Thurston, R. C., Karvonen-Gutierrez, C., Waetjen, L. E., & Matthews, K. (2019). The menopause transition and women's health at midlife: a progress report from the Study of Women's Health Across the Nation (SWAN). Menopause (New York, N.Y.), 26(10), 1213–1227. https://doi.org/10.1097/GME.0000000000001424

Glass, O., Dreusicke, M., Evans, J., Bechard, E., & Wolever, R. Q. (2019). Expressive writing to improve resilience to trauma: A clinical feasibility trial. *Complementary Therapies in Clinical Practice*, 34, 240–246. https://doi.org/10.1016/j.ctcp.2018.12.005

Heijman, J., Wouters, H., Schouten, K. A., & Haeyen, S. (2024). Effectiveness of Trauma-Focused Art Therapy (TFAT) for psychological trauma: Study protocol of a multiple-baseline single-case experimental design. *BMJ Open*, 14(1), e081917. https://doi.org/10.1136/bmjopen-2023-081917

Jallo, N., Kinser, P. A., Eglovitch, M., Worcman, N., Webster, P., Alvanzo, A., Svikis, D., & Meshberg-Cohen, S. (2024). Giving voice to women with substance use disorder: Findings from expressive writing about trauma. *Women's Health Reports (New Rochelle, N.Y.)*, *5*(1), 223–230. https://doi.org/10.1089/whr.2023.0173

Lumley, M. A., Yamin, J. B., Pester, B. D., Krohner, S., & Urbanik, C. P. (2022). Trauma matters: Psychological interventions for comorbid psychosocial trauma and chronic pain. *Pain*, *163*(4), 599–603. https://doi.org/10.1097/j.pain.0000000000002425

Meston, C. M., Lorenz, T. A., & Stephenson, K. R. (2013). Effects of expressive writing on sexual dysfunction, depression, and PTSD in women with a history of childhood sexual abuse: Results from a randomized clinical trial. *The Journal of Sexual Medicine*, *10*(9), 2177–2189. https://doi.org/10.1111/jsm.12247

Moltrecht, B., Patalay, P., Bear, H. A., Deighton, J., & Edbrooke-Childs, J. (2022). A transdiagnostic, emotion regulation app (Eda) for children: Design, development, and lessons learned. *JMIR Formative Research*, *6*(1), e28300. https://doi.org/10.2196/28300

Morison, L., Simonds, L., & Stewart, S. F. (2022). Effectiveness of creative arts-based interventions for treating children and adolescents exposed to traumatic events: A systematic review of the quantitative evidence and meta-analysis. *Arts & Health*, *14*(3), 237–262. https://doi.org/10.1080/17533015.2021.2009529

Parker, C. (2015). An innovative nursing approach to caring for an obstetric patient with rape trauma syndrome. *Journal of Obstetric, Gynecologic, and Neonatal Nursing: JOGNN*, *44*(3), 397–404. https://doi.org/10.1111/1552-6909.12577

Pennou, A., Lecomte, T., Potvin, S., Riopel, G., Vézina, C., Villeneuve, M., Abdel-Baki, A., & Khazaal, Y. (2023). A mobile health app (ChillTime) promoting emotion regulation in dual disorders: Acceptability and feasibility pilot study. *JMIR Formative Research*, *7*, e37293. https://doi.org/10.2196/37293

Qian, J., Zhou, X., Sun, X., Wu, M., Sun, S., & Yu, X. (2020). Effects of expressive writing intervention for women's PTSD, depression, anxiety and stress related to pregnancy: A meta-analysis of randomized controlled trials. *Psychiatry Research*, *288*, 112933. https://doi.org/10.1016/j.psychres.2020.112933

Chapter 13

The Future of Trauma-Informed Occupational Therapy in Women's Health

---

Chapter Objectives

Upon completion of this chapter, the reader will be able to:

1. Examine the systems-level conditions required to embed trauma-responsive practices across healthcare, education, and community environments.
2. Analyze organizational models that support the sustainability of trauma-informed occupational therapy through leadership, policy, and workforce development.
3. Apply strategies for integrating data, research, and client feedback into practice to enhance the effectiveness and accountability of trauma-informed care.
4. Explore the role of occupational therapists as advocates and change agents in promoting structural transformation aligned with equity and dignity.
5. Identify infrastructure elements such as reflective supervision, participatory evaluation, and fidelity mechanisms that support long-term implementation.

Innovation in trauma care has reached a turning point. While new approaches and intervention models continue to emerge, their potential will remain limited unless they influence the systems that shape care delivery. A promising initiative may succeed in one setting yet disappear in another, not because it lacks value but because the institutional structure cannot sustain it. This is the challenge currently facing trauma-informed occupational therapy. The profession has expanded its clinical understanding, but the organizational and policy foundations necessary for long-term implementation have not kept pace.

Women's health offers a revealing lens into this disconnect. Trauma does not only affect individual behavior or emotional wellbeing. It influences how

DOI: 10.4324/9781003658559-13

women interact with health systems, establish identity, and maintain meaningful roles across the life course. Occupational therapy is well equipped to address this complexity, but isolated clinical tools are not enough. The future of trauma responsive practice depends on whether its principles are embedded into the policies, leadership models, and outcome frameworks that define healthcare standards. This is not a call for short-term solutions. It is a call to transform the way care systems recognize and support healing as a shared responsibility, sustained through structural investment and relational integrity.

A 2024 systematic review and realist synthesis by Goldstein and colleagues confirmed this gap in sustainability. While trauma-informed care is increasingly adopted, implementation rarely extends across all levels of a health system. Using SAMHSA's ten-domain framework, the review identified organizational conditions that foster durable outcomes, including leadership buy-in, staff training, policy alignment, and collaborative monitoring. Without these elements, trauma-informed strategies risk becoming temporary programs rather than enduring standards of care.

A future grounded in trauma-informed care will not be built through tools alone. It will depend on how institutions recognize healing as a collective responsibility, not an individual burden. When systems reward regulation over speed, validation over compliance, and collaboration over hierarchy, care becomes safer by design. Occupational therapists are uniquely positioned to influence this shift by modeling what responsive, values-driven, and relational care can look like at every level.

Operationalizing Trauma-Informed Care

When Kelly Garner, a 58-year-old hospital unit coordinator, raised concerns about the way patients with psychiatric histories were being labeled and rushed through discharge, she was told it was "just how things are done." A survivor of trauma herself, Kelly often noticed patterns others overlooked, such as how one patient flinched when nurses entered without warning or how another stopped eating after being moved to a shared room. Despite her role being administrative, she made small changes where she could: flagging charts to alert staff about patient preferences, quietly offering calming routines to those she knew were overwhelmed. Yet without institutional backing, her efforts remained informal and easily dismissed. Kelly often felt like she was swimming upstream in a system that saw efficiency as volume rather than safety.

A turning point came when a new chief nursing officer arrived with a background in trauma-informed leadership. Rather than reprimanding

Kelly for slowing workflow, she asked for her insights. Together, they initiated a staff listening session series and began developing trauma-informed protocols that integrated Kelly's frontline knowledge. Charting templates were updated to include emotional safety needs, patient feedback was used to co-design room layouts, and onboarding included narratives from both patients and staff who had experienced trauma. Kelly's lived awareness became a catalyst for system redesign—not because she held a formal title, but because a structure finally existed to honor and amplify the wisdom of those closest to care.

When trauma-informed care is confined to the skill set of individual clinicians, its reach remains limited. While powerful at the client-provider level, transformation is unsustainable without structural reinforcement. Embedding trauma-informed care into the DNA of healthcare institutions, whether academic programs, hospital systems, or community networks, requires a shift in culture, language, and accountability. It also requires reimagining how policies, funding structures, and interprofessional roles align with principles of safety, trust, and equity.

A growing body of research supports this broader shift. A 2024 realist synthesis by Goldstein et al. identified mechanisms that drive successful trauma-informed implementation across healthcare systems, highlighting the importance of leadership, cross-sector collaboration, workforce training, and evaluation aligned with SAMHSA's ten trauma-informed care domains. These domains function as levers for organizational change, yet few institutions have developed fidelity metrics or sustainable models for embedding them. Without systems-level infrastructure, even well-intentioned efforts risk becoming performative rather than transformative.

The path forward lies in operationalizing trauma-informed care beyond the treatment room. This means defining what it looks like at the policy table, in reimbursement contracts, and within organizational onboarding processes. It also means identifying when trauma-informed care is truly embodied—when it shifts hiring practices, redefines productivity, and shapes the built environment to reduce retraumatization. Occupational therapists, with their systems thinking and functional lens, are uniquely positioned to guide this integration.

Models of Institutional Change

In recent years, the pressure to embed trauma-informed care within organizational systems has intensified—not just for the benefit of clients but for the sustainability of the workforce. A 2024 study published in *The Permanente Journal* argued that burnout in health care is not simply a matter of occupational stress but is intertwined with unaddressed trauma within systems themselves (Elisseou et al., 2024). Elisseou and colleagues (2024) urged a shift toward trauma and resilience-informed leadership that centers neurobiological regulation, staff connection, and systemic healing. This study reframes the Great Resignation as a Great Reevaluation, challenging institutions to become well-regulated ecosystems that foster safety and healing for both staff and clients.

Trauma-informed care is no longer just a clinical framework; it is a leadership imperative. SAMHSA's four core principles for trauma-informed organizations (realize, recognize, respond, and resist retraumatization) are increasingly being translated into operational structures. This includes organization-wide trainings, onboarding modules rooted in trauma science, TIC-informed performance review tools, and even physical environment changes such as recharge rooms for staff. Institutions like the Institute for Trauma-Informed Care at University Health in Texas have launched full-scale initiatives, while state-level resources like Trauma-Informed Oregon provide interactive roadmaps for organizations to assess policies, practices, and culture through a trauma lens.

In education, trauma-informed pedagogy is being embedded into curricula through faculty training, student wellness models, and inclusive design practices that validate diverse learning needs. Certification programs for trauma-informed systems are expanding, offering a blueprint for clinics and schools to operationalize these principles. However, fidelity requires more than surface compliance. Effective implementation is iterative and participatory, led by both leadership and those directly impacted by trauma. Without that bidirectional input, systems risk performative allyship rather than true transformation.

The most effective models of institutional change are those that reconfigure power, invite reflexivity, and design for sustainability. Leadership cannot delegate trauma-informed care to a single department or initiative. Instead, trauma-informed values must be embedded into hiring, supervision, documentation, evaluation, and strategic planning. When organizations begin to behave like living systems, adapting, regulating, and repairing, trauma-informed care becomes more than a framework. It becomes an ethos.

Infrastructure for Sustainability

At a mid-sized community health center in the Midwest, trauma-informed care began as a pilot program in the behavioral health department, led by a passionate occupational therapist named Monica Flaa. She introduced staff trainings, created sensory-friendly waiting areas, and developed intake forms that included questions about safety and identity. The changes were well received, but when Monica left for a new role, the energy around trauma-informed practice quickly faded. New hires were unaware of the initiative, the modified protocols were inconsistently followed, and leadership shifted priorities to billing metrics. Within a year, the program had effectively vanished.

It was not until a former patient filed a complaint about retrauma-tization during a routine visit that the organization reconsidered its approach. This time, they invested in infrastructure. A trauma-informed care committee was formalized, with representatives from clinical staff, administration, and patient advocacy groups. Trauma-informed com-petencies were added to job descriptions and performance reviews. New staff orientation included case-based training modules, and reflec-tive practice huddles were held monthly. Rather than relying on a sin-gle advocate, the center built a durable framework that could adapt across roles and endure beyond individual staff turnover—ensuring that trauma-informed care became not a phase, but a foundation.

Sustaining trauma-informed care within institutions requires more than well-mean-ing policies or isolated training sessions. It demands durable infrastructure that can weather leadership turnover, funding shifts, and the slow erosion of culture change over time (Bacchus et al., 2021). Many organizations launch trauma-informed ini-tiatives with enthusiasm, only to watch them fade when the original champions leave or the urgency dissipates. To prevent this drift, systems must invest in formal structures that embed trauma-informed principles into the DNA of operations.

One foundational element is interprofessional collaboration. Trauma is a mul-tisystemic phenomenon, so its solutions must be interdisciplinary. Sustained col-laboration across clinical, administrative, educational, and community-facing departments is critical to building systems that reflect collective ownership. This may take the form of integrated care teams, cross-sector task forces, or reflective practice groups where diverse professionals share insight, language, and accountability.

Another pillar of sustainability is continuous learning. Organizations often view trauma-informed training as a one-time event, but sustained change requires ongoing education, case consultation, and leadership development. Embedding trauma content into supervision, performance evaluations, and onboarding helps to normalize it as a standard of care, not an optional add-on. Some institutions are developing internal mentorship structures or rotating "trauma champions" to keep energy and engagement high across all levels of the organization.

Finally, sustainability hinges on how trauma-informed efforts are tracked and evaluated. Metrics of fidelity must be defined and measured—not only through outcomes but also through process indicators. These might include staff psy-chological safety scores, retention rates in marginalized populations, or quality improvement data tied to trauma-specific adaptations. Without infrastructure to support reflection and recalibration, even the most promising trauma-informed strategies can stall. When systems invest in collaborative scaffolding, shared lan-guage, and adaptive metrics, trauma-informed care becomes less vulnerable to fluctuation and more likely to flourish across time and transitions.

Embedding Research and Data Into Practice

Despite growing adoption of trauma-informed principles, the field still lacks consistent data infrastructures that capture the complexity of recovery, especially for women and gender-expansive clients. Most healthcare systems are built to track performance, not transformation. As trauma-informed occupational therapy moves toward systems-level relevance, its evolution must be tied to how we generate, use, and translate data. This does not mean relying solely on traditional metrics. It means expanding what we measure, how we measure it, and who gets to decide what counts as success.

Recent advances in artificial intelligence and narrative analysis illustrate the untapped potential of interdisciplinary collaboration. A 2024 study published in *Research Square* explored how AI models like ChatGPT and the ADA text embedding model could identify signs of childbirth-related PTSD by analyzing women's birth stories. The findings were striking. The ADA model outperformed six other domain-specific language models in classifying PTSD symptoms through narrative features, offering a noninvasive, scalable approach to early screening (Bartal et al., 2024). This breakthrough is not just technological—it is epistemological. It challenges the idea that trauma must be directly disclosed to be clinically visible. It suggests that the language women use to make sense of trauma holds diagnostic insight long before a standardized assessment is ever administered.

For trauma-informed occupational therapists, this kind of research opens new possibilities. It points toward data practices that are relational, contextually grounded, and centered in lived experience. Therapists can begin to document not just outcomes but linguistic shifts, affective tone, and narrative markers of identity integration. These qualitative dimensions may offer earlier indicators of change than traditional scores ever could. Integrating these insights requires new partnerships between researchers, technologists, and practitioners. It also demands that therapists stay literate in emerging tools without losing sight of the human story behind the data.

Embedding research into trauma-informed interventions also means creating feedback loops within care (Brunner et al., 2022). Therapists can implement session-based outcome measures that track emotional regulation, safety perception, or occupational engagement through open-ended check-ins or visual analog tools. Rather than relying only on pre-post comparisons, they can use these data points to co-regulate, adjust, and realign goals in real time. When clients see that their voice is actively shaping the course of therapy, not just captured in a chart, it reinforces trust and shared authorship.

Additionally, therapists can participate in practice-based evidence models by documenting real-world adaptations, cultural modifications, and trauma-responsive strategies that may not yet be reflected in published literature. These insights can be shared through clinical case studies, community reports, or collaborative research with academic institutions. When aggregated across settings, these experiential data sources can begin to inform broader frameworks for what works and why in trauma-informed care (Nemeth et al., 2023). This not only advances the field but ensures that future innovations are grounded in lived experience rather than abstract theory.

Advocacy as Clinical Praxis

Trauma-informed care requires more than therapeutic technique—it calls for structural advocacy. When trauma is embedded in systems, policies, and social conditions, recovery cannot be confined to the treatment room. For occupational therapists working in women's health, advocacy becomes a clinical responsibility. It is the act of identifying where clients are constrained by external forces and working to alter those conditions, not just adapt to them. This is especially urgent when clients face intersecting vulnerabilities such as poverty, racism, disability, or gender-based violence (Lwamba et al., 2022). Advocacy is not a separate task. It is a form of clinical reasoning applied at the level of policy, programming, and systems design.

Traditional advocacy has often been framed as speaking for others. Trauma-informed advocacy shifts that lens. It asks therapists to notice power dynamics, share platforms, and help clients build the skills and confidence to advocate for themselves. Sometimes this looks like helping a mother write a letter to her landlord requesting repairs after a traumatic injury. Other times, it may mean participating in coalitions that push for Medicaid reimbursement of trauma-responsive perinatal care. In both cases, the therapist is not only addressing a functional barrier but disrupting the conditions that perpetuate harm. Advocacy, when done relationally, reinforces the client's sense of agency and authorship over their environment (VanPuymbrouck et al., 2024).

This integration of advocacy into clinical practice is supported by a growing recognition that systems themselves can be dysregulating. A clinic with long wait times and fluorescent lighting may trigger the same physiological stress response as a past trauma. Insurance denials, child welfare investigations, or school discipline policies can reproduce cycles of shame and control. Trauma-informed occupational therapists are positioned to translate these patterns into institutional language. They can collect case examples, identify trends, and bring forward recommendations to leadership, boards, or policymakers. In doing so, they transform anecdote into data, and data into systemic feedback.

To make advocacy actionable in practice, therapists benefit from tools that connect everyday observations to larger levers of change. This may include an Advocacy Integration Map—where clinicians track patterns across clients (e.g., recurring access issues, housing instability, diagnostic bias), match them to relevant policy domains, and identify concrete points of influence. See Table 13.1 for a sample tool that can be used in supervision, team meetings, or continuing education settings to integrate advocacy into routine practice planning.

Table 13.1 Advocacy Integration Map for Trauma-Informed Occupational Therapy

Clinical Observation	Underlying Structural Issue	Advocacy Opportunity
Client avoids health services due to past dismissal of pain	Medical gaslighting and gender bias in care	Advocate for provider training on gendered pain response and support inclusive care guidelines
Client drops out of care due to lack of transportation	Geographic inaccessibility and underfunded public infrastructure	Partner with community coalitions to expand mobile health access or advocate for vouchers
Client discontinues therapy after insurance caps sessions	Insurance policies that undervalue mental health and trauma care	Submit data-driven appeals and contribute to coalition advocacy for parity laws
Client feels unsafe in shared housing or shelter environment	Gaps in trauma-informed housing or transitional support	Collaborate with social workers and housing agencies to develop trauma-informed policies
Client reports workplace triggers after returning to employment	Lack of employer education on trauma recovery and accommodation	Provide documentation that supports workplace modifications and participate in DEI committees (Schmidt et al., 2020)

Advocacy in trauma-informed occupational therapy is not an extracurricular task—it is a clinical skill rooted in ethical care. When therapists notice patterns of harm, inaccessibility, or marginalization, they hold insight that many systems lack. This makes their role in advocacy particularly powerful. The table above illustrates how moments that arise organically in clinical encounters, such as a client losing services due to benefit restrictions or feeling unsafe disclosing their trauma history, can become entry points for systemic action. When therapists bring these patterns into interdisciplinary meetings, collaborate with legal or policy partners, or even help shape program design, they move beyond treating symptoms and begin to address the structures that sustain them.

To make this actionable, therapists must have institutional support and protected time for advocacy as part of their role. Documentation that highlights systemic barriers can be anonymized and aggregated to inform funding applications, public comment, or quality improvement projects. Client goals can include community participation or policy engagement, reframing advocacy as occupation (Schmidt et al., 2020). Therapists can also co-write op-eds, participate in legislative advocacy, or design interventions that equip clients to advocate for themselves. These practices shift the frame of occupational therapy from service delivery to systems change, where healing is supported not only by sessions but by the environments in which people live, work, and recover.

Advancing Workforce Development Through Reflective Supervision and Mentorship

Larissa Kelce, a newly licensed occupational therapist working in a women's health clinic, was passionate about providing trauma-informed care. She prided herself on building rapport, adapting interventions with sensitivity, and creating spaces where clients felt seen. But after six months, Larissa began to feel a constant heaviness after sessions. She found herself second-guessing her clinical decisions, struggling to disengage after work, and feeling numb during moments that once moved her. When a client disclosed a trauma history that echoed her own, Larissa froze, not visibly, but internally, and later felt ashamed for not knowing how to respond.

Her clinic's standard supervision model offered little room to explore these reactions. Time with her supervisor focused on documentation errors and productivity targets, leaving Larissa's emotional experiences unspoken. It was not until she was paired with a mentor trained in reflective supervision that things shifted. In their monthly meetings, Larissa was encouraged to explore the emotional terrain of her work, including what was being stirred, when she felt out of alignment, and how her own history shaped her therapeutic presence. These conversations did not solve every challenge, but they restored her sense of clarity, affirmed her instincts, and reminded her that showing up fully human was not a liability, it was part of the work.

In trauma-informed care, the emotional labor of clinicians is often invisible but foundational. Occupational therapists who work with women and gender-expansive clients navigating trauma must attune not only to what clients do, but how they feel, what they remember somatically, and what they cannot yet name. Doing this work over time requires a system of care for the therapist—not just their clients. Yet most institutions invest far more in frontline productivity than in clinician well-being. Without structural reinforcement, even the most committed trauma-informed therapists risk exhaustion or detachment.

Traditional supervision models often prioritize compliance, documentation, and risk mitigation. These are important, but they do not address the internal shifts that come from bearing witness to trauma day after day. Reflective supervision offers a different frame. It supports the therapist as a whole person, making space for processing, integration, and ethical discernment. It also helps surface countertransference, trauma resonance, and areas where clinical decisions are shaped by unexamined emotional material. This is not an indulgence—it is essential to ethical care.

Mentorship, similarly, must move beyond checklists of skills and competencies. Trauma-informed mentorship is a practice of shared presence, where the goal is not perfection but sustainability. New clinicians may struggle to find their voice in complex environments, particularly when working with clients whose stories mirror broader systems of oppression. Effective mentorship names those dynamics and offers guidance without shame. It also models boundaries, emotional regulation, and the courage to stay human in systems that often ask clinicians to shut that part down.

Reflective Supervision as a Core Practice

Reflective supervision is not a therapy session, nor is it a performance review. It is a structured space where therapists are invited to slow down and examine the meaning behind their clinical choices, reactions, and emotional fatigue. Rooted in principles of curiosity and nonjudgment, reflective supervision encourages therapists to notice when they feel stuck, activated, or disconnected. These moments often hold valuable clinical information. Rather than being signs of incompetence, they are invitations to grow in relational depth and ethical clarity.

In practice, this might look like a supervisor asking, "What came up for you in that session?" rather than "Did you complete the documentation on time?" It means noticing when the therapist's nervous system feels dysregulated and helping them explore what that might reveal about the client's story—or their own history. In trauma-informed systems, reflective supervision is not optional. It is built into the calendar, valued in job descriptions, and integrated into the culture of clinical teams (Williams & Farley, 2024). Institutions that normalize this practice often report higher clinician satisfaction, better retention, and deeper therapeutic engagement with clients.

Trauma-Informed Mentorship Models

Effective mentorship in trauma-informed settings is based on mutuality and shared learning. It moves beyond hierarchical advice-giving and instead centers co-regulation, contextual awareness, and cultural humility. In this model, mentors do not need to have all the answers. They need to create space for questions that matter: How are you making sense of this client's story? What parts of this work are resonating personally? Where do you feel aligned, and where are you pushing through dissonance?

Mentorship can be formal, with structured pairings and ongoing learning plans, or informal, through reflective dyads, affinity groups, or narrative rounds. Some institutions are implementing rotating mentorship models to reduce power imbalances and increase exposure to diverse leadership styles. Others are supporting peer-led mentorship programs where emotional literacy and trauma understanding are the cornerstones of professional development. The goal is not just clinical competence, but emotional sustainability. When mentorship is relational, reflexive, and values-based, it becomes a protective factor against burnout and a catalyst for embodied, ethical practice.

Building Accountability Structures for Long-Term Change

Institutional change does not sustain itself through good intentions. Trauma-informed care often begins with energy, commitment, and alignment—but without infrastructure for accountability, its momentum fades. This is especially true in women's health, where trauma is often obscured by stigma, misdiagnosis, or systemic neglect. To ensure trauma-informed occupational therapy is more than a fleeting emphasis, systems must establish structures that make care quality visible, traceable, and responsive over time.

Accountability in trauma-informed systems is not about surveillance or punitive oversight. Instead, it is about feedback loops that elevate lived experience, track meaningful outcomes, and guide decision-making at all levels. When organizations invite honest reflection and co-ownership, they create space for course correction and innovation. The future of trauma-informed care depends on mechanisms that measure what matters, such as connection, regulation, role fulfillment, and equity, not just throughput or productivity.

Fidelity Mechanisms and Trauma-Informed Audits

Fidelity is the anchor that holds trauma-informed care to its principles when scale, time, and complexity threaten to pull it off course. In many healthcare settings, trauma-informed practice begins with training but falters in follow-through. Providers return to routines shaped by billing structures, documentation demands, and cultural norms that reward efficiency over presence. Fidelity mechanisms counter this drift. They translate values into observable behaviors, track alignment between intent and impact, and offer a shared language for evaluating quality across roles and settings.

Traditional fidelity tools in health care often center on task completion, checklists, or compliance with evidence-based protocols. While these tools are essential for safety and standardization, they are insufficient for trauma-informed care. Trauma-informed fidelity requires a more nuanced lens, one that captures relational attunement, emotional safety, and client agency. This may include observational rubrics that assess the tone of therapeutic interaction, audits of whether spaces reduce sensory threat, or reflection tools that explore how providers interpret and respond to nonverbal distress. These are not soft metrics; they are measurable elements of care that shape outcomes.

One emerging strategy is the use of trauma-informed environmental audits. These audits assess how physical space either supports or disrupts regulation. Lighting, sound, seating arrangements, visual cues, and signage are evaluated for their sensory and psychological impact. For example, women who have experienced sexual trauma may feel less safe in spaces with poor sightlines or clinical posters depicting pain without context. Environmental audits often reveal patterns that go unnoticed in daily operations but significantly affect how care is received. When paired with collaborative walk-throughs or narrative walk-throughs (where clients guide staff through their emotional response to a space), these audits become powerful teaching tools for teams and institutions.

Another underutilized fidelity mechanism is parallel process tracking. Trauma-informed care cannot exist for clients if it is not practiced internally among staff. Parallel process tracking invites organizations to examine whether their supervision practices, meeting structures, and leadership communication reflect the same principles they expect providers to offer clients. Are staff invited to name what feels unsafe? Do teams model collaborative regulation during conflict? Are power dynamics acknowledged and navigated intentionally? By building in structured reflection on these questions, institutions not only increase fidelity, they deepen integrity. Trauma-informed care becomes more than a service model. It becomes a way of being, both in the treatment room and across the system.

Co-Created Feedback Loops and Participatory Metrics

Most healthcare systems are built to monitor outcomes from a top-down perspective. Success is typically defined by institutional benchmarks, accreditation standards, or payer requirements. While necessary, these metrics often fail to reflect the lived experience of clients, especially those navigating complex trauma. Trauma-informed occupational therapy challenges this imbalance by embedding participatory feedback into the clinical ecosystem. It invites clients not just to receive care, but to shape it.

Co-created feedback loops move beyond satisfaction surveys. They prioritize qualitative, in-session data collection that captures shifts in safety, voice, and engagement. For example, therapists might use visual analog scales where clients mark their sense of emotional presence at the beginning and end of each session. Others may co-design end-of-session check-ins that prompt reflection on pacing, relevance, or triggers. These tools do not just help therapists adjust in real time. They also reinforce to clients that their perspective is critical—not only to the therapy process, but to the design of care itself.

Participatory metrics can also extend to program-level evaluation. Focus groups, storytelling workshops, and community-based participatory research methods allow women and gender-expansive clients to name what mattered in their recovery. This shifts the center of gravity in data collection. Instead of asking whether a program met its predefined goals, organizations ask whether it honored the identities, needs, and aspirations of those it was built to serve. In doing so, they generate a form of accountability rooted in dignity, not just documentation.

By embedding client voice at every level of evaluation, trauma-informed systems move toward a model of shared governance. Therapists are no longer the sole narrators of progress. They become co-authors, responsive to the evolving priorities of those in their care. These feedback loops do not eliminate the need for traditional metrics, but they complicate and enrich them. They ask a different question, one that systems rarely pose: not "Did we deliver care?" but "Did our care feel like it belonged to you?"

Adaptive Supervision and Reflective Infrastructure

Supervision in occupational therapy has traditionally focused on clinical skill development, productivity, and regulatory compliance. While these are essential components, they fall short in trauma-informed environments that require therapists to continuously navigate emotional labor, attunement, and system-level challenges. Trauma-informed practice is not just cognitively demanding, it is relationally and physiologically taxing. Without structured reflection and relational support, therapists may unknowingly replicate the very dynamics they are working to disrupt.

Adaptive supervision reframes the supervisory relationship as a space for co-regulation and mutual growth. It emphasizes emotional safety, transparency, and meaning making in the supervisory process itself. Supervisors in trauma-informed systems are trained not only in clinical expertise, but in nervous system literacy, power-awareness, and the facilitation of reflective dialogue. They ask not just "How are your goals progressing?" but "Where did you feel disoriented or unsettled this week?" or "What is surfacing in your body when you reflect on that session?"

In addition to one-on-one supervision, systems can invest in reflective infrastructures such as case consultation groups, debriefing circles, and interdisciplinary peer support pods. These formats allow clinicians to explore uncertainty, rupture, and repair within a shared container. They also normalize the complexity of trauma-responsive care. Therapists are not pathologized for feeling stuck or overwhelmed. Instead, those moments are seen as opportunities for insight and recalibration. This shift has organizational impact. Clinicians who feel supported in making meaning of their work are more likely to stay engaged, avoid burnout, and embody the principles they are being asked to practice.

Finally, reflective supervision models help surface patterns that may not be visible at the level of a single session or clinician. If therapists across a department report increased emotional fatigue when serving a particular population or working under certain documentation pressures, those insights can guide systemic change. In this way, supervision becomes not just a support mechanism, but a channel for organizational feedback and ethical alignment. Trauma-informed care cannot be sustained in silos. It flourishes when the people who provide it are resourced, seen, and heard.

Summary and Implications

The future of trauma-informed occupational therapy in women's health will not be shaped by theory alone. It will be defined by how practitioners and institutions translate principles into structure, reflection into evidence, and care into sustained culture. This chapter has explored the path from individual innovation to systemic implementation, underscoring that trauma-informed care is not a single intervention or training. It is a durable shift in how safety, power, and healing are understood and practiced across settings.

To sustain this shift, occupational therapists must act as both disruptors and architects. This means challenging systems that reinforce disconnection or harm and helping to build new ones that prioritize regulation, equity, and collective responsibility. From redefining outcomes that reflect lived experience to embedding trauma-informed practices into education, supervision, and data systems, the profession is moving toward a model of care that values dignity as much as function (McKinney et al., 2024). Success will be measured not just by what changes on paper, but by what changes in people.

At its core, trauma-informed occupational therapy is not just a clinical approach, it is a relational practice. It honors the complexity of recovery, the strength of adaptation, and the importance of belonging. The future will depend on collaboration across disciplines, communities, and institutions, grounded in the belief that healing is possible when systems are designed not just to treat, but to understand.

References

Bacchus, L. J., Alkaiyat, A., Shaheen, A., Alkhayyat, A. S., Owda, H., Halaseh, R., Jeries, I., Feder, G., Sandouka, R., & Colombini, M. (2021). Adaptive work in the primary health care response to domestic violence in occupied Palestinian territory: A qualitative evaluation using extended normalisation process theory. *BMC Family Practice*, *22*(1), 3. https://doi.org/10.1186/s12875-020-01338-z

Bartal, A., Jagodnik, K. M., Chan, S. J., & Dekel, S. (2024). OpenAI's narrative embeddings can be used for detecting post-traumatic stress following childbirth via birth stories. *Research Square*, rs.3.rs-3428787. https://doi.org/10.21203/rs.3.rs-3428787/v2

Brunner, J., Farmer, M. M., Bean-Mayberry, B., Chanfreau-Coffinier, C., Than, C. T., Hamilton, A. B., & Finley, E. P. (2022). Implementing clinical decision support for reducing women veterans' cardiovascular risk in VA: A mixed-method, longitudinal study of context, adaptation, and uptake. *Frontiers in Health Services, 2*, 946802. https://doi.org/10.3389/frhs.2022.946802

Elisseou, S., Shamaskin-Garroway, A., Kopstick, A. J., Potter, J., Weil, A., Gundacker, C., & Moreland-Capuia, A. (2024). Leading organizations from burnout to trauma-informed resilience: A vital paradigm shift. *The Permanente Journal, 28*(1), 198–205. https://doi.org/10.7812/TPP/23.110

Goldstein, E., Chokshi, B., Melendez-Torres, G. J., Rios, A., Jelley, M., & Lewis-O'Connor, A. (2024). Effectiveness of trauma-informed care implementation in health care settings: Systematic review of reviews and realist synthesis. *The Permanente Journal, 28*(1), 135–150. https://doi.org/10.7812/TPP/23.127

Lwamba, E., Shisler, S., Ridlehoover, W., Kupfer, M., Tshabalala, N., Nduku, P., Langer, L., Grant, S., Sonnenfeld, A., Anda, D., Eyers, J., & Snilstveit, B. (2022). Strengthening women's empowerment and gender equality in fragile contexts towards peaceful and inclusive societies: A systematic review and meta-analysis. *Campbell Systematic Reviews, 18*(1), e1214. https://doi.org/10.1002/cl2.1214

McKinney, J. L., Clinton, S. C., & Keyser, L. E. (2024). Women's health across the lifespan: A sex- and gender-focused perspective. *Physical Therapy, 104*(10), pzae121. https://doi.org/10.1093/ptj/pzae121

Nemeth, J., Ramirez, R., Debowski, C., Kulow, E., Hinton, A., Wermert, A., Mengo, C., Malecki, A., Glasser, A., Montgomery, L., & Alexander, C. (2023). The CARE health advocacy intervention improves trauma-informed practices at domestic violence service organizations to address brain injury, mental health, and substance use. *The Journal of Head Trauma Rehabilitation, 38*(6), 439–447. https://doi.org/10.1097/HTR.0000000000000871

Schmidt, E. K., Faieta, J., & Tanner, K. (2020). Scoping review of self-advocacy education interventions to improve care. *OTJR: Occupation, Participation and Health, 40*(1), 50–56. https://doi.org/10.1177/1539449219860583

VanPuymbrouck, L., Chun, E. M., Hesse, E. D., Ranneklev, K., & Sanchez, C. (2024). Developing client self-advocacy in occupational therapy: Are we practicing what we preach? *Occupational Therapy International, 2024*, 1662671. https://doi.org/10.1155/2024/1662671

Williams, H. N., & Farley, B. (2024). Trauma-informed care. *Seminars in Pediatric Neurology, 50*, 101139. https://doi.org/10.1016/j.spen.2024.101139

Index

Note: Page locators in *italic* indicate a figure, and page locators in **bold** indicate a table on the corresponding page.

abandonment, result 82
ableism: cumulative impact 289; impact 25, 93; legacy 128
academic fatigue 47
academic pressures, trauma pathway 79–81
accountability: shift requirement 330; structures, building 338–341
activities of daily living (ADL): proficiency 248; retraining, therapist observations 188–189; sensitivity 206; training 256; training, intervention strategies 283–284
adaptations, emotional weight (validation) 253
adaptive responses 5
adaptive supervision, usage 340–341
adaptive survival strategies, trauma responses (equivalence) 11–12
ADA text embedding model, usage 333
adjusted care routines, initiation 243
adolescence: brain plasticity, developmental neuroscience research (emergence) 34; caregiving roles, continuation 234; dependence, shift 36; developmental considerations 35–40; emotional cost, accumulation 36; occupational disruption 34; physical/digital landscapes 58; reactivated/unresolved trauma, risk 76–78; trauma, neurobiological imprint 45–46
adolescent girls: behaviors, indicators 57; body, reconnection 52; boundaries,

ignoring 39; classroom transitions (case example) 66; concentration, difficulty 57; contextual inquiry, usage 55–56; cyberbullying 58; daily life, problems 55; daily routines, disruption 56–57; dependency, patterns reinforcement 58; developmental tasks (disruption), relational trauma (impact) **37–38**; digital engagement, occupational therapy perspective 58; digital environments, adolescent trauma (relationship) 58–59; digital environments, transformation 58–69; digital peer violence 58; dissociation 50–52; dissociation, support (occupational therapy approaches) **51–52**; dysregulation patterns 46–48; emotional numbing 50–52; emotions, reconnection 52; external expectations, internal capacity (mismatch) 46; fear, reinforcement 59; foster placements 57; grouping structures, advocacy 55; inequity, impact 60; late-afternoon shutdowns 47; LGBTQ+ girls, trauma (layers) 61; marginalized girls, trauma (contextualization) 59–62; microaggressions 59; multiple transitions, intersection 40; neurological changes 42–48; numbing, support (occupational therapy approaches) **51–52**; occupational therapists, assistance 48; occupational therapy approach 41–42; peer withdrawal 52–55; performance, boundaries 58; psychological changes 42–48; reengagement 53; role development, disruption 56–57; routines, disconnection 47; safety/regulation (creation), occupational therapy (usage) 62–64; school refusal 52–55; self-expression, boundaries 58; self-harm 50–52; self-harm, support (occupational therapy approaches) **51–52**; self-worth, erosion 59; social hierarchies, negotiation 58; space (creation), occupational therapy (impact) 50; stress, internal experience 56–57; stressors 34; surveillance, boundaries 58; survival-based behaviors, acting out (contrast) 48–50, **49**; top-down strategies, usage 42; trauma-informed youth wellness program, outpatient OT usage (case example) 67–68; trust, building 61; withdrawal, support (school-based occupational therapy strategies) **54**; world engagement (shaping), trauma (impact) 55

adolescent girls, avoidance 52–55; reframing 53; support, school-based occupational therapy strategies **54**

adolescent girls, trauma: exposure, racial/socioeconomic inequities 60–61; exposure/response (shaping), systems (impact) 57–58; histories 44, 46; meaning, shaping 60; navigation 62; recovery, technology/media (usage) 64–65; responses 48–55

adolescents: case vignettes/reflections 65–68; clinical decision-making, therapist reflections 68; emotional expression, activity-based approaches 64; LGBTQ+ youth, trauma risk 61–62; occupational disruption, environmental/systemic influences 55–59; occupational therapy (trauma-informed principles) **63**; pain, reality 34; relational stress 33; trauma 33; trauma-informed care, meaning 64–65; trauma-informed occupational therapy, usage 62–65

adult-onset diabetes, development 181

adverse childhood experiences (ACEs), long-term health outcomes (connection) 266

advocacy: clinical praxis, equivalence 334–336; integration map **335**; strategies **322**

affect, change (documentation) 320

affective dysregulation, risk 87

affirming goals 273–275; examples **274**

affirming language, usage 310

affirming lens, usage 272–276, 278

age-incongruent occupations, presentation 276

agency: loss 112–114, 137; prioritization 308

agency, sense 167; expression 320; reestablishment 214

aggression, emphasis 13

aging parents, caregiving 142

aging, trauma/occupational transitions (navigation) 136

allostasis, maintenance 275

American Occupational Therapy Association, Guidelines for Trauma-Informed Care 16

Americans with Disabilities Act: protections, alignment 259; usage 93

amygdala: development 42; emotional regulation 53; hyperreactivity 5; prefrontal cortex, connections (weakness) 75; size/function/connectivity, alteration 4; trauma vulnerability 5

ancestral practices, usage 128

anti-oppressive practice 93

anxiety 197–198; client signs 299; elimination 98, 133; history 12; increase 27, 89; labeling 194; reduction 147; test anxiety 96

anxious urgency, bursts 90

Asian American women, emotional silence/stoicism (presumption/damage) 215–216

assignment deadline, missing 90

attachment: disruption (women of color) 220–221; experiences, impact 107

attachment-based responses 8

attendance-related disciplinary action, reduction 176

Attention Deficit Hyperactivity Disorder (ADHD) 173; Individualized Education Plan (IEP), usage 65

audio-guided breath work, usage 325

authentic ambition, over-functioning (differentiation) **80**, 81
authentic occupation, focus 275–276
autoimmune diseases, development 182
autoimmune disorder: diagnosis 141–142; invisible illness, development 183
autonomic dysregulation 245
autonomic instability 206
autonomic regulation 244–245
autonomic response, patterns 21–22
autonomic tracking, usage 181
autonomy: body autonomy, respect 123–124; control 97–98; delay 277; growth 34; navigation, difficulty 36; relational autonomy 256; requirements 203; respect 100; shaping 74–75; transitions 85; violation 166; women, autonomy (occupational therapy approaches) 202–204
avoidance: appearance 248; emotional self-protection, comparison 53; reframing 133; survival strategy 75; trauma-related behavior 265
avoidance (adolescent girls) 52–55; reframing 53; support, school-based occupational therapy strategies **54**

bathing, reframing 177
behavioral accountability, emphasis 75
behavioral resistance, trauma sign 173
belonging: loss 301; sense 71–72
biased diagnostic practices 216
bilateral taping, usage 259
binary decisions, extension 292
biofeedback, integration 313–315
biofeedback-supported strategies **314**
biological disruption, long-term effects 182
Biopsychosocial Framework 16
biosensors, usage 308
birth: agency, loss 112–114; consent, absence 112–114; emergency procedures 112–114; trauma 112–114
birth-related trauma 112
Black populations, care access barriers 27
Black women: culturally responsive care/structural advocacy 127–130; enslaved Black women, experimental surgeries 218; faculty, first-person accounts 212; healthcare experiences 201; intergenerational trauma/ substance use, impact 219; medical

settings, perceived discrimination 216, 217; pain treatment, inadequacy 216; physical function, declines 152; trauma exposure 211; trauma recovery, barriers 222
blindfolded games, avoidance 71
blood flow, promotion 139
bodily autonomy 226; violations, experience 25
bodily cues, interpretation 288
bodily violation, experience 124
body: autonomy, respect 123–124; awareness, intensification 41; check-in rituals 312; composition (disruption), chronic activation (impact) 41; distrust 183; experiences, visual mapping (usage) 42; pain, constancy 125; reconnection 62; tenseness 21; trauma existence 60–61; trust, reestablishment 181; wear and tear 269
body-based anchoring 97
body-based anchors, usage 312
body-based care 161
body-based check-ins, therapist usage 232
body-based engagement 228
body-based grounding, usage 77
body-based habits, disruption 40
body-based occupations, reframing 41
body-based routines, struggle 40
body-based survival responses 8
body scans: display 312; usage 283
boundaries: absence, impact 151; initiation, ease (improvement) 325; personal boundaries, establishment (difficulty) 219; setting 256; setting (trauma-related behavior) 265
boundaries, violation: body-based reminders 166; experience 219
boundary rituals, usage 99
bowel regularities, provider management 246
brain: architecture (rewiring), trauma (impact) 4; changes 105; health, estrogen (role) 139–140; hypoxic brain injury, occurrence 189; traumatic brain injury (TBI) 160–161, 188–190; wear and tear 269
brain-body mechanisms, understanding 5
breastfeeding, frustrations 253
breath-led transitions, usage 258

breathwork, importance 124–125
burnout 211; connections 330–331

calligraphy, usage 284
calming routines, offering 329
campus-based occupational therapy 96
Canadian Model of Occupational
    Performance and Engagement 16
Canadian Occupational Performance
    Measure, usage 89, 155
Canadian Practice Process Framework 16
cannabis, usage (increase) 265
capacity map, co-designing 187
capacity/willingness, contrast
    (examination) 77
cardiometabolic conditions, invisible
    illness (development) 183
career: pressures, trauma pathway 79–81;
    trajectories, shift 140
caregiving: demands, convergence 142;
    expectations, trauma (relationship) 24;
    fatigue 149; responsibilities, impact
    254; roles, focus 324
caretaking, cultural expectations 221
ChatGPT, usage 333
chest, tightness 78, 107
childhood: reactivated/unresolved
    trauma, risk 76–78; rhythms,
    changes 72; sexual trauma, history
    307–308; social hardships 41; trauma
    histories, autonomic responses
    (examination) 22
chlamydia 193
choice-based activity engagement 181
choice, trauma-informed occupational
    therapy usage 28–29
cholesterol: levels, elevation 185; profile,
    problems 180
Christy, Kayonne 218
chronic fatigue 81–82; occupational
    therapy recommendation 180–181;
    report 245
chronic fatigue syndrome, invisible illness
    (development) 183
chronic health decline 206–207
chronic illness 231
chronic inflammation 204
chronic invalidation 38; impact 22
chronic joint pain, occupational
    therapy 171

chronic pain: disorders 185–187; impact
    257; occupational therapy referral 3–4;
    postpartum period 254; presence 211
chronic pelvic pain 190
chronic sleep disturbances 130
chronic stress: exposure, impact 107;
    impact 72; navigation 126; result 219
chronic survival mode 77; neurobiological/
    functional consequences 10;
    occupational impact 9, 11; stress
    response system, involvement 7
chronic tension headaches 228–229
chronic trauma exposure 140
cisgender norms, neutrality
    (relationship) 265
classism, cumulative impact 93, 289
classrooms, overstimulation
    (identification) 55–56
class, skipping 72; suspension 55
client-led regulation 313
client voice, embedding 340
clinical care, fragmentation 3
clinical innovation (bridging), policy/
    advocacy (usage) 321–322
clinical pitfalls, avoidance 289–291
clinical reasoning, problems 265
clinical spaces, misrecognition (women of
    color) 222–223
clinical strategies, examples 274
co-created feedback loops, usage 339–340
coercion: body-based reminders 166;
    long-term coercion, interrupted roles
    (reclamation) 167; manifestations 241;
    sexual coercion, history 190; sexual
    violence, relationship 163–164
Cognitive Behavioral Frame of
    Reference 16
cognitive capacity, assumptions 240
cognitive clarity, support 86
cognitive disruption 258–259
cognitive efficiency, sacrifice 199
cognitive flexibility 140
cognitive fog 258; amplification 137, 140
cognitive health consequences, violence
    (impact) 197–198
cognitive impacts 199–201
cognitive inefficiency 154
cognitive load 251, 268
cognitive reappraisal, prefrontal structure
    reliance 42

cognitive reframing strategy, usage 97
cognitive rehabilitation, need 161
cognitive screening scores 228–229
cognitive shifts, management 154–155
cognitive strategies 183; usage,
    insufficiency 77
cognitive symptoms, emergence 182
coherence, loss 140–141
cold sweats, experience 2
collaboration, trauma-informed
    occupational therapy usage 28
collaborative planning 292–294
collaborative playlist building, usage 284
collaborative scaffolding 332
collaborative sensory regulation,
    facilitation 43
collective memory (women of color)
    224–228
collective ownership, reflection 332
colonialism, legacy 128
colonization, impact 226
community: reengagement, complex
    trauma (effects) 283–284; support,
    trauma-informed occupational therapy
    usage 29; systems, historical trauma
    226–227; usage 303
community-based health navigator
    program, referral 177
community-based interventions 66
community-based technology, usage 323
community-driven innovation
    315–317, **316**
compassion fatigue 142
compensatory energy conservation
    techniques, training 204
compensatory perfectionism 232–233
complex developmental trauma, history 317
complex regional pain syndrome 186
complex trauma, psychiatric outcome
    197–198
compliance: dismissal 222–223;
    functionality, appearance 47
concentration, difficulty 57, 258
confusion: expression 122–123;
    internalization 38
consent: checklist, creation 177; posture,
    relationship 123
constipation 191
continuity, sense: impact 141;
    reestablishment 156–157

continuous learning, importance 332
continuum of care, trauma-informed
    practice **293**; tools 288
continuum of disability, occupational
    disruption 251–253
control, sense (restoration) 113
coordinated care, need 176
coping anchors, usage 284
coping strategies, prescribing 148
coping tools, usage 156
co-regulated breathing, usage 283
co-regulation 124–125; intervention 77;
    role 100; strategies 36
cortisol: reactivity, increase 45; shift 45
creative nonfiction 285
creative pursuits, reintroduction 86
creative tasks, shared playlist
    (initiation) 317
creativity, reconnection 62
Crenshaw, Kimberlé 24
cross-sector task forces, usage 332
crowded spaces, toleration (struggle) 9
cultural affirmation 324
cultural betrayal 213
cultural humility, education
    (commitment) 217
cultural invisibility, impact 171
culturally anchored rest strategies 233
culturally discordant care (women of care)
    216–217
culturally responsive care 127–130
culturally responsive occupational
    therapy, case vignettes/reflections
    130–133
culturally responsive practice (support),
    prompts/reflective questions
    (usage) **129**
cultural misrecognition, impact 217
cultural responsiveness, trauma-informed
    occupational therapy usage 29
cultural scripts, usage 227
cultural stereotyping 213
cultural stigma 27, 221
culture, shift (requirement) 330
cumulative brain injury, possibility 207
cumulative microaggressions,
    experience 25
cumulative stress 142; impact (women
    with disabilities) 253–256
cyberbullying 58

daily energy map, co-creation 211
daily functioning: decline 98, 176; logs, flare tracking (usage) 185
daily functions concerns, occupational therapy referral 3–4
daily life: continuity factures, trauma (impact) 232; engagement, shift (unawareness) 301
daily roles (inconsistency), hormonal sensitivity increase (impact) 44
daily routines: disruption (adolescent girls) 56–57; management, difficulty 307–308; management, disruption 268
daily tasks, survivor-centered adaptations 169–170
data, embedding 333–334
"day in the life" storyboard, usage 43
Dayo, Elizabeth 218
decision-making framework, usage 292
decision making, requirement 39
deep pressure, usage 22
deflection, appearance 166
depression 197–198; increase 89; risk, increase 41
depressive symptoms 39
developing brain (shaping), trauma (impact) 2
developmental disruptions 37
developmental milestones, return (absence) 276–277
developmental pathways, disruption 276–279
developmental readiness 77
developmental reality, importance 277
developmental timing (disruption), chronic activation (impact) 41
developmental trauma 142; addressing 73
diagnostic criteria, usage 74
diagnostic overshadowing (women with disabilities) 242–243
diaphragmatic breathing, usage 132–133
digital abuse 165
digital confidence (rebuilding), occupational therapy (usage) 165
digital engagement, occupational therapy perspective 58
digital environments: adolescent trauma, relationship 58–59; transformation 58–59
digital interventions, emotional/cultural/relational safety (evaluation) 310

digital peer violence 58
digital regulation maps, co-creation 312
digital storytelling, usage 313–315, 323, 324
disapproval, avoidance 12
discharge: planning 298–304; post-discharge, change (sustaining) 300–303
disconnection, recognition 163–164
Discrimination in Medical Settings scale, usage 216
disease (catalyst), violence (impact) 182–183
disenfranchised grief 116–118
disengagement: appearance 40; reflection 77
dismissal, acts 112
disorganization, feelings (compounding) 72
disorientation 5; feeling 104
displacement, impact 226
disruption episodes 284
dissociation, definition 50
distress: ignoring 24; occupational masking 231–232
dizziness, medical history 189
documentation: completion 337; errors, focus 335; pressures 341
domain-specific language models, usage 333
domestic violence, witnessing 173
dormant aspirations, uncovering 285
dorsal vagal state, associations 22
dressing/grooming, self-expression (opportunities) 146
dual coding 246
dual occupancy, concept 133
dual-task sequencing 207
Dunn's Sensory Processing Framework 16
dyadic narrative activities, design 43
dysautonomia, management 206
dysfunctional occupation, toll 230–231
dyspareunia 190
dysregulated cortisol patterns 204
dysregulated diurnal cortisol rhythms, display 44
dysregulated perinatal nervous system, trauma (relationship) 106–112
dysregulation: patterns (adolescent girls) 46–48; tracking 308

early adulthood: demands, unprocessed
trauma (collision) 73; developmental
pressures, understanding 74; trauma, crisis
appearance (rarity) 78; trauma-informed
occupational therapy 90–96
early adversity, reemergence 74
early morning temperature intolerance 206
early postpartum journey, images
(selection/annotation) 131
early postpartum period, trauma-related
responses (occupational therapy
strategies) **113–114**
economic barriers 221
economic inequity, trauma
(relationship) 24
economic insecurity, uncertainty
(prolongation) 81
economic marginalization, impact 239
education, transitions 85
elevated arousal signs, recognition
(absence) 9
embodied learning 110
embodied safety, augmentation 312–313
emergency cesarean, case example
130–132
emergency contacts, list (availability) 168
emergency healthcare workers, study 23
emerging adulthood: developmental task
87; developmental window, criticality
88; occupational disruption 85–89;
stability, routines (impact) 86
emotional abuse, experience 83, 219
emotional accessibility, factors
(impact) 310
emotional burden, increase 217
emotional closeness, independence
(balance) 36
emotional compartmentalization 219
emotional connection, maintenance 36
emotional depletion 154
emotional detachment 198; feeling 104
emotional distance, mistakes (impact) 35
emotional distancing 225
emotional dysregulation 36–37; episodes
258; hormonal sensitivity, increase
(impact) 44; labeling 94–95
emotional endurance 225
emotional enmeshment 83
emotional flatness 233; functionality,
appearance 47; trauma-related
behavior 265

emotional lability: amplification 140;
report 245
emotional labor 255; cultural expectations
221; expectations 88
emotional neglect 38
emotional numbing 50, 51, 144
emotional presence, promotion 48
emotional processing 324;
enhancement 43
emotional reactivity: emphasis 13;
increase, hormonal surges (impact) 41
emotional regulation 94–96, 307–308;
challenges, interpretation 290;
outcome, flexibility 91; support 86
emotional rigidity 166
emotional safety: focus, care plan
(building) 2; support 324
emotional self-protection, avoidance
(comparison) 53
emotional strain 230
emotional stress: experiences 79;
reactivity 22
emotional suppression, cognitive load 268
emotional survival, strategies 39
emotional validation 117
emotional volatility 138, 161; patterns,
emergence 45–46; reduction 325
employment, transitions 85
empowerment, trauma-informed
occupational therapy usage 28–29
endometriosis, history 257
energy-conservation protocols,
avoidance 257
energy contour map: co-creation 184;
development 185
energy depletion (postpartum period) 254
energy mapping 98
engagement: barriers 140; low level 267
environmental adaptation, therapeutic use
23–24
environmental adversity, experience 41
environmental orientation cues, usage 104
environmental stressors, puberty
(intersection) 40–42
episodic conditions, trauma-informed
occupational therapy **252**
equity-focused occupational therapy 205
estrangement 82–83
estrogen: role 139–140; shifts 45
evidence-based protocols, compliance
338–339

executive dysfunction 199–201;
    struggles 268
executive functions: amplification
    140; collapse 206; modulation 139;
    outcome, flexibility 91; screeners,
    usage 154–155; shift 75–76;
    solidification 72; support 76; trauma
    sign 173
exhaustion 210–211; display 217;
    feelings 140
exposure, gendered patterns 4
expressive technology, usage 313–315
eye contact, avoidance 40

failure: feelings, struggle 130–131;
    language 284; perception 77
fall risk 161
familial rupture 82–83
family: estrangement 283; systems,
    historical trauma 226–227
Fantastic Reality Ability Measurement
    Scale 281
Fantastic Reality Ability Measurement
    (FRAME) study 281
fatigue: assumption 65; chronic emotional
    labor, impact 152; chronic fatigue
    81–82; compassion fatigue 142;
    functionality, appearance 47; onset
    182; participation fatigue 266–267;
    postprandial fatigue 206; worsening
    12, 257
fear, reinforcement (adolescent girls) 59
felt-sense indicators, identification 283
female nervous system, dysregulation 8–9
female reproductive health, trauma
    (impact) 90
fibromyalgia 162, 257; diagnosis 206;
    emergence 186; invisible illness,
    development 183
fidelity mechanisms, usage 338–339
financial insecurity, trauma pathway
    81–82
financial vulnerabilities 144
fine motor skills 248
fine motor tasks 229
first-generation professional, burnout/role
    overload (case example) 98–99
flare tracking, usage 185
flashbacks: emphasis 13; reemergence 74
focusing, difficulty 161
forced displacement 163

forced sterilization 118, 216
forgetfulness 5; manifestation 138
foster home, changes (impact) 78
foster placements 57
framework, definition 16
frontline knowledge, integration 330
functional decline, chronic pain
    (impact) 257
functional dependence 240
functional-dysfunctional continuum 230
functional-rhythm profiling 257
future care, avoidance 119
future-oriented approaches, usage 149
future-oriented occupational engagement
    137–138
future visualization series, therapist
    implementation 285

gastrointestinal discomfort, experience 98
gastrointestinal dysregulation 191
gender: bias, experiences 177; identity,
    assumptions 263; responsiveness,
    trauma-informed occupational therapy
    usage 29; sexual minority women,
    relationship 262
gender-based oppression, trauma
    (entanglement) 24
gender-based stressors, burden 211
gender-based violence, cumulative impact
    93, 289
gendered differences 23
gender-expansive clients, story
    minimization (avoidance) 300
gender-expansive youth, trauma
    (layering) 61
gender women: affirming goals,
    co-creation 273–275; affirming goals,
    examples **274**; autonomy, delay 277;
    case vignettes/clinical reflections
    283–285; clinical strategies **274**;
    developmental pathways, disruption
    276–279; diagnostic overshadowing
    265–266; elevated risk, elevated
    visibility (contrast) 264–265; health
    system prevalence/risk/erasure
    264–267; identity, scaffolding 263,
    279–283; imagination, clinical tool
    281–283; milestones (rethinking),
    affirming lens (usage) 278; neutral
    care, myth 265–266; nonrecognition,
    trauma 268–272; occupational

futurity 279–283; occupational
identity 267; occupational therapy
(OT), nonlinear transitions 278–279;
occupation, identity affirmation
270–272; participation fatigue
273–275; physical environment,
safety (centering) 272–273; queer time
276–279; regulation (restoration),
authentic occupation (usage)
275–276; role exploration 277;
role fragmentation 267; split roles,
navigation 269–270; trauma-informed
intervention, affirming lens (usage)
272–276; trauma-informed practice
273; visibility (absence), opportunities
(missing) 264–265; volition/visibility,
clinical practice usage 280–281
*Global Advances in Integrative Medicine
and Health*, self-identified women
(well-being examination) 88–89
goal-corrected partnerships 36
goal-directed activity, therapeutic use
23–24
goals: alignment/adaptation matrix **294**;
setting 273–275; setting, reframing
298; therapist co-creation 293
gonorrhea 193
green energy hours 187
grief: disenfranchised grief 116–118;
emergence, school-based OT (usage)
65–66; experience 140–141;
processing, paintbrushes (usage) 64;
surfacing 117; unprocessed grief,
resurfacing 137; widowhood grief
147–148
grooming habits, fluctuation 166
grounding protocols, usage 283
group activities, attendance (refusal) 243
grouping structures, advocacy 55
guided mediations/storytelling, usage 155
Guidelines for Trauma-Informed Care
(American Occupational Therapy
Association) 16

habits (disruption), trauma impact/
analysis 16
Habte, Ruth 218
harm: misalignment 310, 312; reduction,
impossibility 308; re-experiencing 222
harm-reduction strategies,
requirement 128

Hashimoto's thyroiditis 185
healing: indicators, recognition 318–320;
nontraditional indicators, examples **319**
health: avoidance 217–219; behaviors,
scaffolding 186; conditions,
non-trauma presentations
(differentiation) **192**; equity 204–205;
services, access 171
healthcare: access/quality, racial
disparities 144; engagement, reluctance
162; mistrust 119; neglect, impact 195;
system navigation 201–202
health system: harm 215–217; prevalence/
risk/erasure (sexual minority women)
264–267
heart rate variability, tracking devices 313
heteronormative bias, impact 25
heterosexism, cumulative impact 93, 289
heterosexual norms, neutrality
(relationship) 265
high-functioning behavior,
appearance 120
high-risk deliveries/medical
complications 112
hippocampus: blood flow, promotion 139;
size/function/connectivity, alteration 4;
trauma vulnerability 5
Hispanic populations, care access
barriers 27
Hispanic women, language barriers/
cultural misunderstandings/pain
tolerance assumptions 215
historical responsiveness,
trauma-informed occupational therapy
usage 29
history-gathering 226
home-based occupational therapy,
referral 177
homecoming script, usage 233
hormonal balance (disruption), chronic
activation (impact) 41
hormonal changes, impact 303
hormonal cycles, impact 4–5
hormonal feedback loop 8
hormonal fluctuations 8
hormonal function, alteration 4
hormonal sensitivity: HPA axis,
relationship (adolescent girls) 44–46;
increase, impact 44
hormone levels (change), trauma
(impact) 4

housing insecurity, trauma pathway 81–82
human connection, displacement (absence) 309
Human Immunodeficiency Virus (HIV) 193
Human Papillomavirus (HPV) 193
human stress response, design 8
hygiene tasks, performing (ability) 205
hyperactivation, experience 44
hyperarousal 8
hypertension, diagnosis 185
hypervigilance 8, 144; existence 91; feeling 104; occurrence 130; patterns 142; recognition 163–164
hypoactivation, display 44
hypoarousal 8
hypothalamus-pituitary-adrenal (HPA) axis: activity, increase 107; dysregulation 275; hormonal sensitivity, relationship (adolescent girls) 44–46; impact 8; patterns, occupational implications **45**; priming, trauma (impact) 140; sensitization, early trauma (impact) 138; trauma vulnerability 7
hypoxic brain injury, occurrence 189
hysterectomy: hormonal decline 137; total hysterectomy, experience 155

identity: affirmation, usage 100; consolidation 74–75; development, trauma (relationship) 35; diffusion, incidence (elevation) 87; disruption, trauma impact/analysis 16; erosion 166, 227–228; exploration, disruption 87–88; foreclosure 270; fragmentation, risk 87; integration 97; invalidation 285; rebuilding 137, 283–284; reconnection 62; reconstruction 132–133; repair 92; shattering 137; support (occupation usage), clinical applications **111**; timelines, usage 274; work, usage 99
identity-affirming actions 229
identity-affirming goals 275
identity-based discrimination 275
identity-based harm 264
identity-based marginalization 308
identity-centered practice, trauma-informed care (intersection) 253

identity-congruent content 310
identity formation 34, 36; vulnerability, relationship 38–39
imagination, clinical tool 281–283
imagining, right 279–283
immediate dependency 110
immigrant populations, care access barriers 27
immigrant women, healthcare experiences 201
immune function, alteration 4
immune responses (disruption), trauma (impact) 4
immune system, impact 184–185
Impact of Events Scale, usage 104
impersonal study tips 79–80
Implicit Association Test (IAT) 223
implicit bias: experience 201; reference/operation 223
impostor feelings 89
impostor phenomenon 79
impulse control 42
incarceration 2823
in-class discussions, freezing 73
incontinence 190
independence, emphasis 318
Indigenous women, healthcare experiences 201
Individualized Education Plan (IEP): deviations, absence 68; trauma-informed sensory plan, addition 173; usage 65–66
infant massage 131
infant routines, focus 254
inflammatory diseases, development 182–183
inflammatory markers, elevation 180
information processing, deceleration 138
infrastructure: investment 332; reflective infrastructure, usage 340–341
initiative, requirement 39
injustice, addressing 93–94
inner struggle, obscuring 89
insomnia, experience 79
institutional abuse 165
institutional barriers 239
institutional betrayal 284–285
institutional change, models 330–331
institutional displacement: navigation 156–157; trauma, recognition 157
institutional harm, impact 195, 197

institutional retraumatization, signs 177
institutional scaffolding 72
institutional settings, surveillance
    acuteness 244
institutional trauma 258–259
institutional violence, challenging 172
instructions, memory (struggle) 9
instrumental activities of daily living
    (IADL) retraining, intervention
    strategies 283–284
insula: emotional regulation 53; size/
    function/connectivity, alteration 4;
    trauma vulnerability 5–6
insular shrinkage 5
intellectual disability: IPV context 256;
    women with intellectual disability
    255–256
intergenerational conflict, experience 219
intergenerational load (women of color)
    224–228; psychological/occupational
    weight 225–226
intergenerational routines, co-creation
intergenerational trauma 219
internal mentorship structures,
    development 332
internal stress systems: function 44;
    management 43–44
interoceptive awareness 181; building
    248; promotion 48; support 97
interpersonal feedback, consistency 38
interpersonal trauma, history 27–28
interpersonal violence, experience 25
intersectionality, trauma (relationship)
    24–27
intersectional lens, application 27
intersectional trauma lens, application
    25–26
interstitial cystitis 191
interventions: alignment, importance 297;
    planning/implementation 295–298;
    standardized sequence, avoidance 28
intimacy: interpretation 83; transitions 85
intimate partner violence (IPV) 160–161,
    164; chronic health decline/fragmented
    recovery 206–207; dysregulated
    cortisol patterns 204; histories,
    diseases (appearance) 182; history 184;
    likelihood 239; survival 180–181;
    survivors, patterns 161
intrinsic motivation, lower levels 87
invisible burdens 240

invisible injury, navigation 258–259
invisible labor 217–219
invisible trauma 118–120; signaling,
    client presentations **119**
irritability, increase 242
irritable bowel disease, invisible illness
    (development) 183
irritable bowel syndrome, diagnosis 206
isolation: reduction 43; risks 195; sense,
    worsening 324–325

job, hollowness (feeling) 140
job-simulated tasks, functional
    observation 207
journaling, usage 310
justice-driven occupational responses 145

Kawa model 16

labor period, trauma-related responses
    (occupational therapy strategies)
    113–114
land-based roles, disconnection 283–284
language: domain-specific language
    models, usage 333; exclusion,
    experience 201; shift, requirement 330
language barriers 27; encountering
    215, 216
late-afternoon shutdowns 47
late life see older adulthood
later life, violence 165–166
Latina women: sexual harassment/cultural
    stereotyping 213; trauma recovery,
    barriers 222
Latina workers, trauma recovery groups
    (offering) 259
layered assessment model,
    implementation 257–258
laziness, appearance 34
leisure-based tasks, avoidance 225
leisure bonding 127
LGBTQ: participants, PTSD criteria
    (meeting) 264; professionals,
    workplace trauma recovery 285;
    women (occupational engagement
    support), imagination-based strategies
    (usage) **282**; women, trauma history
    (invisibility) 269
LGBTQ+: clients, sensory/visual cue
    identification 267; individuals,
    physical/social stress 269; survivors,

minority stress/posttraumatic symptom severity (interaction) 265; youth, trauma risk 61–62; youth/young adults, developmental interference 276

LGBTQIA+: advocate, trauma/disconnection recovery 155–156; individuals, medical discrimination 152; women, healthcare experiences 201

life: chaos 231; redesign maps, usage 169; reengagement 113; transitions 75

life, second half: brain health 138–140; case vignettes/clinical reflections 154–157; chronic health conditions 143; hormonal changes 138–140; medical trauma 143; neurobiological/occupational shifts 138–140; occupational identity 140–141; resilience 140–141; role strain 140–141; structural trauma 143–145; systemic trauma 143–145; trauma pathways 141–145

life-threatening pregnancy, occurrence 103–104

light sensitivity 258

limbic system, hyperactivation 75

lived trauma, transmission 225

loneliness, feeling 24

long-held roles, loss 152

longitudinal data, usage 219

long-term change, accountability structures (building) 338–341

long-term coercion, interrupted roles (reclamation) 167

long-term economic exclusion 144

long-term well-being 92

low-demand wins, anchoring 186–187

lower back pain, persistence 262–263

low participation, exhibition 47

lupus 185; diagnosis 184

maladaptive coping 89

marginalization: identity-based marginalization 308; reinforcement 247

marginalized girls: compounded trauma, relationship 59–60; trauma, contextualization 59–62

marginalized women: barriers/occupational therapy advocacy strategies **153**; compounded trauma (addressing) 152

masking, cognitive load 268

maternal agency, promotion 104

maternal bonding 127

maternal deaths (US) 104

maternal health disparities, violence (relationship) 194–195

maternal identity, core domains (impact) *110*

maternal-infant bonding, emphasis 133

maternal mortality/morbidity 194

maternal occupational focus, trauma-informed clinical strategies **126**

maternal occupations, restoration 125–127

maternal recovery, case vignettes/reflections 130–133

maternal self-care checklists, focus 254

meals: planning 232; skipping 90

meaning-making, guidance 224

media, usage 64–65

Medicaid reimbursement, push 334

medical bias 221

medical dismissal 191–192, 266; occupational identity reclamation 257–258

medical experiences (documentation), biomedical blog (usage) 258

medical mistrust: historical context, education (commitment) 217; impact 107; violence, relationship 201–202

medical system navigation, support 201–202

medical trauma 143; history 27–28; impact 147; violence, relationship 194–195

memory: collective memory (women of color) 224–228; exercises 183; recall, dependence (reduction) 155; resurfacing, open-ended art prompt (usage) 272–273; strategies, practice 259

menarche, impact 41

Menopause Cafés, establishment 138

menopause, hormonal volatility 140

menopause, neurobiological changes/occupational impacts **139**

mentorship: evolution 157; usage 336–338

microaggressions: adolescent girls, experience 59; impact, downplaying 224; racial microaggressions 128

micro-interventions 312–313
micro-routine scaffolding, usage 184, 185
midlife: case vignettes/clinical reflections
    154–157; health, culturally responsive
    care/advocacy 151–154; occupational
    disruptions **144–145**; resilience/
    redefinition, opportunities 141;
    stressors **144–145**; trauma-informed
    occupational therapy goals/strategies
    150; trauma/occupational transitions,
    navigation 136; women, barriers/
    occupational therapy advocacy
    strategies 153
midlife trauma: impact, invisibility 137;
    pathways **144–145**
mid-session dips, occurrence 95
migraines: emergence 186; invisible
    illness, development 183; medical
    history 189; presence 211
migration-related stressors, impact 162
migration, survival 213
milestones (rethinking), affirming lens
    (usage) 278
mindfulness-based practices 95
minimization, acts 112
minority stress, posttraumatic symptom
    severity (interaction) 265
mirrors: avoidance 72, 161; discomfort 40
miscarriage: term, medical precision 116;
    work struggles 307–308
missed appointments, patterns 241
missed screenings (women with
    disabilities) 242–243
mistrust, repair (impossibility) 308
mobile apps 310–312
mobility, difficulty 262–263
model, definition 16
Model of Human Occupation (MOHO)
    16, 56–57; usage 98
mood: disorders, impact 197–198; swings
    138; variability 45
moodiness, appearance 40
moral judgment, acts 112
morning disorientation, struggle 204
Mother-to-Infant Bonding Scale
    (MIBS) 107
motivation: absence 34, 174; disruption
    87–88
motivational interviewing, usage 97
motor planning, alteration 244
movement planning 187

multigenerational household, primary
    caregiver role 232
multiple sclerosis 185; chronic fatigue/
    emotional lability report 245
multisystem dysregulation (catalyst),
    violence (impact) 182–183
mutuality, trauma-informed occupational
    therapy usage 28

narrative: approaches, usage 149; clinician
    recognition 211; integration, act
    302–303; internalization 97; mapping,
    usage 274; measures, usage 320;
    ownership 301–302; practice, usage
    284; reframing 92; review 212; shared
    narratives 138
narrative-based inquiry 89
narrative-based tools, usage 42
nausea, experience 798
Navajo woman, presentation case
    283–284
negative body image 230
neonatal intensive care unit (NICU)
    103–104, 114–116; follow-up,
    reaction 120; NICU-related trauma,
    occupational therapy strategies
    115–116; racial microaggressions 128;
    stay, case example 130–132
nervous system: capacity, problem 73;
    cues 120; down-regulation routine,
    practice 97; dysregulation 242;
    literacy 313; regulation 86; regulation
    strategies 124–125; shaping 85;
    shutdown, status 21; stabilization 96;
    stories, presence 4
neural networks, impact 73
neural regions, size/function/connectivity
    (alteration) 4
neurobiological changes, inducing 95
neurobiological growth 36
neurobiological regulation 330–331
neuroception: importance 22; polyvagal
    theory, relationship 21–23
neuroendocrine health, trauma (impact) 90
neuroendocrine shifts, collision 137
neuroendocrine system, impact 184–185
neuroimmune function 245
neurological acceleration 2
neurological maturation 75–76
neuro-sensory anchors 229
neurotransmitters, modulation 139

noise: identification 187; minimization
123; toleration, struggle 9
nonadherence, appearance 166
non-cardiac chest tightness, experience 98
noncompliance: meaning 174;
reflection 77
nonlinear transitions, OT (relationship)
278–279
nonproductive occupation trials 228
nonrecognition, trauma 268–272
non-restorative patterns 231–232
nonspecific abdominal pain,
documentation 176
normative perinatal responses,
trauma-related perinatal responses
(differentiation) 108–109
nutritional re-engagement 187

obedience, demands 219
observational rubrics, inclusion 338–339
obstetric racism 118
occupation: identity affirmation 270–272,
271; violence, long-term ripple effects
166–167
occupational avoidance patterns,
demonstration 243
occupational balance, disruption
85–86, 230
occupational disconnection, recovery
155–156
occupational disengagement 155;
explanation 206–207
occupational disruption 34, 41, 55,
116–117, 251–253; adolescence
34; emerging adulthood 85–89;
environmental/systemic influences
55–59; foundations 1; life, second
half 143; older adulthood 145–149;
patterns 166
occupational dissonance 111
occupational futurity 279–283
occupational identity: disruption
140–141; exploration 92, 97;
reclamation 257–258, 284–285
occupational inheritance 228
occupational justice 13; practice 174;
structural/systemic dimensions 12–15;
system-level advocacy, relationship
171–173
occupational mapping/routinization,
usage 97

occupational participation: shaping 93;
trauma, relationship 35
occupational roles: compression 140;
disruption, trauma impact/analysis 16;
expansion 74–75
occupational strength, episodes 284
occupational therapy (OT): identity
repair 92; impact 90; initiation 104;
intersectional trauma lens, application
25–26; intervention, ability 280;
models 15–16; nonlinear transitions,
relationship 278–279; progress
report, submission 206; questions
3–4; response 198–201; role 23–24;
sessions 207; trauma-informed
approach 15; trauma-informed
care, SAMHSA principles 19–20;
trauma-informed discharge planning
checklist 299; trauma recovery 198;
trauma responsive occupational
therapy, core principles 27–29
occupational therapy (OT) practice:
community-driven innovations/
applications 316; safety planning
template 169
Occupational Therapy Practice
Framework 16
occupational transitions, navigation 136
occupational withdrawal 144; initiation 40
occupation as identity 109–112
occupation-based backtracking 246–247
older adulthood (late life): abuse 148;
culturally responsive care/advocacy
151–154; cumulative loss 146;
dependency 148–149; displacement
148–149; grief 147; medical trauma
148; neglect 148; occupational
disruption 145–149; occupational
erasure 148–149; regulation,
prioritization 149; trauma 145–149;
trauma-informed care, application
149–151; trauma-informed care,
narrative/future-oriented approaches
(usage) 149; trauma-informed
occupational therapy goals/strategies
150; women, barriers/occupational
therapy advocacy strategies 153
one-on-one supervision 340
orthopedic injuries 191–192
orthopedic trauma, recovery 204
orthostatic changes 182

oscillation 8
outpatient occupational therapy (case example) 66–67
outpatient rehabilitation, admission 238–239
overbright lighting, identification 187
over-functioning, reinforcement 227–228
overidentification 225
oxytocin, description 107

paced breathing, usage 104, 186
pacing: importance 100; preferences 288; strategies 225
pain: behaviors, persistence 233; expressions 221; worsening 257
pain management: delay 118; routines, avoidance 213
pain-responsive pacing cues, management 206
panic: attack 96; case example 96–98; episodes 133; revisiting 71–72; wave, feeling 76
parasympathetic activity 22
parasympathetic nervous system, vagus nerve (inactivation) 95
parenthood, experiences 254
parentification 82–83
participation fatigue 266–267
participatory measures, usage 320
participatory metrics, usage 339–340
pathologizing, risk 149
peers: boundary initiation, ease (improvement) 235; check-ins, embedding 43; co-regulator role 43; digital peer violence 58; support, trauma-informed occupational therapy usage 29; withdrawal 52–55
pelvic floor: assessment 190; dysfunction 257; pain 194–195; pain, navigation 127; rehabilitation 193
pelvic organ prolapse 190
pelvic trauma, recovery 204
perfectionism: appearance 120; case example 96–98; compensatory perfectionism 232–233; expectations 88; survival strategy 75; usage 76
performance: difficulties, differentiation 199; expectations 88
performance-based assessments, usage 154–155
performance-based identity, reframing 98

performance-based pressure, reduction 87–88
performance-based roles 92
perinatal care, trauma-informed assessment 120–122
perinatal events, trauma 103
perinatal occupational therapy, trauma-informed assessment strategies **121–122**
perinatal period: breathwork, importance 124–125; co-regulation, usage 124–125; maternal identity, core domains (impact) *110*; nervous system regulation strategies 124–125; restoration 109–112; sensory modulation, impact 124–125; structural/invisible trauma 118–120; structural/invisible trauma, signaling (client presentations) *119*; therapeutic space, creation 122–125; transformations 105; trauma pathways 112–120
Perinatal PTSD Questionnaire (PPQ) 108
perinatal responses, occupation therapy strategies **108–109**
persistent fatigue, hormonal sensitivity increase (impact) 44
persistent threat perception, long-term effects 182
personal boundaries, establishment (difficulty) 219
personalized morning rituals 146
Person-Environment-Occupation (PEO) model 15, 16, 56–57
physical activity, breaks (scheduling) 86
physical closeness, avoidance 71
physical discomfort, ignoring 186
physical education, girls (change refusal) 42
physical environments, examination 248
physical injury: dual-track approach 234; over-functioning 233–234; violence, impact 188
physical mobility strategies 127
physical stress, reactivity 22
physical trauma 191
physiological stabilization, performance goal 181
planning, emphasis 75
poetry reading, usage 284
polyvagal theory, neuroception (relationship) 21–23

positional education, usage 132–133
post-discharge: change, sustaining
    300–303; reengagement 303; role
    integration, collaborative mapping tool
    (usage) **304**
post-exertional symptom exacerbation 206
post-exertional symptoms 182
Postpartum Bonding Questionnaire
    (PBQ) 108
postpartum care, access (difficulty) 27
postpartum complications 114–116;
    Chinese Canadian experience 217;
    occupational therapy strategies
    115–116; violence, relationship
    194–197
postpartum mental health (women with
    disabilities) 253–256
postpartum, neurobiological brain
    changes **106**
postpartum occupational disruption,
    violence (relationship) 195, 197
postpartum period: early postpartum
    period, trauma-related responses
    (occupational therapy strategies)
    113–114; framing 254; medical trauma
    114–116; navigation 254
postpartum psychosis, diagnosis 122
postpartum PTSD, case example 130–132
postpartum recovery 125–126
postpartum trauma, occurrence 116
postprandial fatigue 206
post-therapy identity 303
post-traumatic fatigue, navigation 204
post-traumatic stress disorder (PTSD)
    137; criteria, meeting (absence) 22;
    long-term risk 83; original definition
    13; postpartum PTSD, case example
    130–132; psychiatric outcome,
    violence (impact) 197; symptoms,
    classification 333; symptom, severity
    263–264
post-traumatic stress symptoms, levels
    (elevation) 23
power asymmetries, impact 239
practice settings, systemic advocacy
    opportunities **174–175**
prefrontal cortex: blood flow, promotion
    139; construction 34; development
    42, 72; emotional regulation
    53; size/function/connectivity,

alteration 4; subcortical structures,
    connections (weakness) 75; trauma
    vulnerability 6–7
pregnancy: high-risk deliveries/medical
    complications 112; HPA axis, activity
    (increase) 107; life-threatening
    pregnancy, occurrence 103–104;
    neurobiological brain changes **106**;
    termination for medical reasons
    (TFMR) 116
pregnancy loss 116–118; occupational
    disruption 116–117; occupational
    therapy modifications **117–118**
present-moment orientation, increase 104
privacy, generational denial 226
processing (trauma recovery phase) 295
productivity: absence, perception 232;
    beliefs 231; cultural expectations
    137; patterns, sustaining 91; targets,
    focus 336
progesterone: fluctuations 45; shift 45
progressive conditions, trauma-informed
    occupational therapy **252**
proprioceptive input, usage 22
provider skepticism, experience 201
provider trust, damage 217
psychiatric consequences, violence
    (impact) 197–198
psychiatric histories, labeling (issues) 329
psychoeducational modules, co-leading 43
psychological abuse 165
psychological safety, foundation 38
psychological trauma 244
puberty, environmental stressors
    (intersection) 40–42
public systems, women of color
    surveillance/silencing 214–215
purpose-driven spaces, reentry 156

qualitative interviews, usage 216
queer allostatic load 269, 272
queer identification 324–325
queer identity, discrediting 284
queer time 276–279; LGBTQ+ client
    attunement 276
queer women: experiences 263; PTSD/
    identity-based discrimination,
    navigation 265–266
quiet coloring, adolescent girl usage (case
    example) 66

race-based health data, absence (Canada) 218
racial bias, experiences 177
racial discrimination: impact 25; survival 213
racial equity, education (commitment) 217
racialized stress 221; impact, recognition 155
racialized workplace stress, management 154–155
racial microaggressions 128
racial stressors, burden 211
racing thoughts, experience 2
racism: cumulative impact 93, 289; legacy 128; obstetric racism 118; systemic racism, impact 107
rape trauma syndrome, acute distress (experience) 308
rapport-building: OT prioritization 97; sessions, usage 298
reactivated trauma, risk 76–78
realize (SAMHSA principle) 331
recognition (relational autonomy principle) 256
recognize (SAMHSA principle) 331
recovery see trauma recovery
Recovery Model 16
reengagement, worth (return) 62
referral patterns, examination 248
reflection, mobile apps/self-guided tools (usage) 310–312
reflective decision making, modeling 76
reflective infrastructure, usage 340–341
reflective intake map 290
reflective journaling prompts, usage 42
reflective practice groups, usage 332
reflective supervision: core practice 337; models, impact 341; usage 336–338
reflective transition mapping exercise 302
reflexivity (relational autonomy principle) 256
regression, client signs 299
regulation: building, virtual co-occupation (usage) 324–325; mobile apps/ self-guided tools, usage 310–312
regulation strategies: effectiveness 95; shift, unawareness 301
reimbursement models, examination 248
reintegration (trauma recovery phase) 295
reinvention, episodes 284

rejection: avoidance 12; fear 277; mistakes, impact 35; perception 77
relational anchors, loss 147–148
relational autonomy, principles 256
relational betrayal, impact 22
relational conflict 254
relational dynamics, involvement 246, 288
relational engagement, capacity (growth) 131
relational identity map/tool, usage 228
relationality frameworks, usage 284
relational leadership 233
relational presence, usage 22
relational recovery 256
relational repair 198; integration 167
relational rupture 149
relational safety: rebuilding, therapeutic practice (usage) 83–85; violation 166
relational spaces, reentry 156
relational stress 36; adolescents 33; experience 41
relational trauma 82–85; accumulation 142; gendered exposure 39–40; healing 83–84; histories 137; impact 107; presence 38; recovery, support strategies **84**
relational uncertainty, navigation 75
reproductive transitions, neurobiological/ occupational events 105–106
reproductive trauma: experience 25; impact 22; sexually transmitted infections, relationship 193–194
research, embedding 333–334
residual trauma response 104
resilience, cultural expectations 137
resilience mobile, crafting 131
resistance: client signs 299
resistance, appearance 248
resist retraumatization (SAMHSA principle) 331
respectful care, restricted access 118
respiration, tracking devices 313
respond (SAMHSA principle) 331
rest/laziness, internalized script equivalence 227
restorative occupations: erosion, trauma (impact) 23; usage 99
retraumatization 124; complaint, filing 332; risk 133, 149
return-to-work protocol, avoidance 259

reward compliance, autonomy (relationship) 248
rheumatoid arthritis 185
rhythm-based occupational dosing 185
rhythmic movement, usage 22
risk management 75
Rivermead Post-Concussion Symptoms Questionnaire, usage 207
role: collage, construction 285; collapse 88–89; development, disruption (adolescent girls) 56–57; diffusion (women of color) 220–221; exploration 277, 324; externalization 98; formation, disruption 40; guided exploration 92; identity, audit 234; identity, erosion 252–254; inherited roles (women of color) 227–228; integration, support 86; navigation 92; performance, outcome (flexibility) 91; re-engagement, usage 303; renegotiation 228; satisfaction, change (documentation) 320; strategies, co-creation 89
role-based functional interview, usage 232–233
role-based movements, usage 187
role overload 88–89, 140; invisibility/prevention 89
rotator cuff injury 233
routine activities, micro-patterns (tracking) 242
routine-based interventions, threat (feeling) 164
routines: co-creation 76; destablization 137; disconnection 47; disruption 40, 146; disruption, trauma impact/analysis 16, 145; erasure 146; forgetting 73; impact 86, 141; initiation, struggle 9; management, difficulty 185–186; rebuilding 91–92

safety: planning template **169**; plan/planning 168–169; relational autonomy principle 256; trauma-informed occupational therapy usage 27–28
safety cues, misreading 4
safety/regulation (creation), occupational therapy (usage) 62–64
sandwich generation dynamic, impact 140

scaffolding: collaborative scaffolding 332; micro-routine scaffolding, usage 184, 185; usage 91–92
scar mobilization techniques 132–133
school-based goals, implications 48
school disengagement 39; appearance 34
school refusal (adolescent girls) 52–55
screen-based tension, reduction 325
second half of life *see* life, second half
self: sense, defining 162; sense, shaping 270; suppression 227–228; therapeutic use 23–24
self-advocacy skills, shift (unawareness) 301
self-authorship, opportunities (increase) 87–88
self-blame: feelings 38, 46; language 284; result 210; struggle 130–131
self-care: engagement 307–308; failure, alternative 211; habits, fluctuation 166; maintenance, struggle 9; patterns, sustaining 91
self-concept, disruption 36–37
self-directed life, building 87
self-directed occupations 111
self-directed pause, usage 100
self-directed routines (focus), therapeutic goals (usage) 156
self-direction: practice 75; requirement 39, 198
self-guided tools, usage 310–312
self-harm, definition 50–51
self-identified women (well-being examination) 88–89
self-management, women of color selection 218
self-minimization 136–137
self-regulation: building 43; disruptions 85–86; support 310
self-sacrifice, demands 219
self-sufficiency, appearance (pressure) 254
self-talk, change (documentation) 320
self-trust, developmental scaffolding (relationship) 75
self-worth: erosion, adolescent girls 59; measure 86
sensory-based entry routine, usage 97
sensory-based life story activity, initiation 243
sensory-based self-contact, usage 104
sensory-based stabilization 133

sensory cocreation activities, usage 104
sensory flooding, experience 11
sensory integration, alteration 244
sensory integration tasks, therapist
    usage 228
sensory load 251
sensory modulation 124–125; kits, usage
    185; tools, usage/selection 258
sensory-motor routines 131
sensory processing disorder 242
Sensory Processing Framework (Dunn) 16
sensory regulation 94–96; therapeutic use
    23–24
sensory-safe foods, exploration 232
sensory supports, usage 184
sensory triggers: logging 308; reduction 2
sex-based differences 2
sexism, legacy 128
sexual assault, presence 263–264
sexual coercion, history 190
sexual exploitation 163
sexual harassment, experience 161, 213
sexual intercourse, pain 190
sexually transmitted infections,
    reproductive trauma (relationship)
    193–194
sexual minority women (SMW): adverse
    childhood experiences, long-term
    health outcomes (connection)
    266; affirming goals, co-creation
    273–275; affirming goals, examples
    274; autonomy, delay 277; case
    vignettes/clinical reflections
    283–285; clinical strategies 274;
    developmental pathways, disruption
    276–279; diagnostic overshadowing
    265–266; elevated risk, elevated
    visibility (contrast) 264–265;
    gender, relationship 262; health
    system prevalence/risk/erasure
    264–267; identity, scaffolding 263;
    imagination, clinical tool 281–283;
    imagining, right 279–283; milestones
    (rethinking), affirming lens (usage)
    278; neutral care, myth 265–266;
    nonrecognition, trauma 268–272;
    occupational engagement support,
    imagination-based strategies (usage)
    282; occupational futurity 279–283;
    occupational identity 267; occupational
    therapy (OT), nonlinear transitions

278–279; occupation, identity
    affirmation 270–272; participation
    fatigue 266–267; participation
    pathways 273–275; physical
    environment, safety (centering)
    272–273; queer time 276–279;
    regulation (restoration), authentic
    occupation (usage) 275–276; role
    exploration 277; role fragmentation
    267; split roles, navigation 269–270;
    trauma-informed intervention,
    affirming lens (usage) 272–276;
    trauma-informed practice 273;
    visibility (absence), opportunities
    (missing) 264–265; volition/visibility,
    clinical practice usage 280–281
sexual violence, coercion (relationship)
    163–164
shame 38; reinforcement 55–56;
    triggering, avoidance 186
shared planning role 228
shared virtual co-occupations 325
shyness, exhibition 47
silence: meaning, recognition 163–164;
    structured silence, usage 259
simulation-based sessions 233
single-incident traumas 36
skill acquisition, emphasis 318
skin conductance, tracking devices 313
skin-to-skin contact 107; power 127
slavery, impact 226
sleep: disruption 161, 187; disruption,
    occupational therapy (usage) 171;
    disturbances 138; hygiene 310;
    maintenance, difficulty 122; quality,
    improvement 325; schedules,
    consistency 86; shallowness 162
sleeplessness 9, 78
social complexity, increase 36
social exclusion, impact 239
social hierarchies, negotiation 58
social support, fracture 266
social withdrawal 267
solidarity (relational autonomy
    principle) 256
somatic-cue tracking 258
somatic preoccupation 242
somatic reconnection tools, usage
    132–133
somatic safety: concept 248; restoration
    249–250; usage 248–251

somatic tension 96
spasticity, features 245
spiritual rituals, adaptation (clinician
    support) 224
stabilization (trauma recovery phase) 295
standard assessments, usage 321
startle responses, triggering 5
state surveillance 226
stillbirth: pregnancy 132–133; term,
    medical precision 116
stoicism, dismissal 222–223
story: indirect invitation 292; mapping
    (therapeutic exercise) **291**;
    minimization, avoidance 300
storytelling sessions, facilitation 258
stranger feeling, initiation 1–2
strangulation, impact 189
stress: accumulation 137; body response
    24; cognitive inefficiency 154;
    cumulative stress 142; internal
    expression 9; levels, perception 104;
    regulation systems (disruption),
    violence (impact) 184–185;
    survival 11
stressors, presence 78–85
stress-related dysregulation 9
stress-related symptoms, suggestion 12
stress response system, involvement 7
stress sensitivity, intensification 8
stress-trauma continuum 272
"strong Black woman" trope 220
structural advocacy 127–130
structural invisibility, trauma (link) 24
structural neglect, impact 171
structural pressures 231
structural trauma 118–120, 142; signaling,
    client presentations 119
structure: anchoring 91–92; sense,
    reestablishment 156–157
structured co-occupation planning
    tool 233
structured co-occupations, student
    pairings 43
structured silence, usage 259
structured storytelling, usage 195
Study of Women's Health Across the
    Nation, results 152
Substance Abuse and Mental Health
    Services Administration (SAMHSA):
    framework, replacement (absence)
    22–23; framework, usage 15–21, 329;

principles 331; trauma-informed care
    domains 330; trauma-informed care
    principles 16, 18, 21; trauma-informed
    care principles, operationalization
    19–20
substance use recovery 283
suicidal ideation 39
surface-level intake questions 226
surgical trauma, recovery 155–156
survival-based behaviors, acting out
    (contrast) 48–50, **49**
survival mode 325
survival strategy 35–36
survivor-centered adaptations 169–170
sustainability, infrastructure 331–332
sustainable closure, transition
    mapping **302**
sustainable transitions 298–304
Sustained Occupation Plan, usage
    300, **301**
sympathetic nervous system hyperarousal,
    indicators 96
sympathetic state, body fight-flight
    preparation function 22
symptom-based frameworks, women with
    disabilities (relationship) 246
symptom-based scales 317–318
symptom flares, reduction 181
symptom-impact matrix, usage 206
synaptic plasticity, enhancement 139
systemic advocacy opportunities **174–175**
systemic barriers, addressing 93–94;
    clinical strategies **93–94**
systemic discrimination, occurrence 142
systemic distrust, impact 147
systemic inequities 112, 149, 219
systemic lupus erythematosus,
    diagnosis 206
systemic oppression, impact 22
systemic racism, impact 107
systemic trauma, histories 137
system-level advocacy: occupational
    justice, relationship 171–173;
    occupational therapy, role 153–154
system-level redesign, institutional
    barriers/OT strategies **173**
system-level work, political/policy fluency
    (requirement) 172
systems-led infrastructure, absence
    (impact) 330
systems reinforcement, invisibility 248

tactile-based downregulation routine, development 187

task-based cueing, usage 259

task mastery, emphasis 318

tasks: follow-through, improvement 184; initiation, delay 204; planning/organizing/persisting, difficulty 6; prioritization, teaching 89; recovery 99

teacher, talking back (suspension) 55

technology: expressive technology, usage 313–315; usage 64–65, 308–315

tension, feeling 2

termination for medical reasons (TFMR) 116; occupational therapy modifications **117–118**

test anxiety 96

therapeutic alliance: amplification, technology (usage) 309; restoration, somatic safety (usage) 248–251

therapeutic care, initiation 82

therapeutic practice, usage 83–85

therapeutic silence, difficulty 166

therapeutic space, creation 122–125

threat/safety, distinguishing (difficulty) 5

time-management strategies 79–80

Title Nine rights 93

to-do lists, ignoring 90

toileting, assistance 240

touch, overstimulation 40

trans women, experiences 263

trauma: adolescents 33; biological impact 4; body-based expressions 13; caregiving expectations 24; champions, rotation 332; compounding, migration-related stressors (impact) 162; cues, involvement 246–247; developmental environment, becoming 2; dysregulated perinatal nervous system, relationship 106–112; economic inequity, relationship 24; effects, shaping 24; foundations 1; functional manifestations, occupational therapy response 198–201; gender-based oppression, entanglement 25; healing, occupational therapy (role) 23–24; health conditions, non-trauma presentations (differentiation) **192**; identity development/occupational participation, relationship 35; integration, digital storytelling/expressive technology (usage) 313–315; intersectionality, relationship 24–27; navigation 126, 136; neurological system encoding 76; obscuring 245–247, **247**; occupational choices 23; pathways 78–85; patterns 120, 122; psychological/emotional issue, framing 4; reactions, emotions (coexistence) 77; recognition, absence 264; reenactment 233–234; resonance 3237; responsive occupational therapy 288–289; resurfacing 133–134; risks 195; structural invisibility, link 25; verbal confirmation 243

trauma-affected brain regions **6**

trauma care: innovations 328; innovations, case vignettes/clinical reflections 323–325; strategies, innovation 307

trauma exposure 140, 164; impact 4–5; occurrence 34; racial/socioeconomic inequities 60–61

trauma history: disclosure 336; gathering, questions (avoidance) 291–292; questions, usage 289–290

trauma-informed approach 191; clinical pitfalls, avoidance 289–291

trauma-informed app selection rubric **311**

trauma-informed assessment 120–122; strategies **121–122**

trauma-informed audits, usage 338–339

trauma-informed care: application 149–151; identity-centered practice, intersection 253; importance 229; meaning 64–65; operationalization 329–331; position 90; road trip metaphor 16; role 54–55; SAMHSA principles 16, 18, 21; success metrics, expansion 320–321; sustaining 332; theoretical frameworks 15–23

trauma-informed discharge planning: checklist **299**; initiation 299

trauma-informed efforts, tracking/evaluation 332

trauma-informed environmental audits, usage 339

trauma-informed evaluation, decision making flow 292

trauma-informed evaluation/intake 289–298

trauma-informed frameworks 16–17

trauma-informed gains (sustaining), community/role re-engagement (usage) 303

trauma-informed goal setting 292–294; prompt bank **297–298**
trauma-informed innovation, future 322–323
trauma-informed interventions 221; affirming lens, usage 272–276
trauma-informed leadership, impact 329–330
trauma-informed meaning, addressing (absence) 231
trauma-informed mentorship 337; models 337–338
trauma-informed occupational restructuring 234
trauma-informed occupational therapy 25, 90–96, 128; advocacy integration map **335**; biofeedback-supported strategies **314**; future 328; healing, nontraditional indicators (examples) **319**; models/ frameworks **17–18**; recovery phase framework **296**; role 137–138; support 141
Trauma-Informed Oregon resource 331
trauma-informed organizations, SAMHSA principles 331
trauma-informed postpartum care, independence goal (rejection) 254
trauma-informed practice: energy, fading 331; principles 62; support, prompts/ reflective questions (usage) **129**; tools 288
trauma-informed sensory plan, addition 173
trauma-informed support 142
trauma-informed systems: certification programs, expansion 331; change, advocacy strategies **322**
trauma-informed telehealth practices 309
trauma-informed youth wellness program, outpatient OT usage (case example) 67–68
trauma recovery 95, 198; intervention planning/implementation 295–298; phase framework **296**; phases 295; phases, interventions (alignment) 297
trauma-related disruption 161
trauma-related dysregulation 46
trauma-related responses, addressing 113
trauma-related stress responses, hormonal rhythms (interaction) 45
trauma-related symptoms 137

trauma-related triggers 206
trauma responses: adaptive survival strategies, equivalence 11–12; dysfunction mislabeling 13; physiological states, relationship 21; recognition 12
trauma-responsive frameworks, guidance 22–23
trauma responsive occupational therapy, core principles 27–29
trauma-responsive perinatal care, Medicaid reimbursement (push) 334
trauma-sensitive environment, description 123–124
trauma-sensitive narrative work, usage 77
trauma-sensitive questions 191
traumatic brain injury (TBI) 160–161; domestic alteration, impact 22–229; formal evaluation, initiation 259; intimate partner violence, impact 189; long-term occupational consequences 189; minimization/reframing 191–192; missed diagnosis 207; neurological sequelae 188–190; underdiagnosis, reasons 189
traumatic events, memory encoding (modulation) 8
traumatic temporality 269–270
treatment goals, independence prioritization 247
trust: building 61; intervention role 119; earning 289; violation 166
trustworthiness/transparency, trauma-informed occupational therapy usage 28
Type 2 diabetes, diagnosis 185

unprocessed grief, resurfacing 137
unresolved trauma, risk 76–78
upstream solutions 171

vagus nerve, activation (absence) 95
values-aligned measures, usage 320
values-based activity planning, usage 195
values-based journaling, usage 257–258, 274
values-based planning, usage 97
values-based scheduling, usage 169
values clarification: intervention 92; tools 89
ventral striatum, development 42

ventral vagal state, support function 21
verbal corrections, minimization 189
verbal disclosure, absence 242
vigilance *see* hypervigilance: cycle 11;
    trauma-related behavior 265
violence *see* intimate partner violence;
    later life; sexual violence; women,
    violence: cardiometabolic disorders
    185–187; cardiovascular disease,
    relationship 186; case vignettes/
    clinical reflections 175–177, 205–207;
    catalyst 182–183; chronic pain
    disorders 185–187; cognitive health
    consequences 197–198; cognitive
    impacts 199–201; cognitive impacts,
    occupational therapy strategies
    200; complex trauma 197–198;
    effects, persistence 162; executive
    dysfunction 199–201; fleeing 162;
    forms, occupational impact 162–166;
    healthcare system, navigation 201–202;
    health conditions, non-trauma
    presentations (differentiation) **192**;
    health equity 204–205; indicators 242;
    injuries (addressing), trauma-informed
    approach (requirement) 191;
    institutional harm, impact 195,
    197; interdisciplinary responses
    167–179; long-term ripple effects
    166–167; long-term structural
    damage 188; maternal health
    disparities 194–195; medical mistrust,
    relationship 201–202; medical
    trauma 194–195; mood disorders
    197–198; obstetric complications
    194–197; occupational therapy
    responses 167–170; occupational
    therapy tools/approaches 168–170;
    physical injury 188; post-injury care,
    gender disparities 188; postpartum
    complications 194–197; postpartum
    occupational disruption 195, 197;
    psychiatric consequences 197–198;
    psychiatric impacts, occupational
    therapy strategies **200**; reproductive
    consequences 192–197; reproductive/
    postpartum complications, occupational
    therapy strategies **196**; reproductive
    trauma 193–194; safety plan/planning
    168–169; sexual health consequences
    192–197; sexually transmitted
    infections 193–194; system-level
    advocacy 204–205; system-level
    dysregulation, occupational therapy
    strategies **203**; system-level redesign,
    institutional barriers/OT strategies
    173; trust/autonomy/relational safety,
    violation 166
Violence Against Women study 11
violence-related harm, perpetuation 205
violence survivors: advocacy
    organizations/health providers,
    collaboration 167; aftereffects
    194; clinical care 204; executive
    dysfunction 199; medical mistrust 201
virtual platforms, relational use 323
virtual reality (VR) tools, exploration 312
virtual settings, embodied safety
    (augmentation) 312–313
visibility, clinical practice usage 280–281
visual anchors, display 312
visual cues 189
visual journaling, adolescent girl usage
    (case example) 66
visual mapping, usage 42
visual planning tools: implementation
    155; introduction 186
visual sequencing activity (adolescent girl
    case example) 66
visual shutdown checklist, usage 99
visual storyboards, usage 274
visual tools, usage 91
visual tracking delays 207
voice: reclamation, digital storytelling
    (usage) 324; restoration 113;
    trauma-informed occupational therapy
    usage 28–29
volition: clinical practice usage 280–281;
    demonstration 228; disruption 87–88
volitional engagement, improvement 92
voluntary engagement 198
vulnerability: compounding 239–242;
    identity formation, relationship 38–39;
    intensification 254; shaming, family
    legacy 226

weathering effect 218
weekly occupational mapping activity,
    usage 97
wholeness, sense 268
widowhood: grief 147–148; navigation
    156–157

withdrawal: emergence, school-based
OT (usage) 65–66; patterns,
reinforcement 142
women: assault, experience 161; autonomy,
occupational therapy approaches
202–204; bodily autonomy, violations
25; bodily violation, experience
124; chronic stress, navigation 126;
cumulative microaggressions 25; danger,
responses 182–183; disempowerment/
punishment 13; infantilization 241;
interpersonal violence 25; life histories,
structural harm 152; lives, trauma
(continuation) 3; midlife, changes
143; occupational disruptions 6;
occupational performance, chronic
survival mode (neurobiological/
functional consequences) 10;
occupational therapists, impact
183; occupational therapy (phases),
somatic safety (restoration) 249–250;
occupational therapy, trauma-informed
care (SAMHSA principles) 19–20;
relational adaptations 12; reproductive
trauma 25; reshaping, violence
(impact) 161; stability, occupational
therapy approaches 202–204; story,
minimization (avoidance) 300;
structural/invisible trauma 118–120;
trauma-informed occupational therapy,
usage 318
women, health: community-driven
innovation/co-creation 315–317;
evidence/impact, reimagining
317–321; occupational disruption,
foundations 1; trauma, foundations 1;
trauma-informed app selection rubric
311; trauma-informed occupational
therapy 14; trauma-informed
occupational therapy, future 328
women of color: attachment disruption
220–221; bias reflection 223; case
vignettes/reflections 232–234;
collective memory 224–228;
compounded burden 213–214;
culturally discordant care 216–217;
cultural pressures 219–221; cultural
roles 213–214; cultural silence
223–224; erasure, experience
213; expected strength, cost 220;
harm, continuation 216; harm,

re-experiencing 222; healing 214;
healing, barriers 221–224; health
avoidance 217–219; healthcare
experience, safety/healing (absence)
215–216; health system, harm
215–217; identity 213–215; inherited
roles 227–228; intergenerational
load 224–228; international
violence/institutional betrayal,
experience 211; invisible labor
217–219; medical mistrust 215, 216;
misdiagnoses, experience 216–217;
misrecognition (clinical spaces)
222–223; occupation, problems
230–232; overmedicalization/
criminalization 118; pain, minimization
215; public system surveillance/
silencing 214–215; relational wounds
219–221; representation, weight
223–224; research exclusion 216;
role diffusion 220–221; safeguarding
222; self-management, selection 218;
self, suppression 227–228; strength,
performing (validation) 220; support,
barriers 221–224; survival, vigilance
(cost) 212; trauma 210, 213–215;
trauma exposure, anxiety/depression
(elevation) 212; trauma-informed
interventions 221
women, trauma: misunderstanding/
overlooking 12–13; navigation
126; neurobiology 3–12; recovery,
trauma-informed app selection rubric
311; structural/systemic dimensions
12–15
women, violence: assault 160–161; cases
(Australia/Spain) 163; experience,
invisible illnesses 183; health
implications 180; neuroendocrine/
immune systems, impact 184–185;
participation goals 183; perpetuation
171; personal violation 181; physical
problems, experience 181; recorded
cases (UK) 163; spectrum 160
women with disabilities: access, framing
256–257; advocacy 256–257;
advocacy, documentation (importance)
243; advocacy, scripts (clinician
co-creation) 255; barriers, reporting
243–244; care, fragmentation 246;
case vignettes/clinical reflections

257–259; chronicity 252–254; communication barriers, impact 244; compounded vulnerabilities 240; continuum, occupational disruption 251–253; cumulative stress, impact 253–256; daily life, participation 255; dependency 240–243; diagnostic overshadowing 242–243; documentation, usage 244; episodic conditions, trauma-informed occupational therapy **252**; experiences, underrecognition 239; interdisciplinary communication, usage 244; intimate partner violence, likelihood 239; invisible burdens 240; missed screenings 242–243; participation, emotional labor 255; postpartum mental health 253–256; power imbalances 240–243; progressive conditions, trauma-informed occupational therapy **252**; reframing 244–251; reinforcement, systems navigation 247–248; role identity, erosion 252–254; silencing 243–244; stress/trauma 238; structural change 256–257; surveillance 243–244; surveillance, acuteness 244; trauma (obscuring), diagnoses (problem) 245–247, **247**; trauma-informed lens, usage 244–251; unpredictability 252–254; viewpoint, fixed diagnosis (usage) 245; violence disclosure, shaping 243; violence, reframing 244–251

women with intellectual disabilities, relational trauma/intimate partner violence 255–256
work: discrimination 151; endurance goals 176
workforce development (advancement), reflective supervision/mentorship (usage) 336–338
workload, balancing 154
workplace: assault 207; discrimination 144; dispute/injury 258; injury 262–263; modifications, identification 155; trauma, LGBTQ professional recovery 285
wrist fracture 233

young adulthood: defining 74; developmental tasks 73–78; romanticization 72; trauma, case vignettes/clinical reflections 96–99; vulnerabilities 73–78
young adult women: authentic ambition, over-functioning (differentiation) **80**, 81; chronic stress, impact 72; depression/anxiety rates, increase 72; psychological distress, increase 72; stories, authorship reclamation 72–73; stress/trauma 71; trauma-informed approach, usage 90–91; trauma pathways/stressors 78–85
young women, emotional abuse (experience) 83
Youth Risk Behavior Surveillance data (CDC) 39, 60

For Product Safety Concerns and Information please contact our EU representative GPSR@taylorandfrancis.com
Taylor & Francis Verlag GmbH, Kaufingerstraße 24, 80331 München, Germany